Read
HEAVYHANDS™

"Schwartz is a clear thinker with a good writing style, and he has inserted enough photographs, charts, stick figures and sidebars to keep even those who hate 'exercise books' absorbed." —*San Francisco Chronicle*

"The workouts can burn off eight to twenty-five calories a minute—twice as much as a hard game of racquetball." —*People* magazine

"Scientifically sound and convincing." —*Publishers Weekly*

"More than just a workout schedule. It's a full-grown exercise system with practical and entertaining advice… Heavyhands lets almost anyone move safely toward fitness…" —*American Health*

"Beneficial…helpful." —*Detroit News*

"An entirely new approach to total body fitness not found in any book currently on the market." —*Library Journal*

"Heavyhands chases calories and burns fat at enormous rates equal to, or greater than, those previously enjoyed only by experienced cross-country skiers, marathon runners, bicyclers and swimmers." —*UPI*

Put
HEAVYHANDS
to work for you.

Three or four 30-minute workouts per week will superbly condition not only your entire cardio-pulmonary system, but also ninety percent or more of your body muscle. Have fun as you aim for your best body—it's a goal you can reach.

HEAVYHANDS™

THE ULTIMATE EXERCISE

Leonard Schwartz, M.D.

WARNER BOOKS

A Warner Communications Company

HEAVYHANDS™ is a trademark
of Leonard Schwartz, M.D.

Before embarking on any strenuous exercise program, including Heavyhands, everyone, particularly anyone over thirty-five or anyone with any known heart or blood pressure problem, should be examined by a physician.

WARNER BOOKS EDITION
COPYRIGHT © 1982 BY LEONARD SCHWARTZ
ALL RIGHTS RESERVED.
THIS WARNER BOOKS EDITION IS PUBLISHED BY ARRANGEMENT WITH LITTLE, BROWN AND COMPANY, 34 BEACON STREET, BOSTON, MASSACHUSETTS 02106.
WARNER BOOKS, INC., 666 FIFTH AVENUE, NEW YORK, NY 10103

Ⓦ A Warner Communications Company

PRINTED IN THE UNITED STATES OF AMERICA
FIRST WARNER PRINTING: FEBRUARY 1984
10 9 8 7 6 5 4 3 2 1

Designed by Susan Windheim

Library of Congress Cataloging in Publication Data

Schwartz, Leonard, 1925–
  Heavyhands™: the ultimate exercise.

  1. Exercise.   2. Physical fitness.   3. Weight
lifting.   I. Title.
GV505.S35   1984   613.7′1   83-21682
ISBN 0-446-38004-0 (U.S.A.)
      0-446-38005-9 (Canada)

To my partner and my love, Millie

CONTENTS

Introduction   3

1   Prelude   7
2   Why Heavyhands?   13
3   The Heart of the Matter   27
4   Getting Into Action   43
5   An Introduction to Heavyhands Levers   69
6   A Repertoire of Heavyhands Calisthenics   75
7   Bellyaerobics and Backaerobics: Heavyhands
        for Abdomen and Back   109
8   Heavyhands Walking   127
9   Heavyhands Running and Heavyhands
        for the Runner   151
10 Heavyhands for Lifters and Body Builders:
        The Strength Specialists   161
11 Shadowboxing   167
12 Heavyhands Dancing   175
13 Heavyhands and Sports   187
14 Heavyhands and Injuries   193
15 Fat: Fact and Fallacy   203
16 Heavyhands Intervals and "Cycles"   227
17 Exerpsychology   233
18 Epilogue   253

Appendix: Workload and Calories   273

HEAVYHANDS

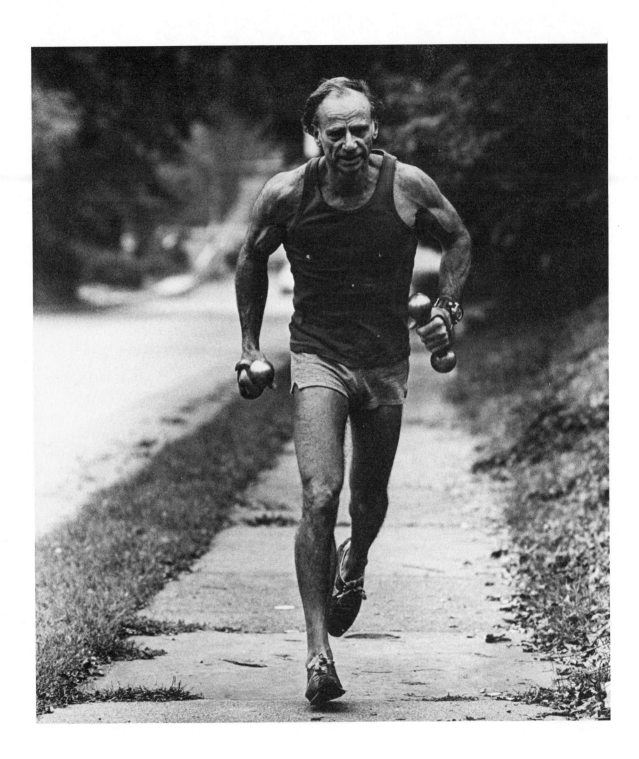

Introduction

ALMOST TWO THOUSAND BOOKS have been written about exercise and almost half of them are still in print. Conceivably we are running out of reasons, or even room, for more of them. But I'm convinced that exercise remains the best bargain in the self-help market. The life-preserving and life-enhancing qualities of exercise have been solidly established during the last decade. The Exercise Revolution, which began about ten years ago, still is, in my view, adolescent: full of spurty and vulnerable enthusiasms — would-be exercisers are ready to start, but quick to quit. A major part of the problem, I think, is that today's various popular methods of achieving fitness are inadequate because they are overspecialized.

The specialization takes several forms. In one, a certain region of the body, usually the legs, gets most of the exercise. In an other, one or two of the elements of fitness, such as strength, endurance, or speed, are neglected. Still another variation of overspecialization finds concern for heart and lung function all but lacking. And, as we shall show, *all* current methods *fail* to exploit the upper torso to the fullest.

Today's popular exercise methods have an either-or ring about them: for reasons that elude me, there is a continuing reluctance to work lots of muscles, lots of ways simultaneously, to the heart's more comfortable cadence. In doing precisely that, Heavyhands comes closest to providing the comprehensive single-package system. The larger workloads generated by the trained Heavyhander inevitably chase calories *fastest,* and with less risk of the injuries that also plague the overspecialized exerciser.

And all this can be accomplished in three or four 30-minute sessions per week, performed not six feet from your TV screen — if you so choose! The practice of Heavyhands will, I hope, whittle away at fickleness, at least where it comes to exercise. To that end, Heavyhands offers a wide selection of movements to intrigue and satisfy the hesitant or "picky" exerciser. I believe that there is an exercise here for everyone; that any one, or combination, of them will produce the largest "training" results possible; and that not one of them neglects the aerobic "musts" the doctor ordered.

Over the past five years I have tried to play devil's advocate, looking for reasons to dislodge any ill-founded enthusiasm for Heavyhands. In my laboratory and in the field I have searched for

---

What it is

Heavyhands is a new kind of exercise. Its claims are explicit: a higher level of fitness than that produced by any known aerobic exercise, and a new kind of fitness. Heavyhands brings strength plus endurance to all of the muscles. No muscle group is neglected; muscles already well trained by other exercise and sports are even further upgraded by Heavyhands. Most exciting of all, the simultaneous movement of many muscles is a superlative way to train the heart. Hard Heavyhands actually feels surprisingly easy. The Heavyhander can become as strong as most lifters, as swift as most runners, and outwork both on smaller investment of time and with far fewer injuries.

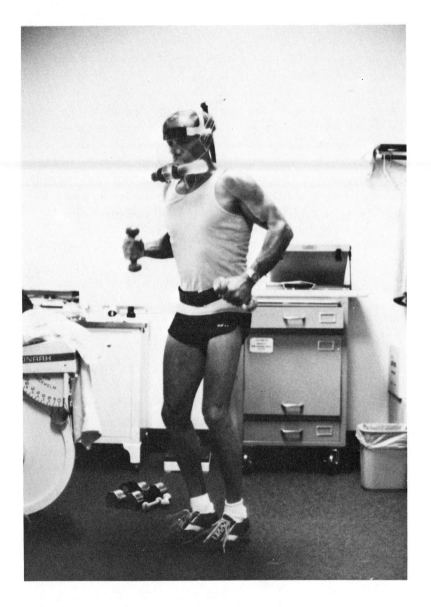

theoretic or practical flaws. I have avoided laying claim to the touted
extras of exercise. I have consciously avoided appealing to what
are for me fuzzy areas — pleasure, body beauty, vague new leases
on life, all states of improvement that defy precise measurement.
The advantages of Heavyhands, which are spelled out in Chapter

2, have been measured and verified. Scattered throughout the book you will find a number of charts that reveal the astonishing workloads and calorie expenditure made possible through the practice of Heavyhands. The data these charts contain have been derived from experiments using the most sophisticated laboratory equipment available.

I've no wish to muscle out the well-entrenched methods of exercise. Heavyhands can complement other methods as a training adjunct, a distributor of special effects to special places on one's anatomy, an antedote to boredom, or simply excellent exercise that works as well indoors as out. Finally, Heavyhands is not only the best way to begin if you've never exercised before; it is also probably the *only* way to improve your overall fitness if you are already a world-class athlete.

It occurs to me that physicians frequently find themselves preoccupied with things apart from what they are supposed to be doing. For me writing is one of those departures and exercise is another. Peter Mark Roget, of Thesaurus fame, was a doctor too, and one who devoted decades to a work that was deviant from his "proper" credentials. *Heavyhands,* far less scholarly, and less apt to shape mountains of muscle than Roget's Thesaurus has shaped language skills since 1852, can do no better than quote from Roget's preface to his first edition:

> Notwithstanding all the pains I have bestowed on its execution, I am fully aware of its numerous deficiencies and imperfections, and of its falling far short of the degree of excellence that might be attained. But, in a work of this nature, where perfection is placed at so great a distance, I have thought it best to limit my ambition to that moderate share of merit which it may claim in its present form; trusting to the indulgence of those for whose benefit it is intended, and to the candor of critics who, while they find it easy to detect faults, can at the same time duly appreciate difficulties.

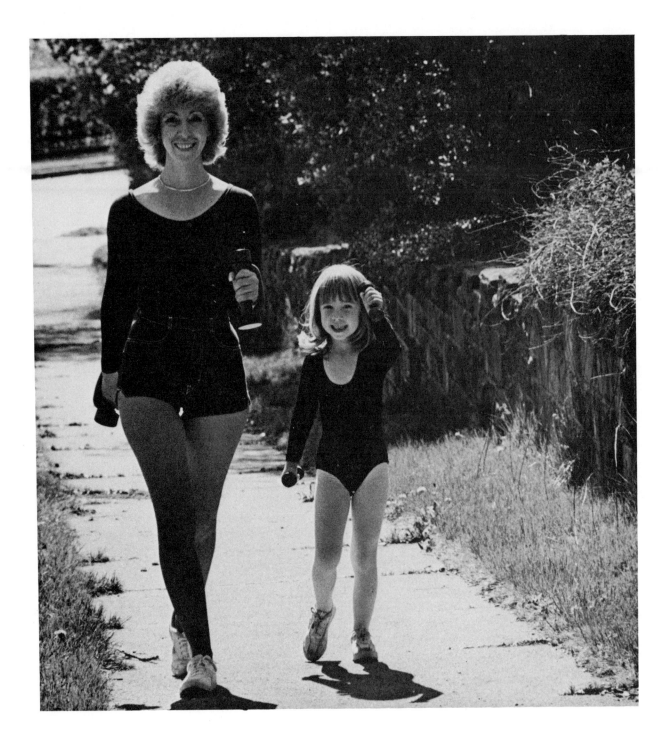

1

Prelude

FIVE YEARS AGO, an educated hunch led me to the discovery of Heavyhands. Two years prior to that, running and swimming had kept me moderately fit. Aside from a bit of weight training during adolescence, and Sunday pick-up softball games, my athletic history was a model of mediocrity. My work as physician, psychiatrist, teacher, and gerontologist was about as sedentary as could be. I don't think I had ever run 300 yards nonstop before my fiftieth birthday. My seventeen years as a heavy smoker, twenty years of high blood pressure, and my chronic back problems seemed to preclude any prospect for superfitness.

Changes in author over a 7-year training period			
	1974	*1976*	*1981*
Age	50	52	57
Weight	147	146	132
Pulse rate (resting)	80	60	38
VO_2Max:			
Legs alone	33 ml./kilo/min^{-1}	54	60
Arms alone	23	38	70
Combined (estimated performance)	33	54	75 +
Body fat percentage	15%	14%	4%
Oxygen pulse		17	20–32
Running speed	5 mph	8 mph	9.2 mph
Grip strength	50 kilograms	52 kilograms	65 kilograms

This five-year experience with Heavyhands has worked some physiologic miracles for me. Indeed, many experts have found my story hard to believe. My oxygen-consumption rate has more than doubled; my resting pulse rate has dipped from 80 to 38. My size puts me in the third percentile compared to all adult American males; but my strength puts me in the ninetieth. Whether working or playing, I tire *after* the kids do. My eating habits resemble those of a small colt. My running times have dropped from a grudging 12-minute mile to a more respectable 6.5 — on about 100 miles per year! And, Heavyhanding, I can use as much oxygen in 2 hours, 8 minutes, and 13 seconds as Alberto Salazar did with his best-ever marathon — though I'll never win in Boston!

When I first began running, the spirit and obvious good sense of Dr. Ken Cooper's *Aerobics* supported my personal health needs and my general interest in exercise and sport. My reading in the field of exercise physiology and sports medicine gained eager momentum. But, after I had pounded the track for a while, it occurred to me that most endurance exercise emphasized one pair of limbs over the other. The legs, having the largest total muscle mass, were chosen as the most effective aerobic drivers; because of their size, it was assumed that the legs would be the most efficient trainers of the heart and lungs. Not one aerobic exercise system stressed strength. Single-package strategies — exercise programs that trained all the muscles, and that included strength as well as stamina — were deemed impossible by many experts. I concluded that current aerobic strategies used too little muscle mass at any given moment, were overconcerned with prolonged endurance and speed, and almost studiously neglected the driving power of the arms.

My hunches went against the grain of traditional experience on the one hand, but were supported here and there by small scraps of evidence, on the other. Convention had it that the arms were relatively poor aerobic drivers, but then cross-country skiers, who used their arms quite vigorously, had posted the highest values of aerobic power ever.

I set up a modest laboratory at home when it became clear that more precise methods were needed to evaluate Heavyhands training effects. I needed to know how much combined exercise involving arm, leg, and trunk muscles (panaerobics) could increase total fitness. And I had to learn how much muscle activity could be fueled by the healthy heart-lung mechanism.

The results have far exceeded my most optimistic predictions. As of this writing there are over one million Heavyhanders. A significant number have been tested in the lab, and the studies continue. Heavyhands offers both the option for a higher *fitness level* and a new *kind* of fitness. Thus far, the injury rate has been astoundingly low considering the intensity of the exercise achieved.

Heavyhands is for the sedentary newcomer as well as for those habituated to activity; for elite athletes and, with proper prescription, for many of the elderly and ailing. It can serve either as your primary exercise or as complement to an assortment of sports. The walkers, runners, skiers, swimmers, bikers, dancers, and rope-

---

Heavyhands compared with other exercise

A few years ago a panel of seven experts were asked to compare some objective and subjective benefits of various exercises. Nine items were selected for comparison and rated on a 0-to-3 scale. A rating of 21 thus indicated that all seven raters gave that item a 3. The ratings are presented in the chart that follows.

Overall ratings (sum of ratings on the nine elements) from greatest to least contributions to fitness were as follows.

Sport	Score
Jogging	148
Bicycling	142
Swimming	140
Skating	140
Handball/squash	140
Nordic skiing	139
Alpine skiing	138
Basketball	138
Tennis	128
Calisthenics	126
Walking	102
Golf with riding cart	66
Softball	64
Bowling	51

RATINGS BY MEDICAL PANELISTS							
ELEMENTS	BASKETBALL	BOWLING	HANDBALL & SQUASH	SKIING ALPINE*	SKIING NORDIC*	TENNIS	JOGGING
Cardiorespiratory endurance	19	5	19	16	19	16	21
Muscular endurance	17	5	18	18	19	16	20
Muscular strength	15	5	15	15	15	14	17
Flexibility	13	7	16	14	14	14	9
Balance	16	6	17	21	16	16	17
Weight control	19	5	19	15	17	16	21
Muscle definition	13	5	11	14	12	13	14
Digestion	10	7	13	9	12	12	13
Sleep	12	6	12	12	15	11	16

*Alpine skiing: downhill and slalom. Nordic skiing: cross-country and jumping.

How might a broad-based Heavyhands program size up against these findings? Scanning the chart we note that jogging received two of the 21 ratings — in cardiorespiratory endurance and weight control, while Alpine skiing received a 21 for balance. Interestingly, jogging received the highest rating, a 20, for muscular endurance and a 17, the highest score for muscular strength. Unexpectedly, handball/squash received a 16 — the highest count for flexibility. Running shared a 14 with Alpine skiing in muscle definition, a dubious category to begin with.

It is doubtful that any group of experts could make accurate assessments of the effects of these sports on themes like digestion and sleep.

Based upon these ratings I would score Heavyhands as follows:

Cardiorespiratory endurance	21+
Muscular endurance	21+
Muscular strength	21+
Flexibility	21
Balance	20
Weight control	21+
Muscle definition	21+

jumpers — the endurance exercisers, *all* can increase their prior best efforts by the addition of Heavyhands to their program.

The female constitution is particularly well suited for achieving fitness through Heavyhands. Almost certainly some lady Heavyhander, probably many in fact, will supersede the terrific workload and oxygen consumption (74 VO$_2$Max) posted years ago by a female Russian cross-country skier — a record not equaled since. And it can only happen with Heavyhands. The day I surpassed my leg-driven workload with *arms alone* using one-pound weights, I knew that Heavyhands, the comprehensive exercise for everyone, would provide the largest fitness increments for women. My reasoning is simple. Men easily outstrip women where it comes to one-shot "ballistic" strength. The average women, trained or untrained, can't lift more than 50 percent of the loads her male counterpart can manage. Fortunately, that's not the kind of activity that spins off huge oxygen consumption, which is what aerobic exercise is all about. When we drop the size of the weights to one that is easily manipulable, women's performances come predictably closer to those of men — within 10 to 15 percent. Thus women's endurance records are typically 85 to 90 percent of men's. In exercise that develops strength-speed and endurance, the size of weights used suddenly becomes very small. In a few of our exercises, such as

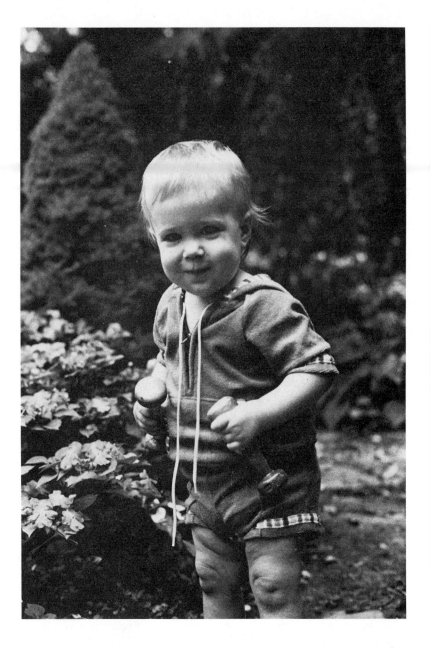

Heavyhands for children

For a long time the wisdom of strength training for prepubertal children has been questioned. Recent literature seems more favorably disposed to it. My pediatric colleagues in the medical community have been enthusiastic about Heavyhands: concerns seem less related to physiologic problems than to the erratic willingness of some children to follow regular exercise programs. I have found children generally most responsive: they slip easily into the most complicated elements of the Heavyhands repertoire as though Heavyhands were designed for them. Indeed it was. Their playful quality and continual willingness to experiment is what children are about. Children enjoy the joint flexibility that makes for exaggerated motion in the best sense of the word.

Skateboards and surfing and roller-skate dancing and hot-dog skiing are young people's territory. So Heavyhands gives the old-timer a shot at childlike spontaneity, and gives children greater fitness to match their unabashed pleasure in motion.

It has been suggested that the increasing early incidence of vascular disease (i.e., diabetes, hypertension) and obesity in children is related in large measure to diminishing activity.

rapid alternate 3-foot lifts of weighted hands, there is probably no one on the face of the earth who can manage 10 pounds! Probably not one — untrained — in 100,000, who can sustain that particular exercise with 5-pound weights for 5 minutes!

So women come to Heavyhands well equipped to play in the same ballpark with men. Women athletes have always been able to excel at the speed-power-endurance complex: in the racquet sports, in endurance-dominated sports, in golf — where small muscle mass can drive distances that humble large men. All of which suggests that the Heavyhands format is a natural for enhancing both the overall fitness and athletic prowess of women.

The reader should scan the contents to get the gist of the text, then read Chapters 2 through 4 carefully. These chapters provide a base of understanding of the principles of Heavyhands, a self-test, and a beginning exercise prescription. From there you can move through the book at a pace comfortable for you, adding new items whenever you choose.

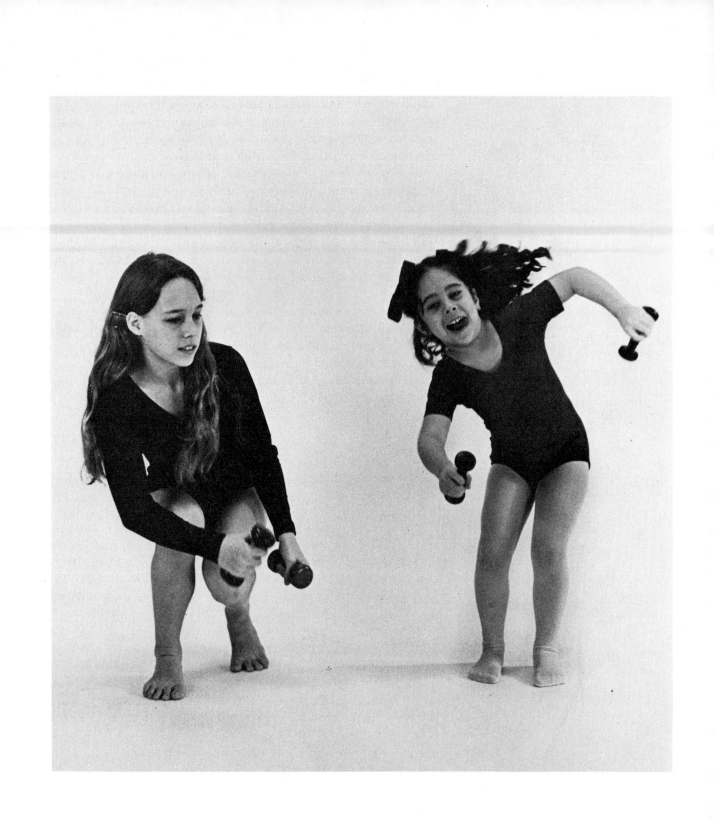

2

Why Heavyhands?

BEFORE DESCRIBING and defining Heavyhands, I think it is useful to explain some of the fundamental physiology of exercise. If you have already done some reading in the field, much of this information will be old hat. If you are a newcomer to exercise (and its theories), you may find some of this material heavy going at first. But a short review of a few basics will help provide a foundation for the new ideas we have to cover.

WHAT IS EXERCISE?

Exercise is *work*. More accurately, exercise is *overwork*. Since most of us are either frankly sedentary or just moderately active, our hearts and other muscles rarely, if ever, get a chance to live up to their inborn capabilities. Even the most arduous jobs don't always approach our bodies' potential, because work usually consists of short bursts of activity with frequent interruptions. Exercise is a kind of elective addition to our usual chores, calculated to make us healthy.

The work we heap upon ourselves when exercising is called workload, and good exercise is a kind of *overload*, meaning, beyond what's typical in our lives. All workloads are composed of two general components — *intensity* and *duration*: how *hard* we work and how *long* we remain at it. So if we're throwing bricks into a truck bed, the number of bricks we throw, say, each minute would represent the *intensity* of the work; how long we continue doing it, the *duration*. Immediately it is clear that intensity and duration tend to seesaw a bit: increasing the intensity will probably shorten the duration. We may throw a hundred bricks a minute for ten minutes. At two hundred bricks per minute we may have to settle for a two-minute burst, at which point either our breathlessness or aching arms and back, or both, call things to a halt.

HOW DO WE MEASURE EXERCISE?

Clocks are all you need to determine duration of exercise. Intensity is somewhat more complicated. Exercise physiologists have invented methods for measuring work intensity and units for describing these intensities. All bodily work burns "fuel" (releases heat), and that exertion requires, as does all combustion, oxygen. Experts can thus measure the heat produced through work by determining how much oxygen is used, or "consumed," while the work is happening. Through experimentation it was learned that a 70-kilo (154-pound) man, at rest, uses just 3.5cc of oxygen per kilo (2.2 pounds) of his body weight each minute. And so physiologists decided to make that amount of oxygen a standard unit for describing work intensity.

Such units are called METs — an abbreviation derived from the word *metabolism*. We say we are using 1 MET at rest, 2 METs while standing, or 3 METs walking at such-and-such pace. Or, we say that running a mile in 10 minutes requires 10 METs of work intensity. The larger the exerciser, the more work is involved at any MET level. A 300-pound man working at 10 METs produces about twice the heat as does a 150-pound person also performing at 10 METs. That really means that our 70-kilo hypothetical man is using 10 METs (or 35cc) of oxygen times 70 kilos of body weight per minute.

Some people have an understandable difficulty in grasping the MET concept. Keeping gravity in mind is often a help. All work, unless it's done in an orbiting space module or its laboratory-based equivalent, takes place in a gravitational field that remains relatively constant. When we *weigh* more, there is more of us to contend with the constant drag presented by gravity, and that boils down to greater metabolic work, i.e., the combined labor of the heart-lung apparatus and the voluntary muscles attached to our bones. That's what creates the small enigma for some. If a 100-pound person and a 200-pound person are both working at 10 METs — translated as ten times as much work as simply dozing in our gravitational field — why does the 200-pounder release twice the heat expressed in calories as does his pint-sized counterpart? METs refer to work per unit of body mass, as though we're saying each piece of a whole person working at 10 METs accomplishes, on average, 10 METs of work — that is, uses up 35cc of oxygen for each 2.2-pound piece! Larger people merely have more pieces working at a given intensity. It will be immediately obvious that some pieces of us contribute little directly to the actual labor of exercise — hair, bones, toenails, large bowel, etc. But the average holds true enough to make the numbers useful in assessing the energy cost of similar work for differing bodies. Here are a few rules of thumb to keep the concepts of MET and calorie loss per minute coupled in mind:

METs

We measure the intensity of workloads by a standard unit called a MET, a term derived from the word *metabolism*. One MET is the amount of oxygen used per kilo by a 70-kilo (154-pound) man each minute while at rest. It has been discovered through experimentation that our hypothetical 70-kilo man uses 3.5cc (cubic centimeters) of oxygen each minute for every kilo he weighs, or a grand total of 245cc of oxygen per minute while resting.

Fifty-seven kilos (about 126 pounds) is the place where MET numbers and calories-per-minute numbers coincide. Thus, if you weigh 126 pounds and run 10-minute miles you'll be working at 10 METs and losing 10 calories per minute. As your weight varies, upward or downward, from 57 kilos, the numbers change proportionately. Here's a quick rundown for those interested: remember these numbers won't win prizes for precision. Biology is that way — mostly ballpark figures — because there are so many variable factors pushing the averages hither and yon.

Kilos	Pounds	Calories Per Minute Per MET
25	55	0.5
30	66	
35	77	
40	88	
(43)	(95)	0.75
45	99	
50	110	
55	121	
(57)	(125)	1.0
60	132	
65	143	
70	154	
(71)	(156)	1.25
75	165	
80	176	
85	187	1.50
90	198	
95	209	
100	220	1.75
105	231	
110	242	
(114)	(251)	2.0
115	253	
120	264	

All of which merely tells you how to relate the number of METs of *intensity* — how many bricks per minute you're tossing into the truckbed — to calories per minute. So if you weigh 80 kilos (176 pounds) and are working at 8 METs, you're using between 1¼ and

---

MET equivalents (approximate) of a few activities

Activity	METs
Sleep	1
Typing	2
Walking (2 mph)	3
Mowing grass	4
Walking (3 mph)	5
Tennis	6–7
Shoveling snow	7–11
Racquetball	8
Canoeing (4 mph)	9
Cycling (15 mph)	10
Running (7 mph)	12
Walking upstairs	15

1½ times 8 calories per minute — about 11 calories per minute of exercise. Can one predict, knowing the MET level, how *difficult* the work will feel? Not unless we know the person's maximal work capacity, i.e., his or her aerobic power. For some, 10 METs of activity is totally out of reach; for others, that workload doesn't generate a pulse rate of 90! So while 10 METs are 10 METs whether performed by a world-class endurance athlete or a victim of heart disease, the impact upon the individual is a very different matter.

When we consider how much exercise we need or wish to do, we can calculate the total work simply by multiplying the intensity of the work (the METs achieved) by the number of minutes we continue it. (MET measurements have been worked out and charted for hundreds of activities.) Or, if we prefer, we can speak of work in terms of calories expended: oxygen-consumption figures are readily converted to calories lost, since every 1000cc of oxygen used represents heat release of about 5 calories.

FITNESS

Fitness is the general term for the complex changes that take place as a result of good and sufficient exercise. If you question a number of people on the subject, you'll find that each has a somewhat different option as to just what fitness is. Some focus on the body's shape, others look to strength and obvious muscularity. Still others refer to the capacity to perform hard and well. The noted exercise physiologist Dr. Herbert DeVries analysed fitness into nine components:

1. Strength
2. Speed
3. Agility
4. Endurance
5. Power
6. Coordination
7. Balance
8. Flexibility
9. Body Control

Some of these components are obviously related to workload, i.e., strength, power, speed, endurance. In the others, the relation to workload is a bit more obscure. (In Chapter 3, for example, we

More on METs

Naturally as your training progresses in each dimension — strength, speed-power, together with both heart and skeletal muscle endurance — the variety of exercises you can expect to tackle successfully will widen. If, for example, your work intensity is limited to 5 METs, jumping movements, which require 8 to 12 METs without the addition of arm work, will be too much for you. If 10 METs is where you are, Heavyhands work involving jumps or hops intermittently will be fine. And when you're at 12 to 13 METs or more, continuous endurance work involving jumps along with arm movement will find you well able to pay as you go where it comes to oxygen transport. All of which should surprise no one. New sources of energy, viewed either psychologically or physiologically, open new vistas. Training effects can yield more than "just" more; they yield more *possibilities*, more qualities as well as quantities of activity. It would be difficult to imagine the differences between a race of humans with work capacities averaging say, 3 METs, as compared with 18 METs. Simple arithmetic, the factor of 6 times, wouldn't begin to describe the gap between 3 and 18 METs. Numbers followed by 4 to 6 zeros might be more accurate, my rudimentary math tells me.

I study the movement abilities of people who live within the crushing limits of 3 METs. The species gap between 3 and 18 METs is at least as wide as the one separating earthworms from eagles.

The components of workload

The performance of work requires strength, speed-power, and endurance. Strength is the force of individual contractions — how much weight can be lifted once. Power, which is used in throws and swings, requires strength and speed to act in concert. Power is work divided by time. Endurance is the number of contractions or repetitions a muscle can accomplish before exhaustion.

Fitness elements

Freud once noted that the "structures" of personality as he labeled them — id, ego, and superego — were not identifiable as such unless the host human was in trouble. Strength, speed-power, and endurance of both heart and skeletal muscle varieties mix during most continuous movements so that none is isolated, though all are plainly present.

shall discuss cardiopulmonary, or heart-lung, fitness, which is crucial but a bit more complicated.) For the moment we want to define the kinds of work that skeletal muscles — the ones attached to our bones — perform.

Strength refers to the *force* of individual contractions. The stronger the muscle, the heavier the weight it can lift *once*.

Power is work divided by time. Power may be thought of as strength combined with speed. Throws and swings — the discus, javelin, or shotput — in which great strength and speed act in concert are examples of power.

Endurance refers to the number of contractions or repetitions a muscle can manage before exhaustion.

All muscle work is accomplished by the release of energy that accompanies certain chemical reactions within the muscle fibers. Two general chemical situations are distinguishable. *Aerobic* work is accomplished when sufficient oxygen allows the chemical reactions to reach completion. In *anaerobic* work insufficient oxygen leads to the build-up of lactic acid in the muscle, which causes the characteristic ache related to work of high intensity and short duration.

WHY EXERCISE?

A veritable mountain of research over the past decade proclaims the wisdom of exercising. Exercise is both preventer and healer of some forms of illness. Its effectiveness in prevention of and rehabilitation in cardiovascular disease has become medical doctrine. It seems to retard the aging process: in Sweden, where physical activity is abundant and universal, the average male outlives his American counterpart by some 5.3 years. Most experts see activity as the best insurance against obesity and perhaps its most effective cure.

Exercise has been found useful in the prevention and cure of certain forms of emotional suffering. Running has proved to be a potent antidepressant, rivaling drug treatment for many victims.

A strong positive correlation exists between academic excellence and fitness levels. My guess is we've only begun to realize the potential benefits exercise can bestow.

WHAT ARE AMERICANS DOING FOR EXERCISE?

Since 1969 when Ken Cooper chose the term *aerobics* to signify the importance of endurance exercise in fitness, literally millions of Americans have tried it. The statistics are ballooning. Perhaps thirty million Americans run; an equal number walk for exercise. It is said that twenty-eight million will take to swimming during the 1980s. Aerobic dancing, popularized by Jacki Sorensen, is claiming new adherents each day. Bikers — both those on the road and those spinning the wheels of stationary models — account for more millions. Countless more faithfully pursue calisthenic routines in the nation's spas and emporia. In all, one hundred thirty-five million Americans are said to be exercising.

Sports, too, are effective means of producing reasonable fitness levels. This is more true of the court games — basketball, racquetball, squash, hockey, and so forth, in which the activity is reasonably continuous. Karate and other martial arts can also be employed as aerobic activities.

All in all, according to various pollsters over 55 percent of Americans are exercising. But all is not as positive as the numbers suggest. The dropout rate is very high, estimated at 40 to 60 percent. Americans who are easily attracted to new ideas may be equally at risk of untimely quitting. Our whimsical nature as a people is amusing and fun when it involves hoola hoops, dance crazes, and faddish clothing; when it involves our health — exercise and diet — it is disastrous.

WHAT IS HEAVYHANDS?

For starters, Heavyhands is an endurance-dominated exercise. Like other aerobic sports, it pushes for duration and intensity, working toward the largest rate of oxygen consumption over the longest reasonable period of time. You will remember, from the previous discussion of how we measure exercise, that oxygen consumption is another way of saying how much work we are doing and how many calories we are losing. As you will see, no other exercise consumes oxygen as rapidly as does Heavyhands.

Favorite American sports	
ACTIVITY	NUMBER OF PEOPLE
Walking	34,500,000
Swimming	27,000,000
Bowling	21,000,000
Bicycling	19,500,000
Jogging	16,500,000
Camping	15,000,000
Tennis	13,500,000
Calisthenics	12,000,000
Basketball	10,500,000
Hiking	10,500,000
Softball	10,500,000
Baseball	9,000,000
Golf	7,500,000
Volleyball	7,500,000
Dancercize	6,000,000
Football	6,000,000
Frisbee	6,000,000
Table Tennis	6,000,000
Slimnastics	4,500,000
Snow skiing (down hill)	4,500,000
Waterskiing	4,500,000
Weight lifting	4,500,000
Badminton	3,000,000
Ice skating	3,000,000
Raquetball	3,000,000
Snow skiing (cross country)	3,000,000
Archery	1,500,000
Boxing	1,500,000
Gymnastics	1,500,000
Handball	1,500,000
Hockey	1,500,000
Karate	1,500,000
Mountain climbing	1,500,000
Soccer	1,500,000
Squash	1,500,000
Track and field	1,500,000
Wrestling	1,500,000
TOTAL:	292,500,000

Heavyhands, oxygen, and calories

No other exercise consumes oxygen as rapidly as does Heavyhands. Since oxygen consumption is just another way of expressing the number of calories used up, no other exercise burns fat as fast as Heavyhands.

Arms versus legs

Because our legs hold us up and our arms just hang down, most people, regardless of how unfit, have relatively "trained" legs and untrained arms. No matter how hard and long they exercise most people cannot improve their legs' workload intensity by more than 25 percent. Using Heavyhands exercises, the arms' workload intensity can be increased by 100 percent or more.

While the muscles of the lower body are much bigger than those of the upper body (about a three- or four-to-one ratio), ounce for ounce the upper-torso muscles can do more work than the leg muscles. Incidentally, the upper torso includes lots of muscle mass that seldom receives adequate aerobic or endurance-type training.

Heavyhands exercises multiple muscle groups simultaneously. Some of the advanced exercises in this book involve virtually every muscle in the body — at the same time. Moving, or working, more of the body's muscle — as common sense would suggest — can produce greater workloads than using fewer muscles does.

Because the legs support and carry around the rest of the body, they are invariably more fit than the arms, which for the most part just hang there. The nonexerciser who over the years has gradually grown unfit and fat has inadvertently been "training" his legs to carry more weight. This means that exercise of the "untrained" arms can produce proportionately greater gains than exercise of the "trained" legs. Equally or perhaps more important, arm muscle can consume much more oxygen than the same amount of leg muscle. (Again, remember that oxygen use means workload and calorie consumption.) For these two reasons — arms are less "trained" than legs; and, ounce for ounce, can do more work (use more oxygen) than legs — exercise of the arms (actually, the whole upper torso and trunk) is emphasized in Heavyhands.

To take advantage of the potential superiority of the arms and upper-torso muscles in exercise, we weight the hands. Do not confuse Heavyhands with weight lifting and weight training, which are strength sports, concerned with lifting heavy weights a few times. Heavyhands is an aerobic exercise system. The weights carried are relatively light, are moved through a high number of repetitions, and are used in conjunction with exercise of the legs.

As you will see, Heavyhands exercises can be enormously varied, but to explain the method quickly, here is a basic exercise: while walking or running, swing (or "pump") a small dumbbell in each hand in an arc from mid-thigh to shoulder level. What seems a simple combination of two well-known forms of exercise produces extensive physiological effects. When increases of speed and movement are introduced, greater effects are achieved.

WHO IS HEAVYHANDS FOR?

Heavyhands is for everyone who can. Physical incapacity or illness is the only real deterrent to beginning Heavyhands. The technique was designed to serve either as a *primary technique* or to complement and extend other aerobic activities or sports.

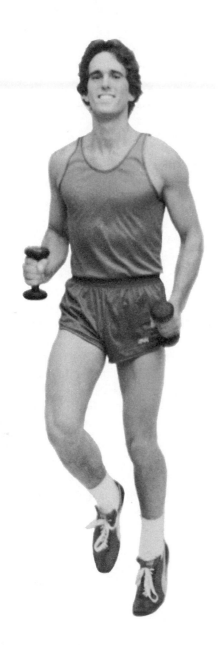

HEAVYHANDS ADVANTAGES

A. *Genderless.* Heavyhands is impartial to the sexes. Though there exist distinct physiologic differences, these are deemphasized by the nature of the method. Strength is promoted constantly, but it might better be termed endurance-strength. Large numbers of movements with moderate weights do not produce bulky muscles in either male or female. The high-repetition option using even tiny handweights also exploits the speed-power option that makes for great endurance and unrivaled body-weight control.

B. *Widest range of workloads (panaerobics).* Five years of experimentation with Heavyhands have shown that four limbs are better than two and can be trained to consume more oxygen per unit of time. Research done almost two decades ago showed that arms and legs working in combination could perform *longer* than legs alone at the same work intensity. It also showed that the exerciser *felt* more comfortable with the arms-legs combinations.

More recent studies have shown the upper extremities to be

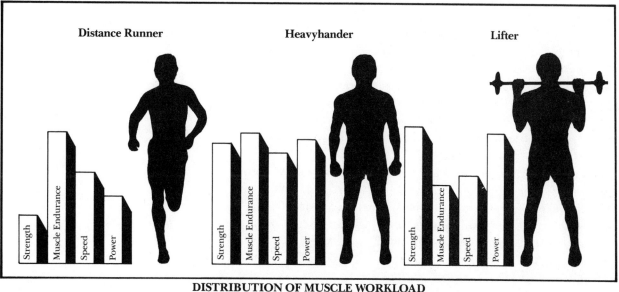

**DISTRIBUTION OF MUSCLE WORKLOAD
COMPONENTS IN VARIOUS EXERCISERS**

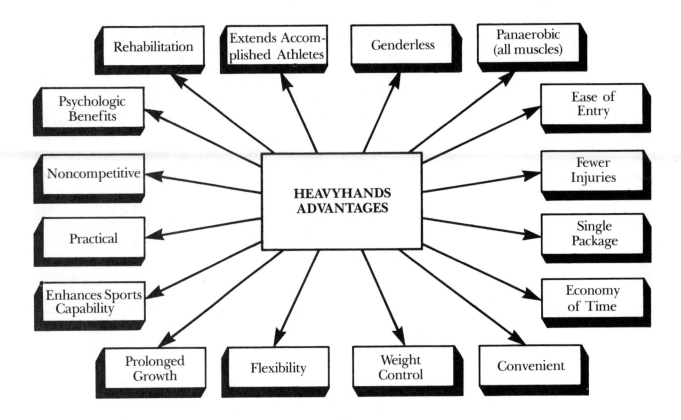

astonishingly effective oxygen consumers — more than legs, per volume of muscle activated. A given piece of arm biceps, for example, can outconsume an equal-size piece of muscle from the front of the thigh. Heavyhands exercise can increase the *total work output* of the upper torso as much as thousands of percent. The legs' development is enhanced at the same time, since they too must support the hands' added weight.

C. Ease of entry for the beginner. For the newcomer to exercise, Heavyhands techniques make starting out easy. Distributing the workload over the entire muscle mass, instead of concentrating it all on one set of muscles, feels less difficult and makes it possible to increase the work intensity gradually and safely. By using weights, you add a variable to your exercise, which allows you to distribute the workload to suit your physique and its level of fitness. Thus, if you find your arms approaching exhaustion, you can use lighter weights and move them faster. Conversely, if your pace produces breathlessness, you simply slow down and/or decrease the weights or the range of motion. The point is that even as a beginner you can accomplish significant and beneficial workloads by distributing the effort over many muscles and by adjusting speed and weight. The important result is that by using Heavyhands virtually anyone — regardless of how unfit — can do 30 minutes of aerobic exercise almost immediately.

D. Fewer injuries. By design, Heavyhands avoids many of the injuries that runners and other aerobic exercisers contend with. The protection is afforded at least four ways: (1) Flexibility training is *included* in the exercise proper. For most Heavyhanders no special "stretch time" is necessary. (2) The wide array of movements and distribution of the workload prevent the overuse typical of most aerobic exercises. For instance, in Heavyhands running the slower pace results in fewer traumatic foot strikes. (3) The high priority given to strengthening muscles and ligaments is probably protective. (4) The development of greater muscle endurance may reduce the risk of injury, which increases in overly fatigued muscles. For a given intensity of exercise, Heavyhands will produce fewer injuries than other endurance training methods. Heavyhands may also be employed temporarily by exercisers hobbled by injuries. By the use of healthy limbs, cardiopulmonary deconditioning is avoided. Because Heavyhands consciously includes muscle groups that are seldom exercised aerobically, a number of typical injuries and maladies associated with flagrant disuse are prevented. This is particularly true of back problems.

E. Single package. Heavyhands delivers *all* of the fitness factors in a single strategy. Additional work may be added for those who wish to specialize in strength, speed, or great flexibility. But Heavyhands, with no additions, will produce outsized values in each fitness category.

F. Economy of time. Because the potential intensity of Heavyhands exercise is greater than that of other training systems, it follows that it will require less total time to maintain a given fitness level. Again, less time is devoted to warm-up and stretching routines, and fewer injuries mean less time lost waiting to "mend."

G. Convenience. Heavyhands technique may be practiced indoors and out, year around. In advanced trainees, workloads equivalent to the running of 4- to 5-minute miles can be achieved while watching TV! Equipment is inexpensive and portable enough to carry on trips. Seasonal weather conditions, which discourage some exercisers, are not deterrents. Some Heavyhanders practice during work hours, doing a number of short "intervals" spread throughout the day.

H. Weight control. I mention weight control (really body composition control) here merely in passing and will deal with this subject at length in Chapter 15. Once you are conditioned, large Heavyhands workloads can mean the largest numbers of calories lost per unit of time — and current research indicates that exercise, rather than diet, is the most important factor in weight control.

I. Flexibility. More so than other aerobic methods, Heavyhands invites growth in many different directions. When one element, such as strength, seems to plateau, others can be emphasized. This very shift of emphasis is the key in Heavyhands. The workload can be shifted from one region of the body to another, either for emphasis or to rest fatigued muscle groups. The large repertoire allows the exerciser to diversify or to specialize without sacrificing central fitness factors. Workouts can and should shift frequently to follow the Heavyhander's changing needs and interests.

J. Prolonged growth. Most endurance exercise generates the greatest improvement within the first six months of intensive training. This generally falls within the range of a 5- to 25-percent increase over the exerciser's original oxygen-consumption rate. Obviously, improvement is apt to be greater among those whose pretraining condition was poorest. After six months, gains in work capacity tend to be insignificant. Since the upper torso is ordinarily relatively deconditioned, its training may continue far beyond what is typical for the legs. I have seen continued increases in the rate of oxygen consumption after five years! Those whose endurance training is leg dominated and who have leveled off may experience some increase in leg-work capacity after beginning Heavyhands training. The extended growth comes from the use of other muscles and increasing the strength component of their workouts.

K. Enhancement of sports capability. Heavyhands will enhance any other sports activity. Sports injuries may be prevented by the increase of strength-endurance in specific areas of the body often neglected by the exclusive practice of the sport itself. Your current program of walking, jogging, running, swimming, biking, or rope jumping can be significantly improved by Heavyhands training. In addition, leisure-time sports, such as tennis, golf, and bowling, can

Travel Heavyhands

I take my weights everywhere. A couple of times when my fantasy life got the best of me, I squeezed 60 or more pounds into suitcases that didn't survive the trip. The weights are indestructible, of course, but your clothes may need intensive care upon arrival. Actually, weights to 5 pounds or more pack beautifully and can be instantly converted to 5- to 20-MET exercise for use in your hotel room; or you can pump 'n' run sightseeing in faraway places.

Heavyhands feels easier — higher anaerobic threshold?

The anaerobic threshold (AT) is that level of work intensity at which the concentration of lactic acid in the blood becomes high enough to turn on certain physiologic mechanisms. The volume of air breathed suddenly increases dramatically, for example, at the anaerobic threshold. Heavyhands training typically increases the anaerobic threshold, or, one might say, *delays* the onset of *metabolic acidosis*. That may be another measurable partial explanation for why the Heavyhander, working harder, feels *less* belabored at given workloads than he would doing conventional, specialized aerobics. We think it's the pitching in of lots of muscle mass as well as the greater *average* contraction and lengthening of individual muscle fibers that raises the hander's AT.

be improved both through the training of specific muscles and by the general "enhancement" of fitness.

L. Practical. Heavyhands training is geared to deal with life's real demands. Its "panaerobic" approach — endurance training for the heart and all of the muscles — makes the typical daily chore easier and new ones a pleasant challenge.

M. Noncompetitive. While competition in sports may be useful, it can complicate, endanger, or even abort an exercise program. Heavyhands' multifaceted, individualized approach helps diminish the unrealistic impulse to compete with those whose skills and abilities are different from ours.

N. Psychologic benefits. Most of the points listed above contribute to the psychological advantages of Heavyhands: large workloads, extended growth, ease of beginning, diversity, safety, flexibility, convenience, practicality — all extend interest and enthusiasm and lessen boredom. The development of skill and the range of possible physiologic rewards reduce the ever-present danger of quitting. Finally, the use of combined exercise makes any Heavyhands workload level seem less taxing than one performed using other methods — an additional psychic bonus.

O. Rehabilitation. One day Heavyhands training will find wide application in the field of rehabilitation. Too often efforts are concentrated solely on resurrecting the disabled muscles while the heart muscle is neglected utterly. So long as even one limb is capable of motion, some degree of cardiopulmonary (heart-lung) training is possible.

P. Extends the accomplished athlete. For the "jocks" who come superbly tuned and trim to Heavyhands, the method will provide exciting improvement to those who have long since reached the zero-growth level. The theory and practice of Heavyhands shows beyond doubt that many elite athletes presently settle for maintenance exercise far short of their best potential.

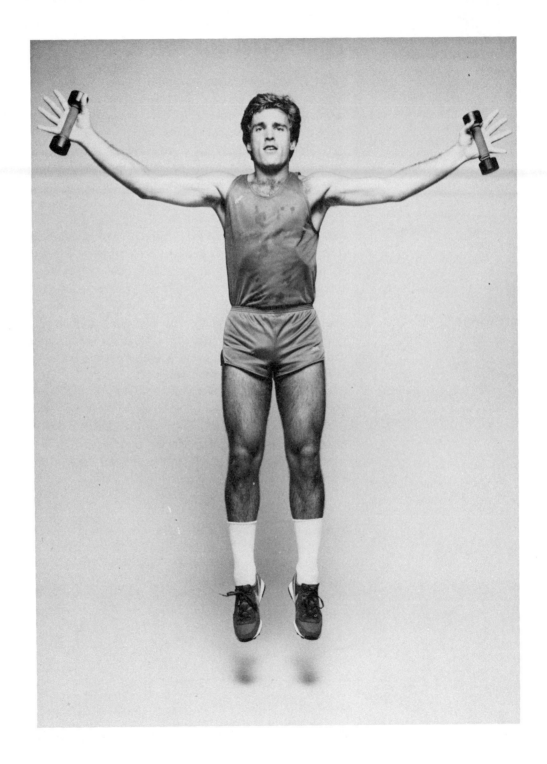

3

The Heart of the Matter

Big hearts and big VO₂Max

It's well known that elite long-distance runners develop large, muscular hearts. Instead of a typical 700cc model, marathon winners measure out about 1200cc. I have a sneaking suspicion that young, advanced Heavyhanders will prove to have smaller hearts than runners with similar oxygen consumption rates (VO_2Max). Why do I think so? Personal experience for one thing. At my age, males typically have coronaries that are about one-third closed. With my five years of training, a relatively high VO_2Max for an old-timer, and with some twenty years of blood pressure that tends to be elevated, one would think my heart would be larger than normal. It isn't. Could it be that a number of duets working simultaneously may not stimulate heart enlargement? Put another way, could overconcentration on few duets have something to do with the heart enlargement we see in some endurance athletes?

THE HEART MUSCLE

HEAVYHANDS IS first and foremost a heart conditioner. The aerobic era, sparked largely by Ken Cooper's work, shifted the emphasis of exercise to the heart, which is central to all endurance conditioning. The heart is admirably suited to that task. Its peculiarly interconnected, branching fibers, viewed under the microscope, are quite different from skeletal or voluntary muscles. While we frequently discuss how many push-ups, sit-ups, or pull-ups we can do, with the heart muscle we don't speak of number of repetitions. We are, however, concerned with the rate of the heart's contractions and the effectiveness of these contractions in pumping oxygen-laden blood throughout the body. For reasons that are all too apparent, when we speak of the heart muscle work we speak only of intensity — never duration! It lasts a lifetime; when it stops, so does life. A skeletal muscle overloaded by hard work will simply quit. When the heart muscle falls behind the workload presented to it, you quickly become aware of it, sense your inability to continue — and soon stop exercising — and the healthy heart muscle continues its beat without a hitch.

STROKE VOLUME

In the case of skeletal muscle, we have all sorts of units by which we describe its work capacity, and most are borrowed from physics. If a 150-pound man steps onto a 12-inch step, we say he has accomplished 150 foot-pounds of work (150 pounds × 1 foot). In the case of heart muscle we speak of the amount of blood the heart can eject either in a minute or per beat. So *cardiac output* is described in terms of liters of blood per minute. Or, dividing that total by the heart's rate, we come up with a number called *stroke volume* — the amount of blood pumped per beat or contraction — of the heart pump. Skeletal muscles, incidentally, may receive enormous increases in blood flow — up to eighteen times what they use at rest — during particularly vigorous exercise.

When we spoke of METs — you'll remember these numbers represented multiples of the resting subject's rate of oxygen consumption — the number of METs gives us a ballpark notion as to how much work is being done during a given exercise. Now, do METs refer to skeletal-muscle or to heart-muscle work? Both. The MET describes the bottom line, so to speak, of what's happening. Ten METs means that the heart delivery system, together with the working muscles at the receiving end, are teaming up to use 10 times as much oxygen per minute as the exerciser would if he were at rest. Since the heart itself is a muscle, it, too, requires oxygen for *its* work.

OXYGEN PULSE

One more slightly technical, but really simple idea, before we go on to more practical concerns. Each heartbeat delivers a certain amount of oxygen to the working muscles. We call that the *oxygen pulse*. I bring it up now because it will be important in your later understanding of the special effects of Heavyhands exercise. Suppose I measured your oxygen use during an exercise and determined that you consumed 3000cc of oxygen during a given minute's work — at a pulse rate of, say, 150 beats per minute. Simply dividing the 3000 by 150 gives us a figure of 20 — the *oxygen pulse* for that workload: 20cc of oxygen delivered per heartbeat. Like METs, this number represents the effectiveness of both heart and skeletal muscle working in concert. While METs tell us how much total work is being done *compared to rest,* the oxygen pulse tells us how efficiently oxygen is being transported at a *variety* of workloads.

The number of METs, representing work intensity, will run a pretty close parallel to heart rate: the higher the MET value, the higher the pulse rate during sustained exercise. Oxygen pulse, on the other hand, remains *relatively* constant throughout a range of work intensities. With some variation, the oxygen pulse is independent of heart rate. Thus, if your oxygen pulse were 15, you would consume 15cc of oxygen with each of 100 beats a minute, and also 15cc with each of 150 beats a minute of the same sort of exercise performed more strenuously. Obviously your MET or intensity level is considerably higher at a 150 pulse. (When the pulse rate falls below 100–120, the oxygen pulse falls off sharply and is lowest when the body is at rest.)

Stroke volume

Stroke volume is the amount of blood the heart pumps with each beat. Stroke volume can be determined by measuring how many liters of blood the heart pumps during a minute and dividing that by the heart rate.

Oxygen pulse

Oxygen pulse is the term we use to describe how much oxygen is used with each beat of the heart. We arrive at the oxygen pulse by determining how many cubic centimeters of oxygen we use in one minute, then dividing that figure by our pulse rate.

More on oxygen pulse

The oxygen pulse tells us much about how well oxygen transport is being managed. Its level is determined by two main factors: the cardiac output and the rate at which the muscles consume oxygen. The artery that feeds a muscle contains blood richer in oxygen than the vein that leads the same blood away from that muscle. If you measure arterial and venous blood for their respective oxygen content, you arrive at what's called the a-v oxygen difference. The pump output and the a-v oxygen difference determine the oxygen pulse.

Trained Heavyhanders enjoy higher oxygen pulses than they would doing other kinds of aerobics. Even though the cardiac output may not increase much, the "hander's" *total work* capacity *does*. That happens because more muscles involved in "duets" with the heart *extract* oxygen from the blood *more efficiently;* i.e. a higher oxygen pulse. The trained Heavyhander, then, can do more work and lose more calories per heartbeat than his untrained fellows. And lots of trained muscles doing a given amount of work do it with less evidence of *strain;* i.e., slower pulse and lower blood pressure than when only a few trained muscles accomplish the same work. The idea, admittedly, is deceptively simple!

Once I measure your oxygen consumption during the exercise, do I know which of your muscles were receiving most of the oxygen? Only roughly. If you were working on a treadmill or bicycle ergometer (work meter) we would simply assume *most* of the oxygen was going to your belabored legs.

Now supposing we take a well-trained runner, seat him comfortably, and ask him to work his arms to a metronome's beat in a simple up-and-down alternate motion. Presuming he's untrained at such odd antics, when we measure his oxygen uptake, we'll find (1) that he's capable of far less work with arms alone than with legs alone; and (2) that his oxygen pulse will be quite low.

He may, for example, use only 1500cc of oxygen at a pulse rate that had zoomed to 200 during the exercise:

$$1500 \div 200 = 7.5$$

A very low oxygen pulse indeed, compared with his legs-alone value of 20. When we think of oxygen pulse, we are considering the relative effectiveness of the heart supplier and the muscle receiver in a "duet" or unity.

THE "DUET"

In the drawing we'll pretend the body is nothing but a shell of muscle surrounding its heart, which supplies oxygen. And I should state in passing that all of the commerce between the central (heart-lung) and peripheral (skeletal-muscle) elements requires a system of interconnecting conduits called *blood vessels*. When these channels are not wide open, not much happens for very long. But for the moment I've left them out simply to avoid confusion.

In the drawing on page 30, the thickness of the two-way arrows passing from heart to muscle region is proportional to the effectiveness of the oxygen *transport system* vis-à-vis that group of muscles. Apparently the heart pumps on cheerfully, heedless of which muscle groups are the most avid recipients of its oxygen-rich offering. The runners' legs and heart have developed a very compatible and efficient "duet." The rest of the runner's muscles, relatively untrained, simply ignore the oxygen-rich mixture coming their way, since they have neither the need nor the capability to accept much of it.

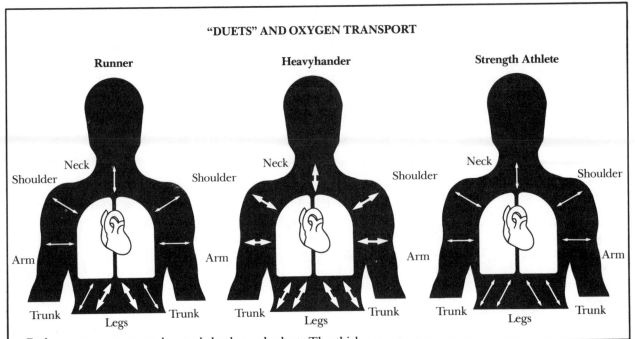

"DUETS" AND OXYGEN TRANSPORT

Runner   **Heavyhander**   **Strength Athlete**

Each arrow represents a heart–skeletal muscle duet. The thickness of the arrow is proportional to the work capability of that particular duet. *Energy* would be another way of expressing a given duet's effectiveness.

Each duet is affected by the training it receives, and each is basically independent of its fellow duets.

Each duet can be described in terms of:

1. *Total workload* — i.e., METs, calorie cost, oxygen consumed, foot-pounds, etc.
2. *Workload components* — strength, speed-power, endurance, range of motion.
3. *Oxygen pulse* — the efficiency of oxygen transport when a given duet is "loaded" by exercise. Oxygen pulse is computed simply by dividing the volume of oxygen consumed per minute by the pulse rate during that work interval. The quotient represents the number of cubic centimeters of oxygen used per heartbeat.

Combinations of simultaneous duets can be described in the same terms — workload totals, contributing components, and oxygen pulse average — as a single duet.

The trained Heavyhander generates the highest workloads for two reasons. He or she employs more duets simultaneously; and, with each duet, the workload can be further increased by altering the range, direction, and variety of movement and by using *all* the workload components — strength, speed-power, and endurance.

VO₂Max

VO$_2$Max is the term used to describe the largest amount of oxygen an exerciser uses during a given period of time. It may be expressed simply as the number of liters consumed or as the number of cubic centimeters of oxygen per kilogram of body weight per minute. For example: if a 70-kilo man's maximum uptake turns out to be 2.8 liters per minute, his VO$_2$Max is 2800cc (2.8 liters) divided by 70 (his weight), or 40 ml/kilo/min^{-1}.

Thus we can say that when a "duet" is capable of great workload it can generate:
- a high MET value: O$_2$ consumed/unit body weight
- a large oxygen pulse: efficient use of oxygen/heartbeat

THE LIMITING FACTOR: HEART OR SKELETAL MUSCLE?

What determines how much total work an exerciser can perform? Is it the heart's work — cardiac output — or the skeletal muscle's oxygen extraction rate? As a matter of fact, we're not quite sure. Research has produced excellent arguments on both sides. For what it's worth and without wasting much printer's ink, I'll present my views as derived from my own experiments and the recent literature.

The largest amount of oxygen that an exerciser can consume in a given period of time is called the VO$_2$Max (the maximum volume

What limits oxygen consumption?

What factors favor the highest possible rate of oxygen consumption? The sustained exercise that mobilizes the largest amount of muscle capable of the greatest total workload — i.e., a combination of strength, speed-power, and endurance. Heavyhands research shows the delivery system is capable of covering more muscle activity than was previously supposed.

Arguments seesaw from delivery-dominant to receiver-dominant theories. Experiments now underway using Heavyhanders may provide the answer. While both delivery system (lungs, heart, blood vessels, and blood) and receiver (muscle) must be limited, *no ordinary sports or exercise programs test these limits during combined exercise of four trained limbs.*

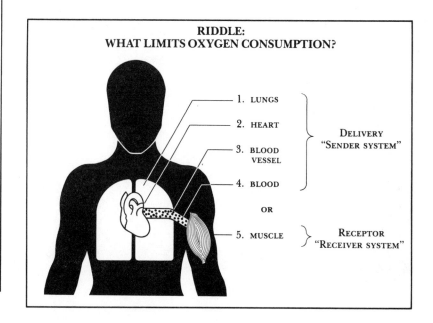

**RIDDLE:
WHAT LIMITS OXYGEN CONSUMPTION?**

1. LUNGS
2. HEART
3. BLOOD VESSEL
4. BLOOD

DELIVERY "SENDER SYSTEM"

OR

5. MUSCLE

RECEPTOR "RECEIVER SYSTEM"

Range of maximal oxygen consumption values for athletes in various sports

SPORT	MAXIMAL OXYGEN CONSUMPTION (CCs of oxygen per kilogram of body weight per minute)
MEN	
Cross-country skiers	70–94
Long-distance runners	65–85
Rowers	58–75
Bicyclists	55–70
Long-distance swimmers	48–68
Gymnasts	48–64
Speed skaters	50–75
Ice hockey players	50–60
Football players	45–64
Baseball players	45–55
Tennis players	42–56
WOMEN	
Cross-country skiers	56–74
Long-distance runners	55–72
Rowers	41–58
Long-distance swimmers	45–60
Speed skaters	40–52
Sprinters	38–52
Basketball players	35–45

Reproduced with permission from J. H. Wilmore, *Athletic Training and Physical Fitness; Physiological Principles and Practices of the Conditioning Process* (Boston: Allyn and Bacon, 1977).

of oxygen). As you read about exercise you'll come across this term frequently. Researchers two decades ago thought that legs and arms working together could *not* outproduce the work (or oxygen consumed) of legs alone. In fact, they believed that if the arms contributed more that 30 percent of the combined effort, the total work level tended to drop. The assumption they drew, naturally, was that the heart was the limiting factor.

Combined benefits

When you stop to think about it, no one should be surprised to learn that an experienced Heavyhander can sustain intensities for a couple of hours that he can only manage for a couple of minutes leg-alone. An elite marathoner runs at about 75 percent of his maximum work capacity. The Heavyhander first increases the aerobic power of the arms that *already* enjoy respectable capability without much practice. Now arms and legs together, working at perhaps 50 percent of their respective capacities, can equal or exceed that 75 percent of maximum load by which legs win marathons. And perhaps that's why it *feels* easier. *Lots* of units, each doing *less,* can add to *more.*

"Sub-duets"

Because all of the muscles of a given body region seldom receive equal work, it is sometimes useful to think of sub-duets between the heart and certain skeletal muscles. For example, the hamstrings, the biceps of the leg, rarely get the opportunity to contract fully during continual vigorous exercise or sport. Thus, a person superbly trained in leg aerobics generally may carry a large hamstring mass that performs poorly given tasks that put the knee joint through a great range of motion. (See *"Heavyhands Kickbacks for hamstrings,"* page 200.)

These researchers did find, interestingly, that combined arm-and-leg work, when equal to the maximum leg-alone work, could be continued *twice* as long. Additionally, the exercisers reported their sense of effort was *lower* during the combined exercise. In view of these two findings — that combined exercise felt easier and could be continued longer — it is curious that these obvious benefits weren't exploited.

New literature, however, tells us that some exercisers *can and do use more oxygen in combined exercise than with legs alone.* Research in the past decade on combined arm-leg exercise has uncovered two interesting facts. If the subject had the benefit of special arm training, such as a canoeist, his combined workloads often exceeded his legs-alone effort. Or, if his leg-alone performance was rather low, there was a good chance that his combined *total* would be *better than his leg maximum.*

Further, from my research and training I discovered: 1. Heavyhands training could produce high leg workloads (mine are in the ninety-ninth percentile for my age). 2. My arm workloads increased to such an extent that combined work *continued to surpass* my large leg capability. What I didn't realize until recently was that *Heavyhands training, without special emphasis, could produce arm totals that surpass even high leg totals.* The effect of such training — accomplished in two to three hours weekly — will be best imagined when I explain that working arms and legs together I can cruise for two hours at workloads my legs can scarcely sustain for two minutes! And I have no reason to believe, as of the moment, that this is out of range for *anyone* who is healthy enough to train at it.

It remains uncertain as to *just how much* the arms and other nonleg muscles can contribute toward increasing the total workload, because few people have embarked upon a stength-endurance training program that involves the arms, much less almost all of the musculature. But having trained with Heavyhands for over five years, I experienced explosive increases in legs-alone work output for half a year, then moderate and decreasing progress. The arm workload, in both duration and intensity, increased far more spectacularly and continued to climb at a *faster* clip than did that of the legs. The point is the heart *continued to cover* all of the additional hard work put to it. A highly trained runner — entering a serious program as a Heavyhander — can expect his total oxygen con-

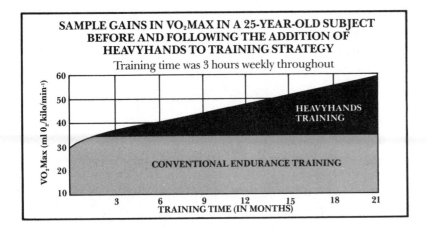

SAMPLE GAINS IN VO₂MAX IN A 25-YEAR-OLD SUBJECT BEFORE AND FOLLOWING THE ADDITION OF HEAVYHANDS TO TRAINING STRATEGY

Training time was 3 hours weekly throughout

y-axis: VO₂Max (ml O₂/kilo/min⁻¹) — 10, 20, 30, 40, 50, 60

HEAVYHANDS TRAINING

CONVENTIONAL ENDURANCE TRAINING

x-axis: TRAINING TIME (IN MONTHS) — 3, 6, 9, 12, 15, 18, 21

sumption to increase, meteorically if he's young. *While the heart muscle, like everything else, has its limits, typical exercise as practiced today simply doesn't take best advantage of those limits.*

ARM-HEART "DUETS" AND VO₂MAX

Exercise literature suggests that at the same pulse rate arm work can consume only about 70 percent as much *oxygen* as leg-driven exercise does. Those numbers are surprisingly consistent. That is to say that a VO₂Max derived from an arms-alone test will, in untrained subjects, yield oxygen uptake rates about 70 percent of those produced during conventional, leg-driven treadmill or bicycle ergometer tests.

If untrained arms — usually less than 30 percent of the leg muscle mass — can generate 70 percent of the maximum workloads, what, I wondered, would they produce if arm-heart "duets" were trained? Further, what would be the combined effect of many such trained duets, involving even "axial" or trunk muscles — heretofore employed only tangentially, if at all, in aerobics?

When arm work equals 80 percent of the legs' best effort, I learned that *combined arm-and-leg work exceeds the legs' highest workload.* So I needed to determine: 1. What percent of the legs' workloads could trained arms produce? 2. What advantage, if any, would these higher work levels confer upon the exerciser? Heavyhands is, in part, a chronicle of that investigation.

An example of Heavyhands oxygen transport efficiency

On a treadmill winding at a 10-minute/mile pace I run off 2100cc of oxygen each minute. For me, that's about 10 METs or 10 times the oxygen I'd use when at rest. Now I do a floor exercise using arms and legs together, like walking in place, while alternately lifting little weights —again to the tune of 2100cc of oxygen — precisely the same workload I generated while treadmill running. What many find hard to believe is that my heart rate after running for 5 minutes is 120–130; after 5 minutes of combined, same workload exercise, it's 65–70! Of course, it takes four trained limbs to do it, but that's what Heavyhands is all about.

Maximum steady state exercise

While the level of one's maximal performance is good to know, perhaps a more practical piece of information is called the maximal steady state. The VO₂Max is measured after the subject being tested has exceeded his or her aerobic limits. The highest rates of oxygen consumption are measured at the limits of aerobic plus anaerobic work. The maximal steady state represents the highest level at which the subject can continue for, say, 10 minutes or more, and might be considered the limit of his or her steady aerobic capacity. An athlete with a VO₂Max of 75 who could continue for only a minute or two at that level might be capable of "steadying out" aerobically for 10 minutes at a VO₂ of 70.

COMBINED "DUETS" AND HIGHER TOTAL WORKLOADS

In terms of oxygen transport we found that the *trained upper torso could actually produce higher oxygen pulses than even well-trained legs.* More surprising, we found that trained arms could consume more total oxygen than trained legs. We learned, too, that "50-50" exercise was quite feasible: exercise in which legs and arms contribute *equally* to a combined total *far above* the legs' maximal work capacity. It is my conviction that the lower oxygen pulses that were once generally associated with the arms and upper-torso activity merely represent the historical neglect of the upper extremity, not their inherent deficiency as working units and certainly not the heart's inability as their supplier.

STRENGTH-ENDURANCE AND OXYGEN TRANSPORT

The quest for a single-package, comprehensive system of exercise has been impeded mostly by the problem of bringing the strength component to endurance-type training. As we have seen, there have been regional exclusions, i.e., neglect of the upper torso as a respectable aerobic "driver." It is evident that strength, a major contributor to the collective effects we call workload, is usually underplayed in endurance training. While the need for strength is generally recognized, strength work is usually added in the form of separate exercises devoted to that purpose. Some runners and swimmers use weight training, for example. But strength work seldom, if ever, is included in the training devoted to upgrading oxygen transport per se. And so we have an interesting paradox: on the one hand, powerful strength athletes (weight lifters) have only a modest oxygen-transport system; and the endurance specialists (elite distance runners) who consume enormous quantities of oxygen are not noted for their strength.

From the viewpoint of oxygen utilization, there are no real contradictions here. The lifters produce gargantuan workloads for a few seconds. Neither their skeletal nor heart muscle can continue long enough at heavy lifting to make "aerobics" a serious possibility.

Advantages of upper-torso duets

1. Upper-extremity "educability" means a prolonged period of growth (training effects) and greater ultimate workload capabilities.

2. Upper-torso conditioning may provide protection against heart attacks precipitated by unaccustomed upper-torso work and the high heart rates this produces in the untrained individual — witness the snow-shoveling tragedies every winter.

3. Greater pulse-slowing effect occurs than with leg-dominated work per unit of training time invested.

4. Work and play activities are facilitated by the beneficial effects related to skill and oxygen transport.

5. Especially desirable in women because the strength-endurance combination can be developed to an enormous degree *without* major addition of muscle mass; male–female differences in strength-endurance are not as great as in the case of "pure" low-repetition strength.

6. Since upper-torso duets can be trained to produce 70 to 100 percent or more of leg duet workloads, these will serve as effective backup for leg-dominated exercise, preventing cardiopulmonary deconditioning due to injury.

At the other end of the spectrum, the runner can continue to pay his way aerobically, by carefully excluding the strength component. He keeps his body mass, in terms of fat and even extra muscle, stripped to the functioning essentials required by his sport. But the runner's excellence at propelling himself long and fast horizontally is won only at conspicuous cost, measured in terms of strength. Finely tuned marathoners are frequently grossly lacking in jumping strength — their heart-leg duets are keyed quite specifically to the act of running.

Our research shows that a compromise — the wedding of strength and endurance — can probably produce the highest levels of oxygen transport of which our species is capable. And incremental increases of strength produce these high work intensities without sacrificing the duration of the exercise.

TARGET PULSE

Enough physiological theory. It's time to begin Heavyhands exercise. Your heart will be the easiest part of your oxygen-transport system to train. Given a healthy heart to begin with, it will not balk, hesitate, injure, or quit on you. There *is* always some risk in exercising, but exercise's growing popularity rests on the solid premise that for most people it is simply riskier *not to*. Your pulse rate, if your heart is healthy, is a dependable replica of your heart rate; each contraction of your heart is accompanied by a pulse wave that travels along the walls of your large arteries, where it can be felt and counted in places where they course near the body's surface. Each of us has a maximum pulse. It has been calculated to average about the difference between 220 and one's age. If you're fifty years old, your maximal heart rate and therefore pulse rate would be 220 minus 50, or 170.

Physiologists have determined that endurance exercise in healthy folks can be safely and usefully carried out within a range of 70 percent to 85 percent of this age-related maximum. So that same fifty-year-old with his 170 maximum should exercise at a level that will produce a pulse rate somewhere between 120 and 145 in round numbers.

Aging and exercise

The literature tells us that the average human loses about 3 to 4 METs of aerobic capacity between the years of twenty-five and fifty-five; then 2 more METs between fifty-five and sixty-five. These numbers are a bit less ominous in the active than the sedentary. Aging is something like driving from Los Angeles to New York: the trip depends upon the road chosen, the condition of your car, and the way you drive. The 2-MET drop that comes in that ten-year "trip" from fifty-five to sixty-five will make less difference if you drive it in a 15-MET model rather than an 8-MET clunker. It also depends on what you expect to do in New York!

Target pulse

Target pulse is the heart rate, or range of heart rates, at which most people can exercise effectively and safely. To find *your* target pulse, subtract your age from 220, which will give you your maximal heart rate. Your target pulse is then 70 to 85 percent of your maximal heart rate. Thus a healthy thirty-year-old has a target pulse of roughly 135 to 160.

$$
\begin{array}{r}
220 \\
-\ 30 \\
\hline
190
\end{array}
$$

70 percent of 190 = 133
85 percent of 190 = 162

PULSE COUNTING

I continue to be amazed at the unwillingness of many people to take their own pulses. I have taught the technique to hundreds of bright people who seem to approach the task with reluctance. Perhaps we instinctively avoid the examination of our own pulsating innards.

My advice to the beginning Heavyhander is to become instantly and aggressively expert at pulse counting. Once you've learned how, practice it. It is the best information about your heart you can get outside your doctor's office. Taking your pulse frequently teaches you all sorts of things about yourself: your heart's response to stress, fatigue, overeating, passion, anger, surprise, overtraining, as well as exercise workloads.

Pulses differ from individual to individual and from time to time. Not only the count, but the quality. Some pulses, especially in untrained people, are so hard to find it may require several minutes with delicately tuned fingertips. Other pulses fairly bound. In fit exercisers a strong, slow pulse usually indicates training has been effective.

I favor counting the pulse of the radial artery that travels along the thumb side of the palm surface of your wrist. Other books will tell you to count your carotids, located in the neck near the angle of the jaw. I'm slightly prejudiced against that method because some people have oversensitive neck arteries that trigger heart rate or rhythm changes when pressed. With practice you will be able to locate your radial pulse within a second or two. Early in the game your speed in finding your pulse is not important because your rate isn't apt to slow rapidly after exercise. Later it will be more important, but by then you'll experience no difficulty. Your fingers will home-in precisely to the "spot" like a typist's return to the home keys — unerringly.

I teach the six-second method for pulse counting. Though a short sample, it becomes more advantageous as training proceeds. A digital watch or one with a second hand is all you need. Count the first pulse beat as 0, not 1. I've known people who have gotten suspiciously high counts for years simply because they didn't understand the difference. And when you're doing a short count that difference becomes more significant. When you've counted beats

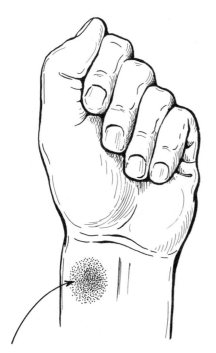

Where to feel for radial artery pulse

Oxygen and heart rate

Most exercise prescriptions are based on the well-documented fact that heart rate and oxygen consumption are proportional. The target pulse — 70 to 85 percent of our maximum heart rate — corresponds pretty closely to 57 to 75 percent of one's VO_2Max.

for six seconds, you need only multiply by ten to have your pulse rate.

After a while you can come within 10 percent of an accurate count just by the *feel* of the pulse and by some other clues. The best of these is your breathing pattern. Soon you will predict your pulse rate accurately enough by the rapidity and depth of your breaths. Later, when beginning new exercises, you will find your pulse rate surprisingly fast at first. This may represent increased muscle tension and the gross inefficiency associated with unfamiliar activity. As your training advances, these fast rates will become slower.

IRREGULAR PULSES

Most irregularities, if present, are readily evident when taking the pulse. A pulse beat may occur earlier than usual in the cycle and be followed by a prolonged pause. This pattern is quite common in anxious people, smokers, and coffee drinkers. If irregularities are frequent or occur in clusters, they can be analyzed by way of a cardiogram and/or a stress test. Sometimes exercise smoothes out the heartbeat. Other times, work precipitates more "premature" beats. In either case, *anyone with irregularities needs a doctor to help decide the place of exercise in his life.*

YOUR DOCTOR'S ROLE

With or without pulse irregularities, if you are thirty-five or over, or if you are not a regular exerciser, you should have your doctor administer a stress test. In ninety-nine out of one hundred cases, you will be cleared to exercise. Even people who have survived massive heart attacks have gone on to run marathons. Indeed, some abnormalities found in stress tests may call for a graded exercise program. In addition, the stress test gives valuable information about your blood pressure response to exertion and may suggest your correct target pulse more precisely than the cruder computation I described earlier. If the stress test does nothing else, it may give you the reassurance and support of your doctor to launch you as a confident Heavyhander.

Even if younger than thirty-five you should know what your

Six-second pulse counting

Count your first pulse beat as *o*, *not* 1. Count the number of pulses for six seconds. Multiply that number by ten. The result is your approximate pulse rate.

Heavyhands for cardiacs

A number of recent studies indicate there is little reason to exclude arm training from the exercise of heart patients. Robert D. Willix, Jr., M.D., Director of Cardiac Rehabilitation and Human Performance in the North Broward Hospital District, Ft. Lauderdale, Florida, is a pioneer in cardiac rehab research using Heavyhands. His findings suggest *less strain* during combined arm-leg aerobic exercise than with conventional training. This exciting effect appears to progress as arm training continues. Dr. Willix's work, still in its preliminary phases as of this writing, emphasizes the fact that circulatory efficiency, i.e., high oxygen pulse, may be a crucial advantage to sufferers from certain forms of heart disease. More total work is actually performed with fewer symptoms and at relatively *slow*, safer heart rates.

Smoking

Excerpt from August 21, 1981, *Journal of the American Medical Association* editorial:

"... Mechanisms whereby cigarette smoking can both accelerate the rate of development of cardiovascular disease and provoke coronary attacks have been elucidated. The chief components identified as noxious to the cardiovascular system are nicotine and carbon monoxide. These have been shown to evoke multiple adverse effects through cardiodynamic influences, atherogenesis, hemostatic changes, and vasculotoxic and inflammatory influences. Nicotine stimulates catecholamine release, increases myocardial irritability and heart rate, and causes vascular constriction and a transient rise in pressure, while at the same time, platelets become more adherent. As all this is taking place, carbon monoxide buildup has reduced the oxygen available to the myocardium. This combination of effects certainly could, and apparently does, precipitate sudden deaths and myocardial infarctions in cigarette smokers with a compromised coronary circulation."

English translation:

DON'T SMOKE!

blood pressure is before you begin to exercise. A rise in blood pressure is a normal response to physical exertion. During endurance exercise, the systolic tends to increase while the diastolic may drop somewhat (these are the names of the upper and lower numbers by which blood pressure readings are recorded), and for your doctor to evaluate these changes, he needs to know the "before" as well as the "after." Any suspected abnormality of blood pressure is another reason for a stress test. Generally, endurance training has a gradual, lowering effect upon the blood pressure, and moderate elevations of blood pressure are not apt to rule out good exercise.

PULSE AND TRAINING EFFECTS

As Heavyhands endurance training proceeds you will be rewarded by evidence of a generally slowing pulse. Both at rest and at a given workload it will be slower. That slowing means your heart's stroke volume, and inevitably your oxygen pulse, are increased. Even

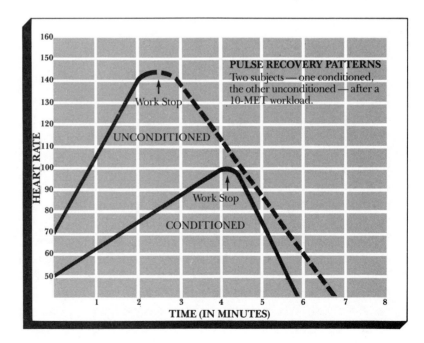

PULSE RECOVERY PATTERNS Two subjects — one conditioned, the other unconditioned — after a 10-MET workload.

without fancy laboratory equipment your pulse will yield excellent evidence of those changing values. If, for example, a given bit of work that produced a 150 pulse two months ago now produces only a rate of 100, you know that for the muscle groups involved the oxygen pulse has increased some 50 percent. Since beginning Heavyhands my pulse has halved itself. That means that 38 strokes a minute supplies my body with the 200cc or so of oxygen it needs at rest. (Remember 1 MET?) For me, it used to require 80 beats.

Another notable effect of training is a rapid slowing of the pulse rate once work stops. This fact becomes apparent in the so-called step tests of fitness. These tests are scored largely on the basis of the rate of recovery of the pulse upon completion of the task. On page 39 are two curves that graphically demonstrate the difference between conditioned and unconditioned subjects. As you can see, the untrained subject's pulse accelerates more rapidly, and returns to normal more slowly after the exertion stops. If you think of the curve as an elastic band you will retain the concept. The "deconditioned" curve is characteristically inelastic; the conditioned curve, yielding less readily, snaps back promptly.

HEAVYHANDS EFFECT ON YOUR HEART

I believe that Heavyhands training has the most telling potential for the cardiovascular system, both quantitatively and qualitatively. Each muscle group apparently exerts its effect upon the heart's activity *separately*. It follows that when various muscles are trained to produce greater overall workloads, there will be a greater number of efficient *duets* — effective cooperation between heart and skeletal muscles. Thus one achieves a greater average slowing of the heart rate — an indication of an enhanced work capacity.

As training proceeds, a given workload is managed at progressively lower pulse rates. The net savings constitute the training effect, and can be expressed in METs. If, say, a year ago, at a pulse rate of 120, when performing a given exercise you produced a work rate of 7 METs, but now, doing the same exercise, a 120 pulse produces 10 METs, the training effect would be 3 METs.

Blood pressure caveat

If you are aware that your blood pressure is frankly elevated or if it rises above the normal now and then, speak with your doctor about the wisdom of exercise for you. Though endurance training has a generally beneficial effect upon high blood pressure, one should not rely on exercise alone. Each case is different: most hypertensives will require medications too. In any event the great majority of those with high blood pressure are treatable: the treatment will seldom rule out endurance-oriented exercise.

Hot showers after Heavyhands

Don't take a hot shower right after hard exercise even though you enjoy hot showers and feel you deserve that pleasure following your honest sweat. Your overheated body continues to work to lose heat by several mechanisms. Hot water applied to your body surface, while courting the touch and temperature nerve endings in your skin, makes the task of losing heat more difficult. A few have died needlessly in hot showers following exercise and there were, as I understand it, no posthumous medals. Stay luke!

THE HEART OF THE MATTER / 41

Now we are ready to discuss equipment and the basic Heavyhands techniques. We will try simultaneous exercise of different parts of the body and observe the muscles' and heart's initial response.

More on pulse-slowing

In a recent class composed of novice women Heavyhanders at Montefiore Hospital, even we were taken aback by the degree of pulse-slowing we found: *90% of the participants' heart rates slowed an average of 2–5 beats per minute per week for the entire 5 weeks of the course (180 minutes of training per week)!* And all slowed at least 1 beat per minute per week. Since many already enjoyed some leg training we are inclined to think that arm emphasis in the combined mode did the trick.

High blood pressure and Heavyhands

It's far too early to be sure, but I believe that Heavyhands training will one day play an important role in the prevention and treatment of certain forms of high blood pressure. The untrained upper torso may create a tourniquetlike effect that tends to keep the pressure in our arteries higher than need be. Herbert de Vries suggested this mechanism in a paper published in the early 1970s. He hypothesized that the arterial pressures generated during exercise were determined not so much by the total amount of muscle mobilized as by localized areas of strain—places where muscular action and oxygen transport were particularly ineffectual. It is known that aerobic exercise tends to lower the blood pressure of those who have essential hypertension (the garden variety of high blood pressure that is estimated to affect as many as 60 million Americans). It is also known that *untrained* arms, pushed to maximal effort in the laboratory, produce dispropor-

tionately high blood pressures and pulse rates in their hosts. Upper-torso training may "release" this "functional" constriction to help to lower the blood pressure. That's the best notion I've come up with so far to explain dramatic pressure drops in a growing number of Heavyhanders with chronic hypertension. I've watched in astonished delight as the pressures of many, including myself, dropped to *below* the normal 120/80 level.

During exercise the normal blood pressure elevation is roughly proportional to the workload—somewhat higher in the untrained than the trained subject. I found that during Heavyhands exercise my pressure increases were about 15 percent of what the literature would predict. Monitoring my pressure regularly I've stopped my medication for the first time in a couple of decades. Incidentally, it is said that one of every two deaths in this country is related to high blood pressure.

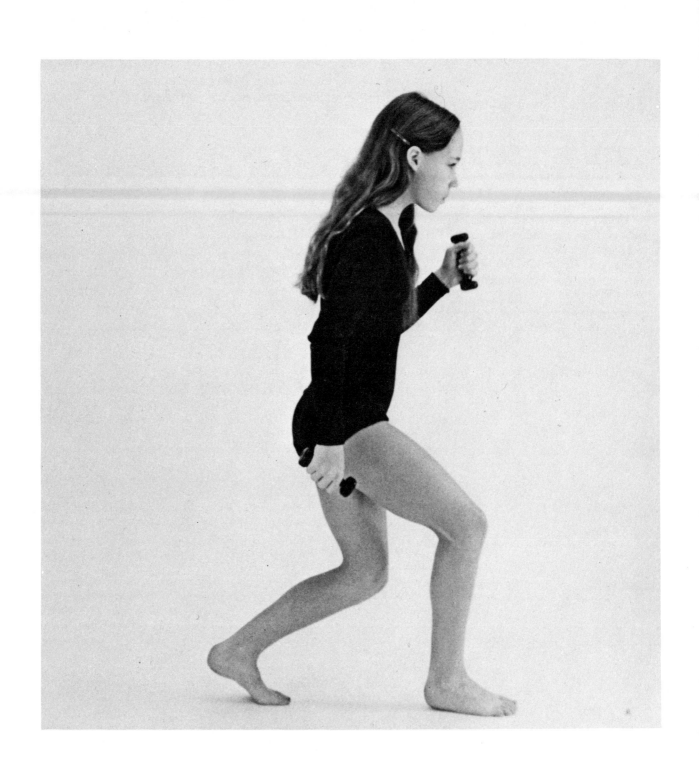

4

Getting Into Action

I'M SURE YOU'RE EAGER to begin Heavyhands exercise. In this chapter I want to accomplish three things: to recap some of the reasoning behind the use of hand-held weights; to cover the matter of Heavyhands equipment; and to get you started with a basic movement that will give you a solid base from which to launch your Heavyhands strategy.

I realize that my readers are a mixed crew when it comes to things like fitness level, motivation, athletic prowess, and innate capacities of all sorts. Those differences don't matter, because Heavyhands is good exercise at *any* level. Training effects are largely independent of the strategy you decide upon. A single movement such as the one I'll show you in this chapter is enough to carry you to superlative fitness. After that it's pure gravy; you can freely pick and choose additional, more complex exercises as you wish. A wider inventory of moves is not essential, but it does make it all the more interesting and fun — an added motivation.

WHY HANDWEIGHTS? A RECAP

As I said earlier, my initial impetus to run with weights came in the form of a hunch that endurance exercises unwisely ignored the arms. When, later, extraordinary changes began to occur in my body, questions arose. How far can arm work go? Obviously, everything has limits. We see evidence of that in the tight clusters of best performances in sport, like Derek Clayton's 2:08:33 marathon time, unequaled, until recently, for better than a decade. So I trained patiently, working my heart and total musculature — conscious of endurance-speed-power and strength. Waiting to hit my limit. Five years later, I'm still waiting . . . and enjoying every blessed minute of it.

Bunches of new questions posed themselves. I had learned that cross-country skiers, both male and female, had achieved the highest levels of oxygen consumption ever recorded. The number of runners far exceeds the number of cross-country skiers. If runners and cross-country skiers were equally conditioned, it would be improbable that the record-breaking oxygen-consumption rates would so consistently go to the skiers. Could it be the skier's arm work that, added to leg exertion, used all that oxygen? Since the poling action itself amounted to 25 to 30 percent of the skier's work, I wondered what would happen if "poles" in the form of dumbbells ten or more times the weight of real poles were used, and in more exaggerated ranges of motion and tempo.

As my workloads rapidly escalated it became increasingly obvious that the arms and upper torso could be useful vehicles for endurance exercise. If so, why had we continued to neglect them? How much oxygen could humans consume working four limbs simultaneously?

As mentioned in Chapter 3, previous research had indicated that arm-plus-leg work could equal *leg work alone* so long as the arm work constituted *no more* than 30 percent of the combined total. I wondered why and how the researchers had come to these conclusions. My first hunch was that subjects they used had better-trained legs than arms. The heart's oxygen output was simply sucked out of the blood best by the trained leg muscles, which are incidentally three to four times larger than the arms!

trained, could duplicate my *trained* arm performance. And that led me to doubt the axiom that held that arms and legs could not outproduce legs alone.

Historically the upper torso, with a few exceptions, had been given short shrift in athletics. Only swimmers, kayakers, and canoeists perform strength-endurance arm work; but water always offers the same resistance to the paddle, and stroke frequency falls within a narrow range, so strength increases are limited. Even so, these athletes produce sizable if not heroic VO_2Max levels, using arms predominantly.

Several recent studies suggest that arms-plus-legs indeed can supersede legs-alone performance. We simply *don't know yet* what workloads combined arm-and-leg work can produce, and how much muscle work the heart's output can adequately cover.

We do know that by young adulthood most of us have already established rather capable duets between our massive leg musculature and our heart-lung delivery apparatus. When we start a running program, for example, unless we lose many pounds of

---

Why arms?

1. Per unit of muscle weight and volume, they can outdo legs. With Heavyhands training, arms can often outdo legs' total work, even though legs outweigh arms by a multiple of 3 to 4.

2. Arms are freer to move than legs and are capable of swifter, more complex, less grooved motion.

3. Arms have greater training potential — leg endurance can be upped only 10 to 25 percent; arm endurance by 100 percent or more.

4. Arms are relatively immune from injury when trained; they are not blighted by the "strikes" that cripple the endurance leg athlete.

5. We need strong arms: our work and play patterns require clever, strong hands attached to a strong upper torso.

6. Hands enjoy a denser network of connections with our brains than do feet and legs. Hand work thus feeds into human intelligence more than does less imaginative leg work.

7. Feet carry *us;* hands carry *everything else.*

8. Hands and arms are nearly indispensable for self-protection.

An example of Heavyhands efficiency

When I run at a 10-minute pace, I ordinarily reach a pulse rate of 120–130. When I perform at the same workload with a Heavyhands exercise that uses four limbs simultaneously, my heart rate, again at 10 METs, is only 65–70! Of course, that doesn't hold true until all of your limbs are trained aerobically.

body weight, our VO_2Max will improve 5 to 25 percent in the course of six months of serious training (about 210 minutes weekly). After that, improvements come slowly — perhaps inching up a few more percentage points during the remainder of a lifetime. In other words, we choose to train the limbs that are *already* better than halfway there. And we are apparently willing to settle for the extra 25 percent we can squeeze from them, defining that as the standard of superlative fitness.

The heart, however, is such an incredible muscle, and so easily trained, that it sometimes supplies more oxygen than the legs can handle, increasing the danger of overuse injury. Only the exceptional serious and well-trained runner can keep pace with the heart's offerings injury free, for long.

So long as the potential for significant arm work remained unrecognized, pushing the legs' natural talent as aerobic drivers seemed to justify the risk of injury and the endless repetitions that characterize most leg-driven endurance exercise. Aerobic dance seems an exception, as its leg movement is more varied, but the fitness levels achieved are, on the whole, more modest.

Leg-driven exercise, again with some exceptions, works *horizontally*. Indeed good form in running dictates minimal upward movement of the body's center of gravity. To use up the heart's exquisite delivery service efficiently and simultaneously, we must run *fast*. But then again, leg speed is associated with more leg injury.

Weighted hands in motion — in contrast — *must* engage the vertical. Since the pull of gravity is always straight down, once we move our hands from the dead-hang position, we must counter that downward drag. Remember, exercise is hard work, overwork. This rather arrogant flying in the face of gravity may be inefficient, but that's precisely what makes it indisputably *good* exercise.

The legs continue to work hard — in fact, as you will discover later on, they work harder in more ways — and the arms now work harder than they ever have. The orchestration of arms and legs produces a higher intensity of work with a delightfully low sense of travail.

Peculiarities of the arm-shoulder anatomy make it especially suited for hard work. Unlike the leg's deeply socketed position, the arms enjoy a special freewheeling quality. Most of us don't realize that the entire upper girdle almost floats in muscle. It is attached to our skeleton only where the collarbone (clavicle) joins the top of the breastbone (sternum)! We may not choose to use this arm-shoulder dynamo, but it is there for the using, as the saying goes.

Doesn't that contradict the physiologists' admonition to use big muscles as aerobic drivers? Arms are definitely smaller; but by adding the mass of muscle that effects shoulder motion — chest and back muscles — we're into respectable bulk. Many ordinary folk will be able to bring their arms to *equal* their leg work but even when that isn't possible, the addition of significant arm work to the legs' strength-endurance experience is what Heavyhands is all about.

EQUIPMENT

You are not apt to risk many dollars outfitting yourself for a Heavyhands program. Outdoors or inside, comfortable shorts or jogging suits are fine. Your present walking or running shoes or sneakers, deck shoes, or shoes used for tennis or racquetball will suffice for starters. As your program takes specific form you may decide on some kind of specially suitable footwear. Because of the "distributed" exercise you're less apt to log the kind of mileage a serious runner would, so you'll not need the four pairs of shoes per year he ofttimes requires. A sweatband is a handy addition.

Weights are the next order of business. The per-pound price of cast-iron weights is climbing fast like everything else, but even at $1.00 or more per pound, your total investment will be small compared with almost any exercise gadgetry you can buy. Several companies make weights in one-pound increments to ten pounds, then twelves, fifteens, and five-pound increments far beyond anything you will move more than a few times. Not more than 1 percent of the population will require weights exceeding 20 pounds, and for the great majority of men 10 pounds will be plenty for most moves. Most women will find pairs of 1-pounders through 6-pounders provide a good range for most Heavyhands work. I would not advise *most* of the available adjustable type dumbbells, the kind that have collars for containing variously weighted plates. They are inconvenient and could be dangerous when used with some Heavyhands routines.

Heavyhands and eyeglasses

About 57 percent of us wear glasses. Without mine I'm helpless as a bug on his back. But glasses have always given me fits. They slide up and down my sweat-slippery nose and fog on cool days when my body temperature has risen. The elastic bands I buy to connect the ear pieces behind have a habit of getting lost. Then I bought a pair of wire rims called "Hunter's frames," the ones with the C-shaped piece that hooks securely around the ears. Those, and antifog pastes, made me happy ever after. Now when I double ski-pole, dance, and shadow-box, my glasses remain fixed to my face.

Sweatbands

Sometimes I think a headband looks as though someone's halo has slipped. They really are a very practical and inexpensive piece of equipment-apparel. If you thoughtlessly try wiping your drenched brow with a piece of cast iron, you may find yourself pump 'n' running toward the nearest sweatband emporium. Save those that have stretched too much: they make colorful waistbands once Heavyhands has trimmed your middle!

Heavyhands hardware

Being different, Heavyhands exercise expectably required special equipment. After much experimentation and hundreds of hours of "road testing," a weight was developed that seems to best implement the "handers'" need for safety and comfort during prolonged workouts oftentimes involving thousands of repetitions. Simply called Heavyhands, the weight includes a strap that cradles the hand, reducing enormously the tendency to overgrip. Both shaft and strap are covered with soft rubber. "Heavyhands" make higher and faster pump-action possible with less conscious concern devoted to hanging on to the weights. Likewise, various throws and punching movements, wherein the hand attains high velocity, don't cause cramping of the fingers. And you can pulse-count, answer the phone, sip a cold drink, and tune your TV without setting the weights down!

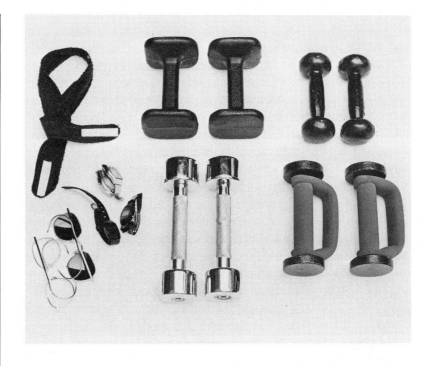

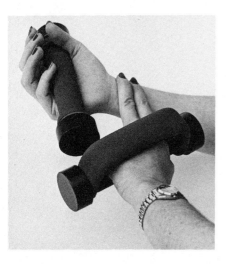

Generally I would choose weights with handles that are rather short, fitting the hand snugly, rather than elongated handles, which tend to slip during prolonged exercise when the hand begins to tire and cramp.

The larger the assortment of weights the better, within reason, to allow for quick shifts during an exercise session. Even one-pound differences are significant in Heavyhands because of the high number of repetitions and the total distance through which the weights must travel. Rough-surfaced cast weights feel better when covered once or twice with glossy paint. If you use heavier weights you will probably develop a small round callus at the base of your thumbs that can come only from Heavyhands. It is better to start with weights that will prove *eventually* too light for you than the other way around. I recall a young physician who decided to try a shadowboxing routine. I suggested 2-pound weights. Unable to find that size, he bought a pair of 12-pounders and promptly developed severe biceps tendinitis while trying to do the impossible with an untrained pair of arms.

It helps if you can buy your weights where you can see and heft them to be sure they feel right. You'll need a pair of 1-pounders for the 1–10–100 test (see page 56). Remember that you're looking for weights you'll be moving hundreds of times. If you buy some you can handle with comfort immediately, chances are that within three weeks they'll not be heavy enough for you. That's good. Weights don't really become too light because you can "fill" by doing faster moves—more reps per minute—and choosing more difficult moves to increase the "felt" workload. Your next purchase would typically be a heavier pair. However many you own, you'll surely make use of all of them. As each pair comes to feel lighter you will spontaneously try more complicated moves with them. If you do outgrow them, they make wonderful gifts for newcomers to the art, a symbolic bestowing of your good exercising fortune.

You'll need a watch or clock with a second hand for pulse counting. And since the number of moves per minute is important, we need some method to control or direct our pace. A good metronome is a wise investment. I like the mechanical kind rather than some of the inexpensive electronic ones, which tend to be less accurate. The metronome provides an even, rhythmic guide to your movements. Later you will want to use it to check your progress against earlier performance.

"Pacer" digital watches are becoming inexpensive, are perfect portable metronomes, and are very accurate. Some don't beep as fast as you might like, but you can double-up on the signal, e.g., move twice per beep with the pacer set at 100 to do a tempo of 200.

Music provides another, though less precise, timer. Heavyhands makes much of the advantage inherent in music, as you shall see.

How much handweight?

People ask what handweight is right. This simple formula is the best I've been able to come up with. *Any weight* is useful while performing the exercises described throughout the book, *so long* as you can continue with it for 4 or 5 minutes at an appropriate exercise heart rate. That's how long it takes our circulations to achieve a steady state. Naturally, as you become stronger and more facile, the range of weights you'll be able to include during workouts will grow.

WARMING UP

Warming up prior to exercise is generally considered not only wise but essential. Warming up is a gradual kindling of the metabolic fires, so to speak. Experienced exercisers do that instinctively, having learned that one risks injury and mars performance by lurching suddenly into near-all-out effort. Moreover, it's likely that cooling off gradually is at least as important, since a significant percentage of cardiac "incidents" occur *right after* stopping maximal exertion.

In any case, a graded entry and retreat from the targeted aerobic session *can't hurt*. As your training progresses, your metabolic gears can shift more quickly and gracefully into "high." Fitness should provide, among other things, the mechanism for safer sudden starts. Life, after all, may make occasional demands upon our circulation and muscles without providing convenient time for warm-up.

PUMP 'N' WALK AND
PUMP 'N' RUN IN PLACE

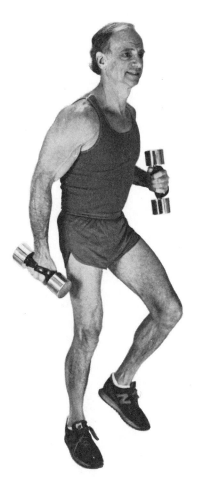

This is Heavyhands' opening gambit. It will pay off handsomely once you've mastered it. The simplest prototype of *combined* exercise, it lends itself nicely to a lot of interesting variations. Through it you will gain the feel of Heavyhands. You will learn how a simple combination of movements can be used in a number of ways to juggle the fitness factors to suit your needs. So even though you've thumbed through these pages and glimpsed pictures and drawings of other movements, bide your time! Pump 'n' walk in place will get you going. Adding to your Heavyhands repertoire should take place gradually, when your body and spirit are prepared.

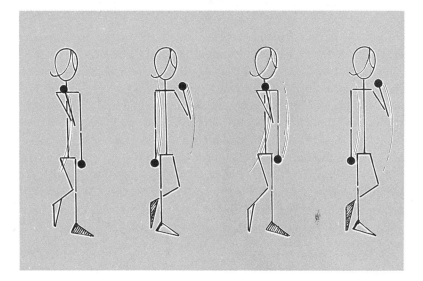

Pump 'n' walk and pump 'n' run in place are not simply slow and fast versions of the same exercise. Running in place means your body is airborne for an instant — both feet off the ground. In walking, one foot remains solidly on terra firma — however fast you're moving. Running becomes onerous at very slow tempos, say 100 steps a minute or less. At fast tempos — at step frequencies above 200 — walking *feels* harder than running at an identical pace. That's because it really *is* harder.

Whether running or walking, lift your feet so that your heels rise about a foot off the floor each time. You can approximate that by looking in a mirror or better still having someone watch and estimate for you. When your foot has been lifted to the proper height, your knee pokes out a certain distance in front. Once accustomed to that position, you'll be very close without thinking about it. It's not important enough to be compulsive over, at any rate.

It is important to stress again that the essential difference between run and walk, as we're using the terms, is not velocity. Walking, one foot is always on the ground; when running, for an instant both feet are off the ground. If speed were the important criterion, the great walking Olympian, Ron Laird, covering a mile in under 8 minutes, would be "running," though both feet *never* leave the ground simultaneously.

Now to try the moves with weights. Pick up a pair of 1-pound weights. If you haven't gotten around to buying them yet, cans of food, or bricks or books make tolerable temporary substitutes. Short lengths of pipe or solid round bars are quite satisfactory. Plastic bottles, the kind with jug handles, can be filled to appropriate heaviness with water (a pint of water weighs a pound).

Standing erect in front of a full-length mirror, if that's convenient, hold the weights at your sides, your palms facing your thighs, your shoulders relaxed, your arms hanging loosely at full extension. Try pump 'n' walk first because it's the easier to learn. These *in-place* moves are "ipsilateral," meaning the arm and leg on the *same side* move at the *same time.*

You will notice in the photograph that the shoulders and hips tilt slightly upward toward the side of the curling limb. You needn't think about doing that. It happens naturally, even more so when you're loose. Try not to clutch the weights tightly. If you learn that at the outset, you'll spare yourself unnecessary hand and forearm muscle cramps when you're into prolonged exercise.

Pump levels

You needn't stick religiously to pump Levels I, II, and III as I described them. Level I½, II½, III½, or even IV — or any other lift level that suits your fancy — is good exercise. More important, you should try to vary these levels by adjusting the tempo and the size of hand-weights used. You can compute the calorie cost of these "tweeners" by extrapolating to the numbers we've supplied. Thus, Level I½, about an 18-inch pump, would well use energy at a rate midway between that required by Level I and Level II. At least it's close enough for folk singing, as the saying goes.

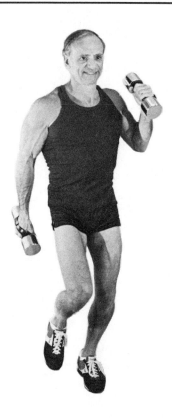

Keep that glottis open!

You'll read that again and again in caveats to exercisers. It applies especially to strength work, where for some reason people feel impelled to suspend free breathing. The lifter or push-upper or snow shoveler may actually breathe against an unyielding resistance — the closed trapdoor atop the windpipe called the glottis. It's recognizable in the flushed face, clamped-shut lips, often bulging eyes of the strainer — along with the absence of breath sounds. Pressure in the chest cavity increases; cardiac output diminishes. When the breath is suddenly released, other changes take place in cardiovascular-respiratory dynamics. It's called a Valsalva maneuver, and though experts disagree as to the extent of its harmful effects in exercise, you can bypass the problem nicely by consciously keeping your breathing unimpeded both in and out, during exercise.

Initial problems with combined exercise

Some find pump 'n' walk and other four-limbed exercise awkward at first. Various complaints are registered. "My legs can't keep up with my arms," or vice versa. Some feel impelled to move their arms only half as often as their legs. I would discourage that simply because the arms will ultimately log your best improvement in oxygen transport. Sacrifice any and every work element — resistance, speed-power, range-of-motion — so long as you preserve the 1:1 ratio of arm to leg movement.

Go slowly and deliberately, continuing until the movement loses its strangeness. Try it faster — still walking — but go back to square one if you get mixed up. Even if it takes you hours of frustrating experiment to learn this — which it won't — it might just be the best single time investment of your life.

There are a few details to be mentioned in relation to the arm pumps or curls. Like learning a golf swing or tennis stroke, it's wise to establish good habits early in the game. There's really not much you can do wrong with arm pumps because the elbow joint is a hinge that keeps your movement lined up.

The biceps and triceps muscles, respectively on the front and back of the upper arm, do most of the arm work. The biceps along with other muscles lift the weight; the triceps work either in *pushing* the weight down or in *resisting its rapid fall.* Strengthening your biceps, by the way, will make you able to open stuck jar lids and turn a screwdriver more effectively.

The pumps are of three varieties determined by the height to which the weighted hand climbs from its starting position at dead-hang at mid-thigh. Thus:

Level I — the weights are lifted to a height of 1 foot.
Level II — the weights are lifted to a height of 2 feet.
Level III — the weights are lifted to a height of 3 feet.

Those heights correspond to navel, shoulder joint, and top of the head, respectively, on *my* 5′7″ body. If you're looking for landmarks on *you,* they'll vary according to *your* height. If you're 6′5″, Level III may hit about the middle of your ear, and if you're 4′11″, Level III will end up somewhere *above* the top of your head. The only advantage to keeping the lift or pump levels standardized is to ensure that the workloads I've measured in the laboratory (and assembled in charts that appear later) will be accurate for you no matter how tall or short you are. Use a tape to find out what corresponds with the three levels on your anatomy and practice a few times until you do it automatically. No need to be scrupulous about it, but the workloads achieved from lifting to these levels vary significantly, especially at the faster tempos. At Level I, the elbows stay pretty much at the side, the angle between arm and forearm about 90 degrees. At Level II the elbows slip forward and upward slightly and the angle becomes more like 45 degrees. At Level III, that 45-degree angle is preserved but the upper arm reaches the horizontal position at the top of its pump. There's

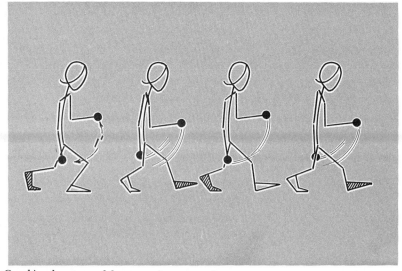
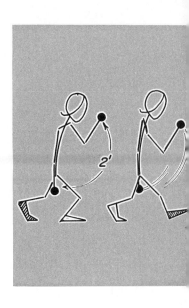

Combined arm-and-leg exercises—on the move—   *Level I*

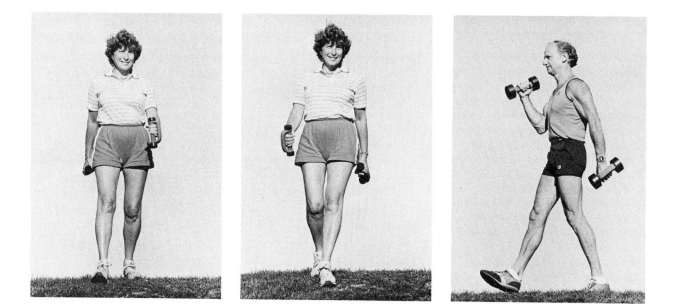

—in place—

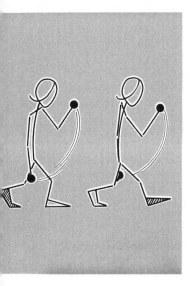

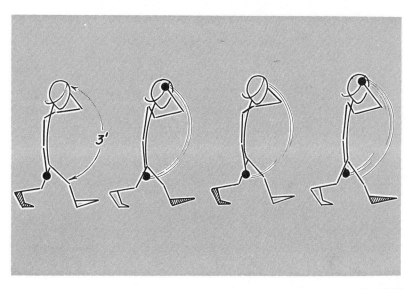

Level II

Level III

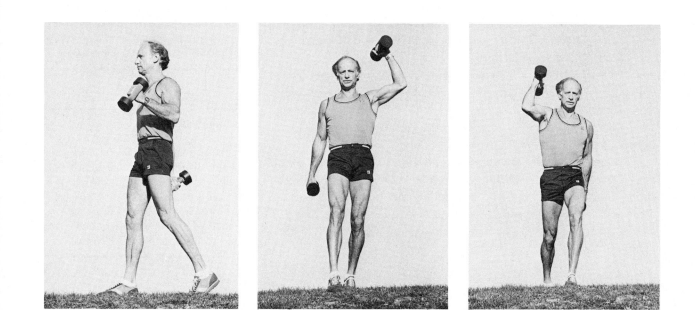

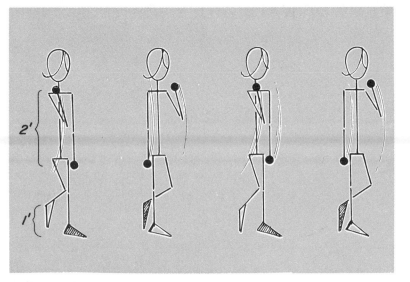

Walking in place with arm lifts (Level II)

Legs or arms?

Heavyhands is a combined exercise, and since arms have been neglected in almost every other aerobic exercise, this book stresses arm and upper-torso work. But almost everyone, including long-distance runners, is an amateur at Heavyhands. When you begin Heavyhands, therefore, let your legs, which, regardless of your general condition, are undoubtedly better trained than your arms, absorb the major part of the workload. As your training progresses, your arms will catch up to, and then pass, your legs' rate of improvement.

Grip

Do not grip your weights tightly or, when you exercise for long periods, you'll suffer muscle cramps in your hands and forearms. Conscious, intermittent relaxation of the grip will help prevent these muscle spasms.

Don't "chop"

Be sure to let your descending arm return to its original mid-thigh position at rest. If you abbreviate the descending arm's motion, you will not receive the full benefit of the exercise. More important, you will tire and cramp rapidly.

absolutely nothing wrong with moving higher if you wish, i.e., to your own "Level IV." But your workloads, should you estimate them, will of course be far larger.

The various levels — really ranges of motion — when mixed in with different weights and tempos provide a wide range of workloads for the upper torso. A heavy weight at Level I could, at the same tempo, produce as much oxygen consumption as a much lighter one at Level III.

It is very important that you not settle for an abbreviated "chopping" motion that stops the weight prematurely in its descent. That spoils the relaxation so useful in avoiding the discomfort and fatigue associated with spasm or cramping. Consciously allowing the shoulder on the descending arm's side to sag exaggeratedly helps avoid that pitfall.

PUMP 'N' WALK AND YOUR BEGINNING HEAVYHANDS STRATEGY

Thirty minutes of continuous exercise is an ideal goal for a beginning Heavyhander. For one thing, most knowledgeable exercise physiologists believe that you must elevate your heart rate to target pulse and hold it there for 20 or more minutes to achieve heart-lung training. Incidentally, once comfortably able to exercise for 30 minutes, you will find that two hours at slightly reduced intensity is surprisingly well within your reach. Thirty minutes makes sense for other reasons. At four to seven times a week it brings you to a healthy weekly minute total, yet leaves time for days off. Many physiologists believe an aerobic session should use at least 300 calories. Since most people will easily manage 10 or more calories per minute, that time frame fits the doctor's exercise prescription handily.

So our initial project is to get you as soon as possible to a 30-minute exercise base. Having accomplished that you can leisurely continue to work through the book at whatever pace is right for you. If you're an old hand at endurance training, you can skim through this section. For newcomers, some explanation will help.

To repeat: all exercise is measurable as intensity times duration — METs times minutes, or calories per minute times minutes. It all means the same thing: how hard you're working and how long you stay with it.

Supposing you were embarking on a jogging program. Starting from deconditioned scratch, you would jog to the point of breathlessness and a relatively fast heart rate, then settle for walking until you paid off your "oxygen debt."

You jog until you feel the first inklings of anaerobic discomfort — when your oxygen transport system isn't quite making it — then lower your workload (walk) until you're "steadied out," when you meet your oxygen needs *as you go.* Analogously, if you spend your paycheck two days after receiving it, that puts you in the fiscal "red," and you must halt the spending. Aerobic exercise is pay-as-you-go exercise.

Why not advise the beginning jogger to go slowly enough to last the full 30 minutes? Because even at its slowest pace, the hard vertical work involved — those little airborne moments — may be

Your first goal

Your first task is to exercise at target pulse for 30 continuous minutes and to do it at least four times a week. Almost all physiologists agree that a four-time-a-week dose of 30 straight minutes of aerobic exercise is the basic prescription for heart and lung conditioning. Many physiologists also believe that each 30-minute session should use at least 300 calories. Heavyhanders don't have to worry about the calories; once into training you will, most likely, lose many more than 300 calories in 30 minutes.

Aerobic and anaerobic work

Aerobic work is the "pay as you go" kind. Steady work that continues for several minutes is fueled adequately by the oxygen in the air the exerciser breathes. Anaerobic work exceeds the aerobic capacity. It overtaxes the oxygen transport apparatus. Lactic acid accumulates in the blood and causes the characteristic ache that occurs at the end of an all-out sprint, or the last of a series of bench presses. Both systems can be upgraded consciously during training by alternating the steady (aerobic) and the all-out (anaerobic) routes.

more than a beginner's oxygen transport system can manage. That's why running at a slow pace, even in place, is hard work.

Some authors suggest some sort of testing procedure at the start of an endurance exercise program. Aside from the stress test done in your doctor's office, Ken Cooper's fitness tests are perhaps the most popular. One is the 12-minute test, the other the 1.5-mile test. The former requires that you determine the longest distance you can travel in 12 minutes — then rate yourself against age-matched peers. With the 1.5-mile test you could run 6 quarter-mile laps at the track and see how your *time* stacks up against others on the charts Cooper provides.

The problem with these and similar tests is that it's hard to determine beforehand how ambitious a given testee is. The tests inevitably push the willing subject into the anaerobic "red." For older subjects, that may introduce some risk factor, however small it may be.

The beginning jogger is usually unable to settle into a 30-minute aerobic workout immediately. He works at it gradually, increasing the amount of jogging and reducing the amount of walking that makes up the 30 minutes. He varies the intensity, we say, in order to accomplish the 30-minute prescribed *duration.*

Heavyhands exercise, employing four limbs and varying hand-weights and frequency of movements, enjoys a unique advantage. We can engineer *work intensity* for each beginner so that he or she can, in short order, stay aerobic — out of the anaerobic "red" — for the full 30 minutes. At the same time, using the same principle, we can *test* the beginner, again avoiding the unpleasant anaerobic state. The test is performed *not* to compare you with others, a dubious preoccupation to begin with, but to help provide a suitable prescription for the initial *intensity* of your 30 minutes of Heavyhands. Once established at 30 minutes, whatever its intensity, your training is aimed at adding, however slowly, to that intensity level.

THE 1–10–100 TEST

This test differs from most exercise tests in that the workload is kept relatively constant. Everyone gets the same task. What's measured is your response to it. Using the heart rate as the most accessible indicator of that response, we merely count the pulse at the beginning and at the end of the test — noting the extent of the

---

Staying aerobic

Using Heavyhands exercises virtually anyone can exercise for 30 minutes without ever becoming anaerobic. By spreading the workload over four limbs instead of two, and by varying the pace, range of motion, and the weight, even the unconditioned beginner can work out for 30 minutes without running out of gas.

Conversely, the superbly conditioned athlete, by taking advantage of four limbs in combined exercise and by increasing weights and pace, can surpass his previous all-time-high workloads.

Target pulse

Target pulse is the heart rate, or range of heart rates, at which most people can exercise effectively and safely. To find *your* target pulse, subtract your age from 220, which will give you your maximal heart rate. Your target pulse is then 70 to 85 percent of your maximal heart rate. Thus a healthy thirty-year-old has a target pulse of roughly 135 to 160:

$$\begin{array}{r} 220 \\ -\ \ 30 \\ \hline 190 \end{array}$$

70 percent of 190 = 133
85 percent of 190 = 162

The 1–10–100 test

1. When extending your 30-minute prescription, first increase the frequency by increments of a few beats per minute.

2. Increase weights when 30-minute exercise has reached either 175 or 200 beats per minute.

3. Increase weight by 1-pound increments, then test using the formula X lbs.–5–100. Or 150 if that is comfortable and preferable.

4. If additional weight increments produce arm-weariness, return to the previous weights and use higher frequencies.

5. With each 30-minute prescription add strength sprints (St — add) and speed sprints (Sp — add), using the following formulas;
Strength sprints—X pounds +2 additional pounds for 3- to 5-minute intervals at the 30-minute prescription frequency.
Speed Sprints—X pounds + 1 extra pound for 3- to 5-minute intervals at 50 beats per minute above the 30-minute prescription frequency.

6. When frequency reaches 150–175, go to pump 'n' run, first with speed-sprint intervals, finally with your 30-minute prescription.

7. If pump 'n' run is painful or otherwise uncomfortable, continue to use the pump 'n' walk option, remembering that it is more difficult at high frequencies and may increase your pulse rate beyond the level pump 'n' run at the same frequency would produce.

Note: These weights, times, and frequencies are suggestions and need not be held to rigidly. Target pulse should receive the highest priority, followed by the 30-minute duration.

increase. The test is purposely rigged to be easy enough for most healthy people with minimal discomfort and next to no risk. Using the 1–10–100 test you can "prescribe" your own exercise. The system is really a series of prescriptions. Learning to listen for the signs of progress, you'll decide just when to change the prescription.

I call it the 1–10–100 test because we pump 'n' walk in place with 1-pound weights in *each hand* for 10 minutes at a frequency of 100 steps (50 left steps per minute). Any prescription for pump 'n' walk or pump 'n' run in place exercise is written this way. Thus a 5–30–150W "script" would simply mean 5 pounds for 30 minutes, walking at 150 steps per minute (the letter W or R next to the frequency obviously refers to either walking or running).

The 1–10–100 can be done *without* weights by increasing the pace to 120 steps.

Conditioned beginners will show smaller pulse-rate responses than unconditioned ones. One subject beginning with a pulse rate of 55 finished up with a rate of 75. The 1–10–100 didn't faze him; it taxed his oxygen-transport system almost nil. He clearly needed a much more ambitious prescription to reach target pulse range.

Another subject starting at a 90 pulse ended with one of 120. Since his target pulse was 130 or so, small additions of either weight or frequency would provide his 30-minute prescription.

Starting with the 1–10–100, the beginning Heavyhander *eases up* to his or her target pulse without using the "off and on" anaerobic-aerobic approach of the beginning jogger. Before trying the 1–10–100, don't take your beginning pulse *while seated*. Your pulse may increase several beats per minute just from standing. Remain standing for a minute or so and begin when your pulse has stabilized.

If your 1–10–100 test brings you to a pulse rate substantially *above* your starting pulse (say, an increase of 30 or more beats per minute), it means you need exercise! If it brings you *within* your target zone you should begin to train at 1–10–100 daily, toward a 30-minute session. How long it takes to get to your 30-minute prescription will vary, of course. Some do it the first day, most within a few days, and three weeks would be exceptional.

If your pulse increase is moderate (10 to 20 beats per minute) and you are *not* yet at target — wait a few minutes, then increase the weights by one pound. You can now shorten the test interval time from 10 minutes to 5 until you find yourself at target pulse.

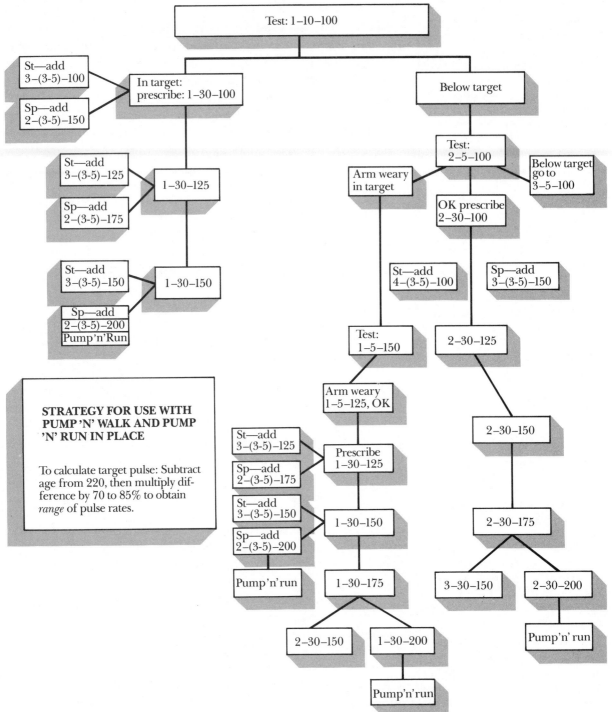

Test: 1–10–100

St—add
3–(3-5)–100

Sp—add
2–(3-5)–150

In target:
prescribe: 1–30–100

Below target

St—add
3–(3-5)–125

Sp—add
2–(3-5)–175

1–30–125

St—add
3–(3-5)–150

Sp—add
2–(3-5)–200
Pump'n'Run

1–30–150

Test:
2–5–100

Arm weary
in target

OK prescribe
2–30–100

Below target
go to
3–5–100

St—add
4–(3-5)–100

Sp—add
3–(3-5)–150

2–30–125

Test:
1–5–150

2–30–150

**STRATEGY FOR USE WITH
PUMP 'N' WALK AND PUMP
'N' RUN IN PLACE**

To calculate target pulse: Subtract
age from 220, then multiply difference by 70 to 85% to obtain
range of pulse rates.

Arm weary
1–5–125, OK

St—add
3–(3-5)–125

Sp—add
2–(3-5)–175

Prescribe
1–30–125

St—add
3–(3-5)–150

Sp—add
2–(3-5)–200

1–30–150

Pump'n'run

1–30–175

2–30–175

2–30–150

1–30–200

3–30–150

2–30–200

Pump'n'run

Pump'n'run

Pump'n' run

Then begin to train toward your 30-minute session using your revised prescription.

Thus if you're seeking a 150 target rate based on 70 to 85 percent of your age-related maximum pulse and your 1–10–100 brings you from 75 to 95, a 20-beat increase, try 2–5–100 (2 pounds each hand for 5 minutes at 100-steps-per-minute frequency). Continue increasing the weight until one of two things happens. 1. If 3–5–100 or 4–5–100 brings you to 140 to 150 pulse at the end of 5 minutes, use that prescription for your daily training. If that's still too easy, continue to add weight. 2. If you are forced to stop from *arm weariness,* or ache, drop back to less weight, one pound at a time, and *up your steps* per minute by small increments until you are at target pulse. (If you hit 150 or more steps per minute, you may feel better running rather than walking. See the next section, Pump 'n' Run in Place.)

To review: It makes no difference how you reach your target. Do whatever is more comfortable. Eventually, you'll move up three ways. The upper torso contribution is exquisitely controllable in Heavyhands. Varying *how much* (weights), *how far* (height level), and *how fast* (tempo), you can fine-tune upper-body steady workloads within ½ MET — "moving up" so gradually that the increase is barely noticeable. So long as you generate sustainable workloads that keep your pulse and breathing steady, and you comfortable, the specific ingredients of your prescription are not important. In less than an hour you ought to know which formula is best for your 30-minute plan. Don't be too eager to use large handweights at first. Allow your experienced legs to help you while your arms are beginning to accumulate aerobic power. That happens at an enormous rate, as you will see.

If for a few days you feel better splitting your 30-minute session into two 15-minute intervals, that's perfectly all right. Or three 10-minute sessions. But do try to get to 30 continuous minutes and to do at least three of those each week.

INCREASING YOUR PRESCRIPTION

Growth will happen in irregular, often unexpected spurts. After a day or two away from exercise you may find that your weights feel light. You'll wish to take on heavier ones. Do it. Your instincts toward change are probably reasonable and stand for training effects reaching your consciousness by whatever mysterious route. Some days you'll hanker for speed and usually your performance will verify your impulse.

As you exercise, whenever your breathing feels unusually hard or easy, stop and check your pulse. These interruptions won't hurt the flow of your exercise, and they will keep you at target pulse and teach you about your body's response to exercise. During the first week, you should check your pulse frequently. I would suggest 5-minute intervals. Again, this is to teach you about yourself and exercise and to insure that you are working at the proper level. Later on you will check your pulse far more infrequently, and much later, hardly at all.

STRENGTH-SPEED DRILLS

Suppose you find your initial training goal is 2–30–100. You can increase the speed of your progress by inserting into your prescription short intervals stressing either strength or speed or both, e.g., 4–5–100 (strength), 1–5–200 (speed). You may insert these into your 30-minute session, or add them as the spirit moves you. That's why a variety of weights help. Strength drills can be of even shorter duration. Alongside a basic 2–30–100 prescription, for example, a 4–3–100 interval might work well. These strength and speed drills will make the basic 30-minute exercise easier to do, and that helps you to higher workloads. Don't remain too long at 100 frequency. Moving on to 150–180 steps per minute is at least as useful as upping poundages.

A last word about strength-speed drills. Most exercisers run into plateaus; they seem to "stick" at a given weight and/or frequency. For some reason, strength-speed drills tend to shake you loose and overcome this problem.

PUMP 'N' RUN IN PLACE

When your walking frequency hits 150 to 175 steps per minute, it is time to pump 'n' run. As I've indicated, running may feel a bit easier and you may enjoy the sense of being briefly airborne during each cycle. Now the foot strike changes. You will probably prefer

---

Grading your 1–10–100 performance

The workload of the 1–10–100 falls very close to 6 METs. Translated into oxygen terms, that means 21cc of O_2 for every Kilo — 2.2 lbs. of the exerciser's body weight. Your heart rate, taken immediately upon completing the test, will give a rough notion of your condition.

Pulse Rate	Condition
< 60–	Excellent
60–80	Good
80–120	Fair
120–140	Poor
>140–	Very poor

The key to progress: strength-speed drills

For unknown reasons, possibly psychological, the body and its various muscle systems tend to get into grooves. A certain level of workload is reached and then mastered, yet surpassing that level becomes exceedingly difficult. By adding on to, or injecting into, your basic — and comfortable — 30-minute prescription short (3- to 5-minute) strength or speed drills, you can get past that plateau. For reasons unknown, these brief sprints are inordinately useful in breaking through the body's resistance to change.

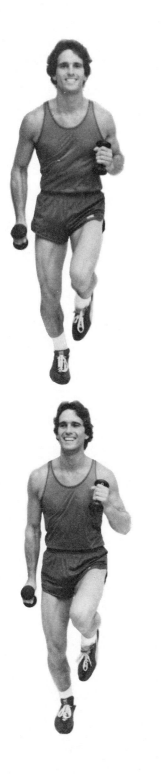

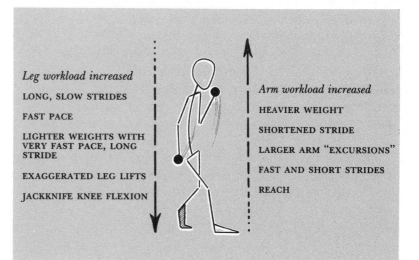

Pump 'n' walk in place

to land on the balls of your feet. If any immediate pain or next-day soreness occurs, you should return to pump 'n' walk. When your feet feel better try some more running.

Leg workload increased

LONG, SLOW STRIDES

FAST PACE

LIGHTER WEIGHTS WITH VERY FAST PACE, LONG STRIDE

EXAGGERATED LEG LIFTS

JACKKNIFE KNEE FLEXION

Arm workload increased

HEAVIER WEIGHT

SHORTENED STRIDE

LARGER ARM "EXCURSIONS"

FAST AND SHORT STRIDES

REACH

Whenever you're below target pulse, add weight or increase frequency. You will soon come to know several means of bringing yourself to your target rate with variations on pump 'n' walk and run in place. Once you are able to exercise continuously for 30 minutes, don't hesitate to shift from fast-light to slow-heavy. These variations add interest to your exercise and versatility to your heart-muscle duets. Remember, one of the biggest advantages of Heavyhands is its flexibility: the freedom to juggle the components of your workload. Whenever you experience undue discomfort or fatigue of the arms (or anywhere in the upper torso, for that matter) alter the poundage and/or your pace. Conversely, any such discomfort or fatigue in your legs calls for a slower pace and perhaps some adjustment of the arm work.

> **Walk or run**
>
> Depending upon your build, and training at somewhere between 150 and 175 paces per minute, walking will become a burdensome chore. At that point, you should switch to running.

ACHES AND PAINS

Little injuries and soreness may blight your progress from time to time. Soreness is of two general kinds: one occurs right after exercise, the other will be evident on awakening the next morning. They are symptoms of overwork and they will lessen generally with experience only to crop up again when you attempt increases that are a bit overambitious. These aches and pains are part of your initiation. A Heavyhands catchword is "gradual" increase: the small signals of discomfort will divert the Heavyhander from excesses that could really injure. In competition those same signs are apt to be ignored because of the strong wish to *win*. I don't tout pain as a virtuous appendage to Heavyhands exercise. The biggest workloads I've generated to date were mostly pain-free. Though increased amounts of lactic acid in your muscles cause the familiar aching sensation, training tends to offset it. The ache begins later and later as training proceeds.

As you work to improve your pump 'n' walk or run technique, its rhythm will grow on you. Soon you can even watch TV while you practice, paying little attention to your cadence.

> **Is pain essential to good exercise technique?**
>
> There's no good evidence that suffering pays off. Some muscle soreness is probably unavoidable simply because the pain signal is usually delayed until after the damage is done. Hurts encountered *during* exercise should, of course, bring those movements to an instant halt. Movements that don't cause pain are ordinarily safe though they involve the injured limb or even the same muscle group contracting at a different angle.

BREATHING AND PULSE

After you have counted your pulse a number of times, your inner sensor will accurately assess your pulse at a given work intensity. Breathing is the best clue, since heart and lungs are so intimately coupled physiologically. After five years at Heavyhands, I now almost never take a pulse except during the resting state, when I'm experimenting with a new move, or when I'm in the lab where my cardiograph counts it for me. Sometimes I take it when I'm curious about the state of my body fluids after a long pump 'n' run in the summer's heat. (It's good to remember that you'll get a higher pulse rate for a given workload when it's warm and humid.) Again, I'd check it when restarting exercise after being under the weather from a cold or overtraining.

I've tarried so long with pump 'n' walk and pump 'n' run because they're prototypes. If pump 'n' walk and pump 'n' run in place get your circulo-respiratory system tuned, they have served their purpose well. Chances are they will have accomplished much more: a goodly chunk of your musculature will have undergone significicant change by the time you've reached that important 30-straight-minute threshold. Now the fun begins because you're ready to build a repertoire. These two exercises will continue to serve as your exercise's bread and butter. Less demanding than most of the other movements, these old friends can be returned to when the going gets rough or you need to be indoors.

PUMP 'N' WALK AND
PUMP 'N' RUN ON THE MOVE

This next stage is logical, I think, because it is at once similar to what you've been doing and a useful departure from it. On the move, pump 'n' step feels different. I find that walking or jogging with arm curls is best accomplished using a diagonal stride. That means that the right arm curls upward while the left leg strides,

---

"Moving up"

That's the expression we use to describe any increase in workload. Your heart rate will respond to the subtlest change: tempo, range-of-motion, and weight, but also the inclusion of new muscle: heart duets, new movements that feel a bit awkward and are performed inefficiently. Subtle increases in the depth and rate of breathing will likely be the first signal that you're working harder than usual.

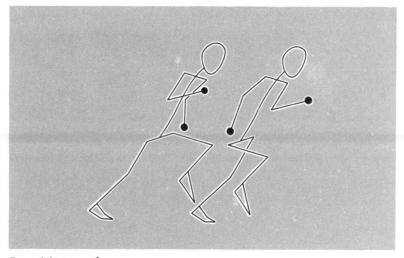

Pump 'n' run on the move

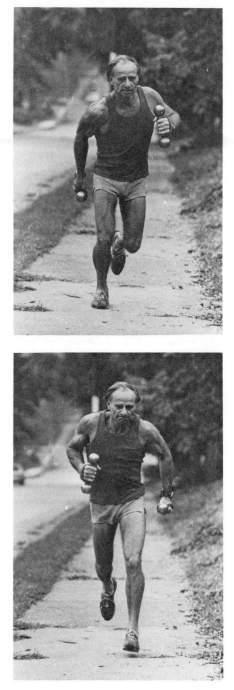

and vice versa. It too will feel strange for a short time, but don't worry about it. In due time you will be able to shift fluidly from the in-place same-side pump 'n' step to the on-the-move diagonal motion.

You can learn the on-the-move pump 'n' walk or run in your living room, basement, or backyard. Only a few feet of space are required to practice their essentials. Some people prefer to run on their heels, other on the balls of their feet. In Heavyhands you will find that when the handweights feel heavy and a bit clumsy you tend to land on the front of your foot. As you become used to those weights, your strike may move toward the flat or even the heel. There is nothing hard and fast about this. Let comfort and balance decide for you.

You will probably notice a difference, an increased speed, in your pulse-breathing pattern when on the move. Part of that obviously comes from the fact that you have undertaken a bigger workload; but part also derives from your use of slightly different muscle combinations of the legs and hips. Finally, part may be due to your unfamiliarity and subsequently reduced efficiency with the new move. This will happen every time you try something new, incidentally. Such responses are apt to be transient. They last longer when some new muscle group — completely lacking in endurance training — is given its maiden voyage in exercise.

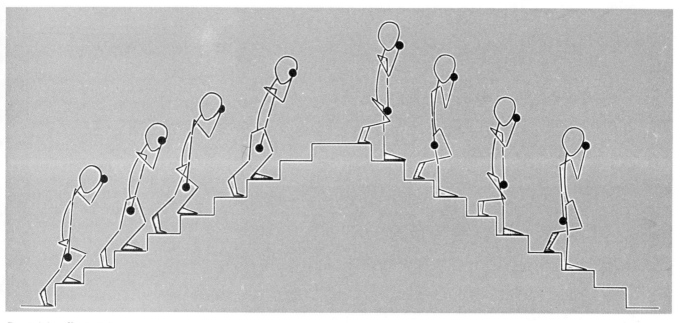

Pump 'n' walk up stairs

USING THE STAIRS

Practice shifting from in place to on the move until it feels right without conscious thought. Working indoors you can bring your stairways into the pump 'n' walk motif. Walking up and down stairs with weights is terrific work. Unlike running and walking, where horizontal forces predominate, on stairs vertical ones are at work. Climbing stairs is tough to begin with, and pumping weights make it a special challenge. *Don't* do this one unless you've come a long way in your training or if you've any reason to doubt the state of your cardiovascular system. Even with good reason for confidence, *go easy and slow* at first so you don't pop over your target pulse range. The workload on stairs is simply astounding. It is marvelous exercise, and does things for your quadriceps (huge anterior thigh muscles) indoors that only pump 'n' walk or run hill work can do outdoors.

When going *up* stairs pump 'n' walk style, use a diagonal stride; going down, same side — "ipsilateral." You'll find this shift avoids a peculiar, clumsy torque of the body.

An indoor workout with pump 'n' walk or run can thus become quite varied. One can shift from in place to on the move, from walk to run cycles, and, ultimately, have a go at the stairs to break the monotony.

STRETCHING

The introduction of systematic endurance exercise created the parallel need for systematic stretching. Muscle stretching is accomplished by elongating a particular muscle or group of them. Stretching helps prevent or annul the muscle spasm or cramp that may come from overuse. Many runners often stretch routinely for rather prolonged periods both before and after their aerobic workouts proper.

Stretching is of two types. In *static* stretching a position is taken and held for 15 to 30 seconds. Any muscle can, of course, be stretched; but the calves, hamstrings, quadriceps, low back, and groin muscles are the ones most often exercised this way. In *dynamic,* or *ballistic,* stretching there is some associated movement along with the elongation.

Stretching increases the range of motion around a particular joint and lends suppleness and freedom to the exerciser's motion. Experts vary in terms of how much they emphasize stretching. The recent books by Bob Anderson and Paul Uram are excellent in-depth treatments of the subject.

In Heavyhands individual needs will vary where it comes to stretching. A significant number of Heavyhands exercises will, by their nature, reduce the need for explicit stretching time. The exercises themselves provide dynamic stretching within the aerobic session itself. But some of us are inherently tauter than others. Individuals exhibit wide differences in muscle tension, range of motion, and vulnerability to the spasm that increases the risk of injury.

At this point in your Heavyhands work it is not likely that you will encounter much need for stretching. If you have considerable aerobic exercise experience you will already know how and how much you need to stretch. If aerobics is new to you, your low work capacity will protect you in most instances from overuse injury.

Exercise soreness after pump 'n' run, as in the calf muscles, suggests dividing your 30-minute sessions into two 15-minute periods, allowing a few hours between them. Later, when the initial discomfort disappears, you can move toward 30 minutes again.

I will discuss stretching again in Chapter 6, including there a trio of dynamic stretches specifically designed for Heavyhanders.

To stretch or not to stretch

Stretching before and/or after exercise can't hurt you, if your muscles have been properly warmed up, but Heavyhands requires less stretching than any other aerobic exercise. Because you divide workloads over your entire musculature, the stress and strain on any given muscle — particularly if you're a beginner — will be too small to cause injuries. As your training continues and you become a more vigorous Heavyhander, the need for stretching still remains negligible because your muscles, particularly those around joints, are constantly being strengthened, and because most Heavyhands moves contain components that *stretch* muscles.

Soreness of the upper extremities ordinarily will be of the mild, short-lived, limited variety and will not require specific stretching. Upper-torso work enjoys some immunity from the discomfort of muscle spasm because arm and upper-body work doesn't involve the "strikes" that produce traumatic overuse as of the feet, ankles, and knees in running.

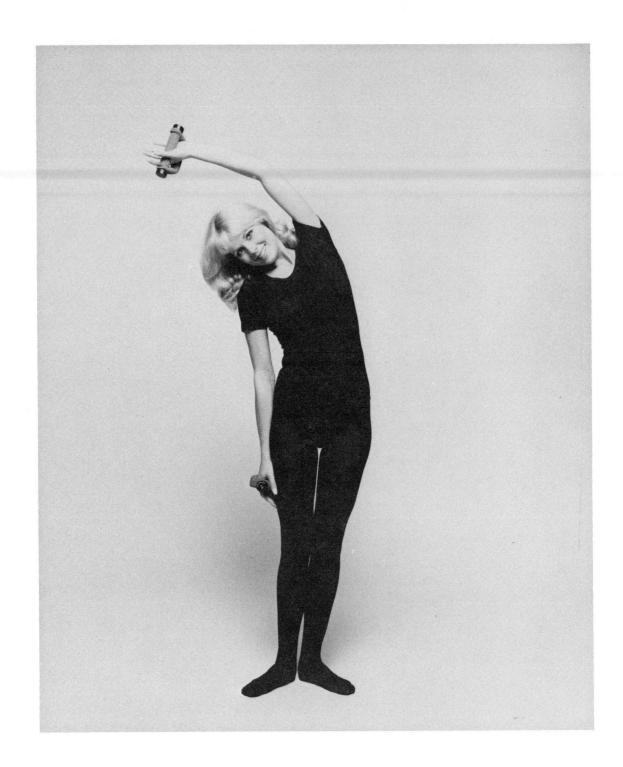

5

An Introduction to Heavyhands Levers

EQUIPPED WITH pump 'n' walk or run exercises that satisfy aerobic requirements and give you the feel of four limbs together in motion, you can choose electives — my suggested ones, or those you contrive yourself. Heart training, in the absence of some real impairment that your doctor would have warned you about, is virtually automatic. Keeping reasonably close to target pulse during three or four 30-minute sessions weekly, you cannot avoid training effect in the heart-lung system. The other fitness components — strength, muscle endurance, speed-power, flexibility — will require more of your conscious attention.

SHORT AND LONG LEVERS

I had a reason for selecting pump 'n' walk or run as a beginning point. While the upper extremity, indeed the entire upper torso, represents uncharted and unused aerobic territory, the biceps and triceps do get some reasonable activity in everyday life. So they're a good place to start. The biceps is probably the best-known muscle; it is the one kids flex to demonstrate their strength. In flexing the arm we use what one might call a *short lever*. The deltoid, a triangular muscle that caps the shoulder joint, is an example of a *long lever*. Its action raises the whole of the arm, its motion pivoting from the shoulder joint. Our musculature is full of such short- and long-lever combinations. And if you recall any of your elementary high school mechanics, you will realize that long and short levers by their nature have various advantages. Even if you're unequivocally bored by the subject of the physics of biomechanics, you will intuitively see how these long and short levers affect the practice of exercise. And in Heavyhands, where we deal with simultaneous use of muscles, knowledge of these so-called levers will be of immense practical importance to you.

SAME WEIGHT; DIFFERENT WORKLOADS

If you curl a 2-pound weight, that accomplishes a certain amount of *work* and *feels* a certain way to you. The work can be both ob-

LEVERS		
Long Levers	**Examples of Long Levers**	
• Shoulder and hip	Deltoid	
• Ball and socket joints	Pectorals	
• Wide range of motion	Gluteii	
• Complex actions	Abductors and adductors of thigh	
• Often underused		
• Usually slow tempo movement at given weight		
Short Levers	**Examples of Short Levers**	
• Knee and elbow	Biceps	
• "Hinge"-type joint limits range and complexity of motion	Triceps	
• Tempos may be faster because of short excursions	Biceps femoris	
• Tend to receive plenty of action because of their great mechanical advantage as compared with long levers		

LL, **SL** (labels on upper silhouette)

Combination Long AND Short Levers (caption on lower silhouette)

Note: Some muscles span two joints and thus activate both long and short levers: for example, quads and hamstrings.

Short lever action helps lessen the inefficiency of long levers by shortening them in a sense. Most moves are performed by combinations of long and short levers. Throws and kicks and ambulatory exercises are examples of such combinations. Examples of pure long levers are the tennis strokes and the stiff left arm of the golf swing.

jectively and subjectively assessed. If you curl 2 pounds to a height of 1.5 feet, that represents 2 pounds × 1.5 feet, or 3 foot-pounds. When you lower it you perform so-called negative work, which is less, estimated at about one-third as much as the upward stroke, in this instance 1 foot-pound. The total excursion then uses 3 + 1 or 4 foot-pounds.

Supposing you laterally raised the same 2-pounder from dead-hang to the level of your shoulder without bending your elbow.

Here the weight travels through a longer arc represented by your whole arm's length. You may laterally raise it 2.5 feet or more if you're very tall. The workload objectively may be 5 to 8 foot-pounds for the whole up-down excursion of your weighted hand — not counting, of course, the weight of your arm itself.

The feeling that goes with this movement will be quite different from the curling motion. It's plain harder for most. The motor requirements of everyday life seldom call for such "lateral" raises. There are other long levers that work from the shoulder, as in raising the weights from dead-hang at your sides straight forward and up to overhead.

So if you did a 1–10–100 using lateral raises, each extended arm moving alternately from dead-hang out to shoulder height, while walking in place at the same frequency, the heart rate response would be significantly greater than in "pumps," a short-levered movement. For one thing, the work is greater, as I've indicated. But also the muscles that activate the odd movement are typically neither strong nor equipped for endurance exercise. The heart-shoulder duet that accomplishes this portion of the 1–10–100 is particularly unprepared and inefficient, and that adds to the surprisingly high pulse rates we get.

WHEN INEFFICIENT MUSCLES ARE USEFUL

While the 1–10–100 test using pump 'n' walk in place can be performed to completion by almost any healthy person between ten and seventy, that may not be true if lateral raises are substituted for curls. Many people will find themselves muscle-weary or too achy to continue. I have watched a strong man whose 100-pace walk in place produced a pulse increase of 40 then escalate to 80 beats per minute after laterally raising 3 pounds for 4 minutes at the same frequency!

I suggest you try a lateral raise, long lever, 1–10–100, noting both the pulse rate you generate and the specific kinds of muscle difficulty you encounter. If your pulse and muscle responses are greater than you anticipated, take heart! The difficulties you have encountered represent greater potential for growth. If the biceps and triceps short-lever drivers are educable, the long-lever deltoids and the other muscles that mobilize the shoulder joint are immensely so.

There are nine shoulder movements actually, all of them yearning for strength-endurance exploitation. The long levers involved will improve more rapidly than any part of your muscular armor, with the possible exception of the lower back and abdominal groups.

These shoulder muscles and their tendons and the ligaments about the shoulder joint are all too frequently blighted by injury, which is another reason for bolstering them with strength-endurance training. They are called upon in all sorts of sports moves, but seldom receive training of the strength-endurance type. As you proceed through this book, you will be struck, I'm sure, by my emphasis on moves that use the upper-torso long levers that revolve about the shoulder joint. In striving for whole-body aerobics, these muscle masses are prime targets. In terms of total work until fatigue, a 1000-percent increase within one year is a modest expectation.

Long levers are inefficient machines, which makes them good for exercise. In other words, it is very hard to oppose gravity's pull by way of the long levers, and that's precisely why they're excellent choices for the thinking exerciser. The logic is simple. They're neglected because they're inefficient, which makes them tend to waste, or "atrophy." That in turn makes them excellent prospects for resurrection and improvement at a meteoric rate. Since the cardiopulmonary apparatus isn't particular about which muscles it nourishes, the whole oxygen-transport system gets a boost when we use long levers.

> **Potential improvement**
>
> Because long-lever movements are usually so awkward, difficult, and inefficient, the muscles that propel them are terribly underused. As a result, in a year you can expect these muscles to increase their total workload by 1000 percent or more. Only the muscles of the lower back and the abdomen can surpass that kind of improvement.

MIXED LEVERS

Many of the movements you are about to learn are not strictly speaking exclusively short or long levered, but are a bit of both. With pure long levers, the limb is completely extended; in those starting with the shoulder joint, the elbow is kept straight; those from the hip have the knee extended (or straight) as in the punter's or Rockette's kicks. Our mixed levers are compromises. We can increase both tempo and weights by allowing some flexion, or bending, at the elbows and knees. Many of the movements of work and play are combinations involving complex flexions and extensions of the joints. Thus the throws, kicks, punches, and swings of many sports moves are mixed short and long levers.

The long-lever option in Heavyhands highlights the difference between competing unrealistically with others and competing essentially with one's own yesterdays. As an exerciser concerned with self-improvement, inefficiency — gross, mechanical disadvantage — is exploited. The inherent mechanical disadvantage of the body's long levers lends them a special usefulness in Heavyhands exercise.

UNUSED MUSCLES, INJURIES, AND GRACE

This special kind of movement is a kind of adventure: the development of strength-endurance capacity in a lot of strange places will have a powerful effect in upping your workload capacity, shedding calories, strengthening muscle parts that are especially vulnerable to injury, and improving the grace and suppleness with which you move.

Some of our muscle levers are used so seldom that it's not difficult to guess why we're so prone to ailments. The long levers of the legs and the great movers of the hip joint are good examples. Our low-back problems or our susceptibility to various hernias, when things poke through weak spots in our muscle armor, results from our failure to strengthen the trunk and abdominal muscles. In addition literally dozens of short-levered muscles that could make for graceful, fluid motion of the spine are rarely used, and almost never in aerobic exercise. That means there's aerobic potential to be realized through working these back and abdominal muscle levers. You will see in Chapter 7 that hand-held weight can allow your back and belly muscles to do what they've *never* done before.

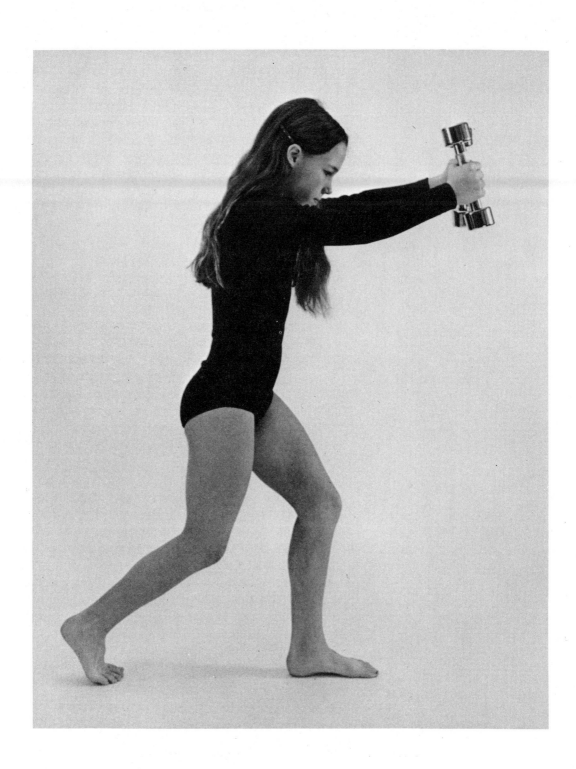

6

A Repertoire of Heavyhands Calisthenics

ONCE YOU CAN pump 'n' run in place or on the move, and understand short and long levers, your Heavyhands technique can begin to expand. Each of the following Heavyhands calisthenics offers something different from the others, and each attacks the fitness problem from a different angle. You should not try to include all of them immediately. If you were to add one of them every two weeks or so, your progress would be more than adequate — it would be sensational. They are not easy; each requires practice; and not one of them is essential to your Heavyhands strategy. Try them all, abandoning, for the time being, those that don't work for you immediately. Later, armed with more strength and endurance, you may be surprised to find you like them the second time around.

Suppose you were starting to play the piano. The first piece you learned might by now represent little challenge. But when more complicated assignments frustrated you, indeed you might resort to it for reassurance of your previous progress. When you reflect on it, that progression is what learning is about: a mosaic of bits of understanding in various stages of completion. To be effective at any skill — and certainly at exercise — you must view yourself as a *practitioner*. The music analogy works because it implies ever-increasing difficulty, continuing self-appraisal tinged with humor, and *practice:* thoughtful training rather than a Sisyphean chore.

Each new move will add some measure of strength and grace to the movements that you acquired earlier. You're not as smooth at pump 'n' run now as you will become. The following moves were selected for their overall workload, for the amount of muscle mass mobilized, for "getting to" often neglected muscles, and for special movement effects such as flexibility, power, and fluidity. They're comprehensive and they will train you in ways that none of the standard aerobic methods can. But they don't begin to exhaust the possibilities. Since I invented them, they are to some extent bound by the peculiarities of my structure and abilities. After learning the basic moves, don't hesitate to modify, embellish, amplify, or exclude outright. There's enough here to improve your fitness substantially, but you should adventure, explore, improvise, refine to your own taste.

Each exercise may be used either in a prolonged aerobic session, an interval of 3 to 10 minutes, or as a brief portion of a sequence of exercises we call medleys. Later, when dancing is discussed, you may want to include some of the calisthenic moves in your routines.

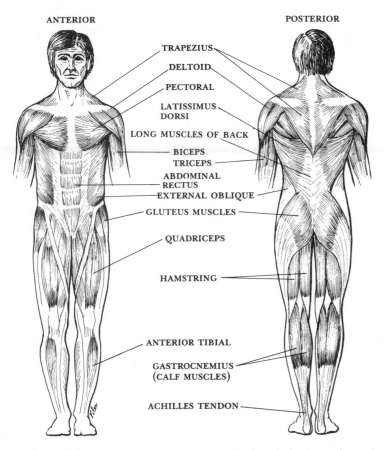

ANTERIOR

POSTERIOR

TRAPEZIUS

DELTOID

PECTORAL

LATISSIMUS DORSI

LONG MUSCLES OF BACK

BICEPS

TRICEPS

ABDOMINAL RECTUS

EXTERNAL OBLIQUE

GLUTEUS MUSCLES

QUADRICEPS

HAMSTRING

ANTERIOR TIBIAL

GASTROCNEMIUS (CALF MUSCLES)

ACHILLES TENDON

For now, the problem is to learn the "feel" of the exercises. Go slowly, think hard about the directions, gain clues from the photos and drawings, and above all, *practice*. I'll mention some of the muscle groups that the exercises emphasize and I've included an "atlas" to point out their locations.

Just as pump 'n' walk leads quite naturally to pump 'n' run, these basic moves will also lead to more complicated variations. I will provide some examples of how simple exercises can evolve into complex ones. Many of you, already spontaneous and graceful, can supply your own variations. Don't allow my choices to stifle your innate creativity. So long as you obey the cardinal rules — keeping your heart cadence where it belongs and establishing growth along the strength, endurance, and speed axes — and so long as you don't hurt yourself — you *can't* go wrong.

Always use smaller weights than necessary when learning the moves.

Safety first

These calisthenics are presented in a rough order of difficulty, easy ones first. It is a very rough order, and it is *my* sense of difficulty. Your sense of difficulty will be based not only on your condition, but the peculiarities of your structure. Many of these exercises are likely to use muscles you didn't even know you had. Therefore, go slow and, most important, go light. Use the smallest weights you have to learn them. If you encounter difficulty learning them, or if muscles fade, ache, or go into spasm, you should learn them and practice them at first without any weights.

Hang loose. I'll suggest some metronome frequencies for starters, but you will vary those depending on the weights you select.

Remember, when you're least aware of it — frequently when you're learning new exercises — you may find yourself clutching the weights tighter than necessary. Loosen your grip. As I suggested earlier, a tight grip tends to diminish blood flow, which leads to spasm and cramp and may cause your exercise to halt prematurely.

I. Alternate Curl (Pump) with Alternate Long-Lever Side Step

This introduces a leg long lever to upgrade your pump 'n' run. Instead of in-place pump 'n' run, you merely kick sidewise from the hip on the same side as the arm that's pumping the weight. Add a hint of a hop as you move from the ball of one foot to the other. Stop and check your pulse when you're mildly winded. Experiment with this one, varying weights, metronome rate, and duration — noting the effects of various combinations on your pulse. You can also vary it slightly by moving the entire body backward and forward by small amounts with each move, e.g., 5 hops in a forward direction and 5 back. Mixing this exercise with pump 'n' walk and run will form your first medley. (120–135 steps per minute)

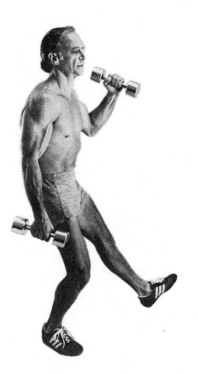

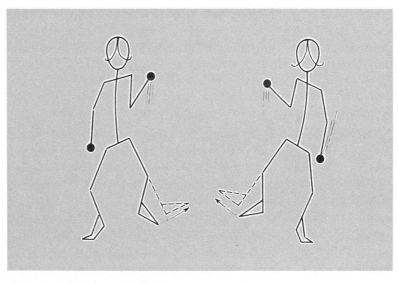

Alternate curl with long-lever side step

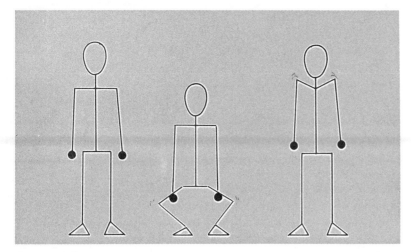

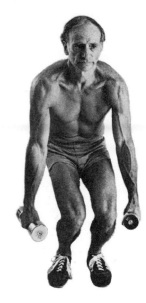

Squat and shrug

II. Squat and Shrug

Stand with weighted hands at sides, feet 12 inches apart. Squat halfway down until your thighs are at about a 45-degree angle to the floor. As you come back to your original upright stance, shrug your shoulders enthusiastically toward your ears, while allowing your hands to hang. Relax the shrug as you slide into the next squat and so on. Keep your back vertical as you move up and down. It sounds easy, but you're doing plenty of leg work and your large trapezius muscles will be in for a workout. This exercise takes weights heavier than you normally use in pump 'n' run. (110–140 steps per minute)

III. Dip 'n' Punch

While we're punching, here's another variation with a very different feel. Stand in a crouch with your hands at the "ready" position: elbows close to your sides, hands about waist level. At the first count punch hard straight in front with the right hand so that it ends its flight with your right arm fully extended out in front of your face. As you throw the punch, the right knee dips slightly along with a slight rotation forward of the right hip. As the left arm duplicates this movement, the right arm is yanked enthusiastically backward, behind the body, the upper arm remaining approximately parallel to the ground. This can be graceful and smooth despite the violent

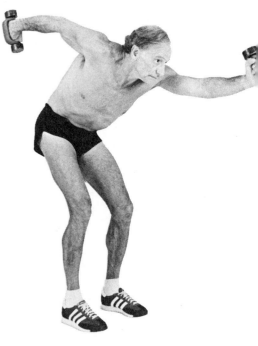

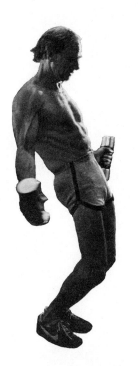

to-and-fro thrusts. Watch your pulse climb; and it will tighten your middle as well. The exercise is a treat for the whole shoulder girdle. (120–140 punches per minute)

IV. Lateral Flings and Heel-Toe Rock

Here's a lovely short- and long-lever combo which cures bad moods for me, not to mention soggy deltoids. It has a jazzy and exuberant aura to it, and is marvelously adaptable to dance. You'll want to start with tiny weights. Stand with knees flexed at about a 45-degree angle. Place your weight back on your heels. With elbows comfortably bent, hold the weighted hands, thumbs up, in front of you at nearly arms' length, at about the level of your navel. On the next count you do a lot of things. Move each hand sharply outward until you seem to feel your shoulder blades bump. They don't really, but they seem to. Simultaneously thrust the pelvis and knees forward and move to your toes. Return to the original position, back on your heels, as your arms close in front of you. That's all there is. Your derriere pokes out rather comically in the hands-forward, "heel" position. The exercise will make a tiger of you, and it will also shake the spasm of a backache. In addition, I've found that it relieves my troublesome hamstrings, which tend to tighten after a long, too-fast-for-me run. It's great for lateral deltoids, pectorals, several muscles about the hip joint. (60–70 full cycles per minute)

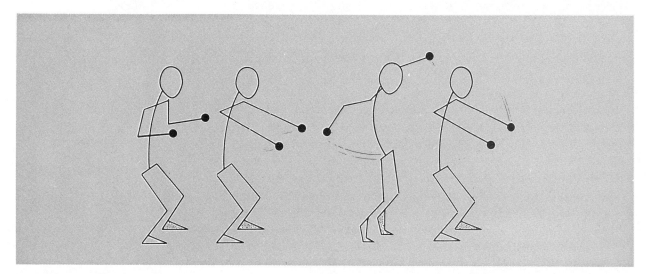

Lateral flings and heel-toe rock

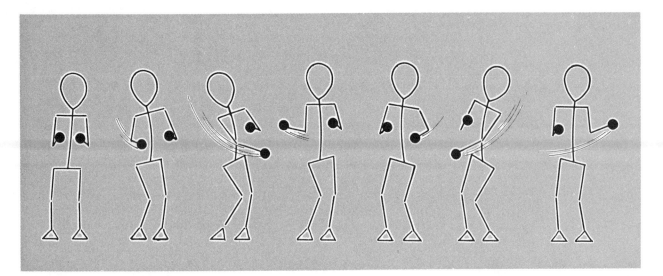

Variations on No. V bag punching

V. Punching the Timing or "Speed" Bag

This is a favorite of mine because I use it when I'm glued to the TV. It's a natural because your head doesn't move enough to divert your vision from the tube. It looks easier than it really is, unless, of course, you've punched a speed bag before, in which case the choice of the weight is the only problem. Standing with the lightest weights you own at about waist level, you're essentially going to swing each hand twice, a kind of forehand and backhand, then repeat the move with the other hand. So, it's done in four counts. (*Read all of this paragraph before you try anything.*) Start with the right hand. Looking straight ahead, sight a spot at about the level of the bottom of your sternum (breastbone). Swing your right hand first in a throwing motion so the weight passes the sighted target, sliding off toward your left side and ending at waist level a few inches to the left of your hip bone. Count 2 finds that weight retracing roughly the first trajectory, traveling back in an upward slope to your right, past your target, then downward angling toward a spot a few inches to the outside of your right hip bone. Looked at from the front, your right hand describes a curve that rises in the middle of its course and passes downward on either side of your body.

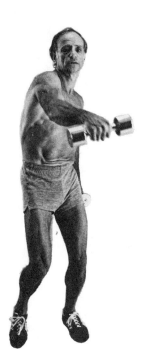

The hand's velocity is, of course, maximal as it passes "through" the target, decelerating as it slopes to the outside. Your elbows should be slightly bent, not rigidly extended. A later variation (or evolution), in fact, is consciously to keep the arm extended, a long-lever variation. Counts 3 and 4 merely repeat the same process with your left hand. Properly executed, the sequence should go smoothly in four counts so that your left forehand starts its moves just as your right backhand has eased to a halt. The metronome will keep you honest.

Another evolutionary extension: to really soup up this exercise, bring your knees into it. This seems a bit difficult at first, but once you've got it, wild horses can't separate you from it. With each count you do a slight, quick dip of the knees — down *and* back up with each arc of each swing. Thus, when you've completed a four-count cycle, you'll have accomplished four complete semibends and recoveries of your knees. As a second phase of the evolution, lean way over to the side, bending at your waist so that your weight is transferred to your left foot. While you lean left, do the two right arm punches — forehand and backhand. Then reverse the procedure, leaning to your right and striking with your left. It will take time to organize all that, but when you have it, it's fun to do and will put the lion's share of your muscle tissue into aerobic synchrony.

It's difficult to say what weights you will eventually use in this exercise. One thing is certain — the total workload will grow both in intensity and duration. Bear in mind that once you master "fully evolved" bag punching you are aerobically exercising *70 percent* of your entire muscle mass. You are working the major muscles of arms, legs, shoulders, chest, abdomen, and back. (80–120 punches per minute as you go from "heavy" to "light")

VI. Kick 'n' Punch

From the "ready" position, merely punch hard straight forward, trying to strike the foot (same side) you've kicked, stiff-kneed, in front. At the top of the kick, the leg is almost parallel with the floor. This one has always been tough for me and I hate it. Dancers and karate practitioners, however, seem to love it. The arm is retrieved briskly to the side at waist level just as the extended leg returns to the floor. It will turn a mean pulse for you. Bending forward with each punch is a useful added touch. (50–70 kicks-punches per minute)

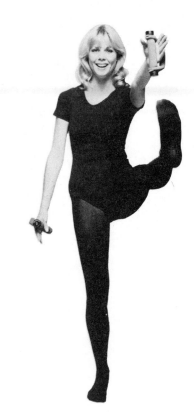

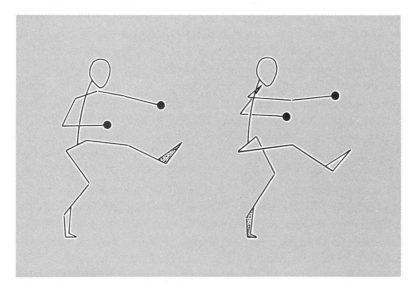

Kick 'n' punch

VII. Double Ski-Poling

Don't be fooled by the seeming simplicity of this exercise. *It's among the best in the book.* (There's much more about this one later.) Simply start with the hands together in front, high overhead. Bring them vigorously down and back. As they start down from the front position, the knees dip and then straighten as the weights proceed downward past the legs toward the rear. As the arms return to the forward up position, the knees repeat the dips and so on, with each sweep of the arms. On the upward swing the anterior shoulder group and the major chest muscles are strengthened. On the down movement as the arms move to the rear, the great swimming muscles — the latissimus dorsi, or "lats" — contract. The dipping action of the leg builds thigh strength and endurance. Don't hesitate to continue as long as your breathing is comfortable and nothing hurts. (30–50 complete cycles per minute)

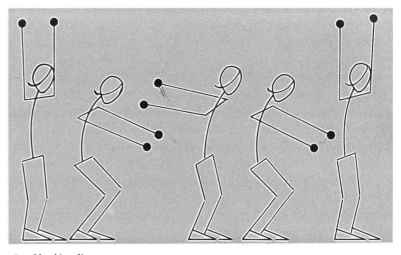

Double ski-poling

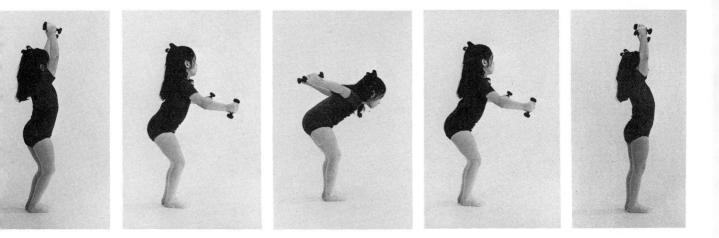

VIII. Alternate Ski-Poling

The same as double ski-poling except that the arms move *alternately*, this is a very special exercise, and one that lends itself to expansion and evolution. Starting with alternate pulls from dead-hang, forward to overhead, the knee dips are added first subtly, then exaggeratedly. The dip is both down and up *with each swing of each arm.* Extend the arms backward as far as is comfortable. As facility develops, the torso can lean a bit *away* from the side of the raised hand. There are few major muscle groups left out of this effort. Your training with it will reward you in obvious ways soon enough. You will notice an increased ease in stair-climbing or in dealing with steep grades in walking or running. As your handweights increase, even slightly, the effects translate themselves into quadriceps (front thigh) strength, the kind that propels you upward. Proficiency in this exercise, because of its muscular and cardiopulmonary benefits, will produce enormous capacity for losing calories at a fast clip. The leaning to the side distinguishes this exercise most from double ski-poling. But that's important because it includes some abdominal groups and tends to protect you from sports injuries involving twisting of the body. (70–100 moves per minute counting both arm swings)

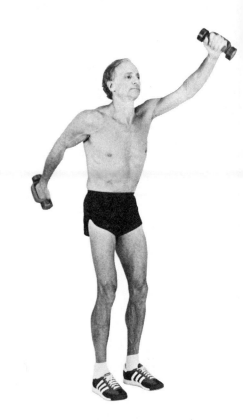

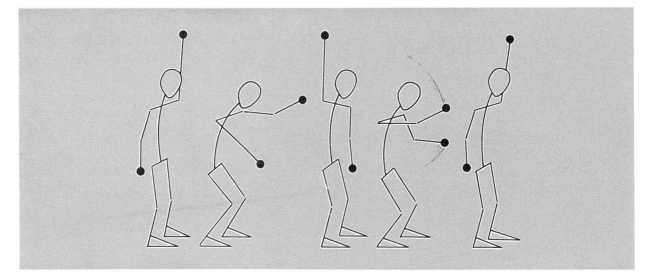

Alternate ski-poling

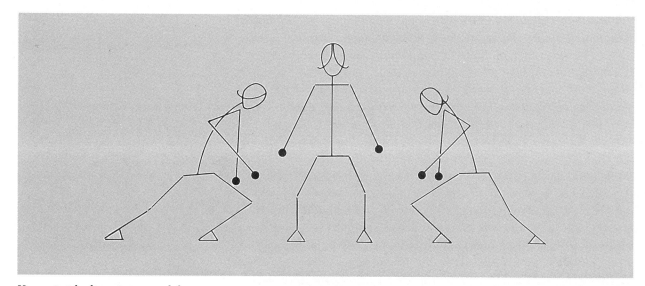

Heavy stretch alternate over each knee

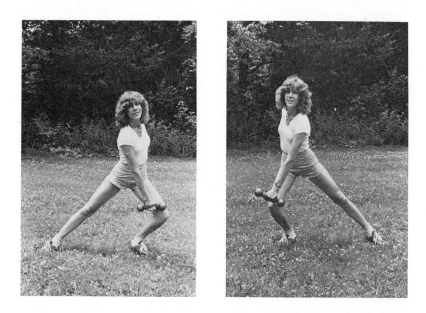

IX. Heavy Stretch Alternate over Each Knee

This one was borrowed from a standard runner's stretch exercise. You've seen it, I'm sure, dozens of times at any track or gym. With feet wider than shoulder width apart, first lean your body over one bent knee, then straighten it while slowly shifting to the other bent knee. The straight limb stretches the hamstring (back-of-thigh) muscles on that side. Plagiarizing from that move, I add the following: assume the above-described spread, holding relatively heavy weights (for you) at hang position at your sides. At the first count bend your left knee so that it travels downward, forward a bit, and outward. At the same instant twist your torso so that your right hand comes to lie just in front of your left knee, your left hand behind it. On two, shift to the opposite position, wherein virtually all of your weight plus the added iron is situated over your right foot. When you're doing this correctly, you will find yourself literally·able to lift the leg that's not flexed at the knee, at least a bit. Later modifications: lean even farther, extending the front-of-the-knee weight even *farther* so that it may lie outside the knee by as much as several inches, depending on your reach, strength, and flexibility. Having gotten that down pat, an additional extension involves jerking the front-of-the-knee weight in an arc up toward your chin and then down, ending behind the opposite knee. If this sounds confusing, the pictures should clear it up for you. This exercise does so much it would take a professional kinesiologist to unscramble and tabulate the total contractile events. You can use relatively heavy weights. You will notice a degree of next-day soreness in the buttocks from it. If you're a golfer, swing a club a few times after this one, noting the easy fluidity with which you shift from leg to leg during backswing and stroke proper. A good bit of your shoulder girdle, latissimus, and abdominals also are pushed by this movement, not to mention considerable cardiopulmonary effect as evidenced by the good pulse level achieved. (40–80 shifts per minute)

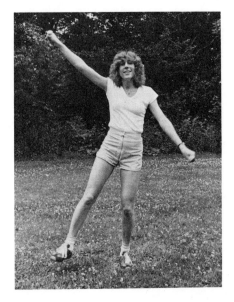

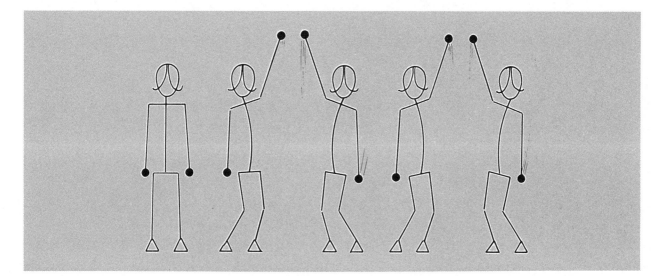

Lateral long-lever raises

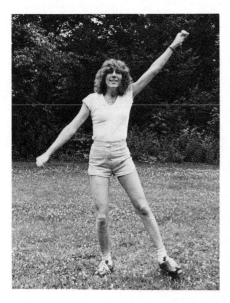

X. Lateral Long-Lever Raises

This starts with leg motion like the knee dip in No. VIII. Each arm is raised alternately, the hand traveling upward and laterally to above-shoulder height. The knees dip while this is happening so that each alternate arm movement begins with the knees flexed and ends, at shoulder-height, with the legs straight. Synchronized, it should feel as though your straightening knee is *helping boost* each arm upward and to the side. Sometimes I add a little "press" at the top of the arm raise: having gotten one arm overhead (your upper body is not listing to the side opposite your raised arm), you allow that weight to drop slowly to shoulder-height, whereupon you thrust it again skyward, fast. The weight is then lowered to your side by the same route it followed when it was elevated and you start over with the other hand. I got the idea while experimenting with shot putting and found the added "press" a fair facsimile of the shot put itself. These alternate lateral long levers can be coupled to a long lever of the lower extremity, kicking sideways from the hip as the arm is raised. This includes two long-lever moves and it's very tough exercise. Start with small weights and experiment with various tempi. (40–70 dips 'n' raises per minute)

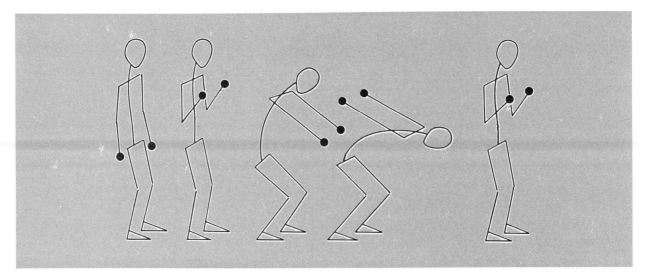

Curls, bends, and triceps extensions

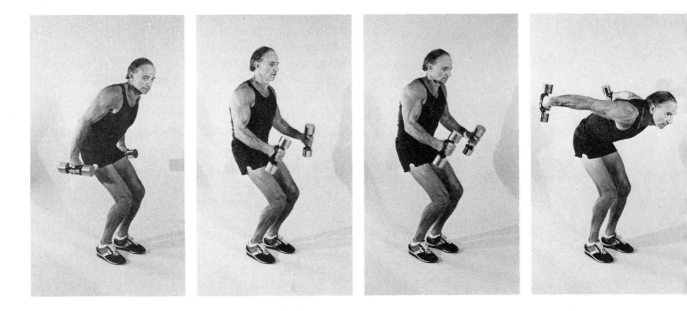

XI. Curls, Bends, and Triceps Extensions

Curl both weights from a dead-hang to shoulder, keeping your
elbows rather close to your sides. As you lower them, dip the knees

and bend forward from the waist. Continue the weights past the vertical to the rear and up so that at the move's end, the weights are jutting backward from extended arms while your knees have meanwhile straightened. The knees dip again as the weights are brought forward. This is similar to double ski-poling. Doing it correctly, every time your hands pass your knees, they will be at the lowest point in their dip. (30–50 full cycles per minute)

XII. Side Bends

An easy one but not to be underestimated from either the aerobic standpoint or the effect on the oft-neglected oblique muscles that wall the abdomen, this exercise will nicely complement the *abdominal aerobics* that I discuss later. One usually can afford to use heavier weights here and/or a brisk tempo to make it aerobic. It will also stretch your neck and trapezius muscles. Standing with feet spread at about shoulder width, weights at dead-hang position, simply tilt sideways, allowing the downside hand to slide to mid-calf or thereabouts. Recover and tilt the other way, etc. There's room for considerable leeway. (40–100 "tilts" per minute depending on weight)

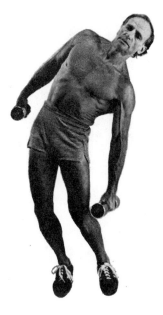

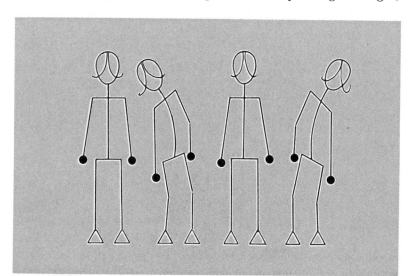

Side bends

XIII. Hand over Hand

Just that: holding your hands in front of you, just below chin level, elbows flexed, simply rotate them vertically around one another. It's a good basic move to learn and to become accustomed to, because we'll use it in both shadowboxing and dancing. Good for the entire upper torso, it is especially excellent for wrists, forearms, and biceps. Use weights small enough that you can gyrate them long and fast. Extend the exercise by doing fairly deep knee dips slowly while you hand-over-hand rapidly. Vary it by leaning to the right and left during the dip cycle. To complicate matters further, alternately raise and lower each shoulder at the same rate as the hand-over-hand cycle. (Any frequency that keeps you at pulse for 3 minutes or more)

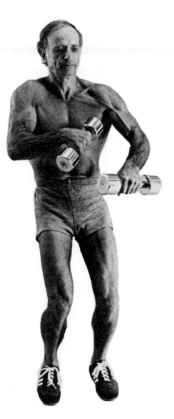

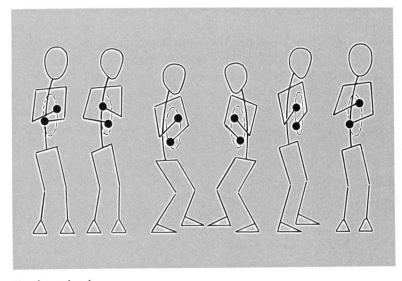

Hand over hand

XIV. Squat Thrusts Heavyhands Style

Here, an old warhorse is reinstated by the simple act of adding handweights. Stand erect, holding weights at dead-hang at your sides, knuckles out. Then bend your knees enough to lower the weights to the ground just outside your feet, which are rather close together. Kick both feet to the rear, leaving you in the final stage

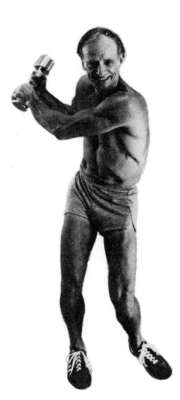

of the push-up position. Return the extended feet to the squat position, then stand *all the way* up. Needless to say, this is an excellent exercise *without* weights, so what you add should be very conservative. This is particularly true if 10 or so cycles, without weights, brings you to target. When that happens, postpone the addition of weights until you can manage 2 to 3 minutes with your pulse within your calculated range. But don't postpone the addition of handweights indefinitely. Train toward their inclusion. (About 20 per minute for starters)

XV. Swing 'n' Sway

Take a heavy weight and clutch it securely in both hands. Swing the weight so it describes a figure eight turned sideways in front of you. As the weight moves to your left, let both knees, slightly bent, move to the left, too; and knees to the right when weight swings to the right. Your golf club or even a 42-ounce bat feels almost weightless after a couple hundred of such movements. And your heart and lungs will verify the hard work involved. If you can't grip one weight comfortably, two separate handweights held close to each other do nicely. (50–90 "swings" per minute)

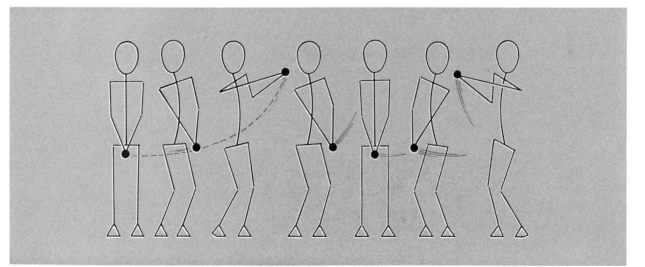

Swing 'n' sway

XVI. Variations of Calisthenics V, Bag Punching with Hops

You're ready for this only after bag punching has become auto-matic. It is not an easy exercise, but it will appeal to those who enjoy the challenges of multiple coordinated movement patterns. Since the exercise actually consists of three different components, it's best to learn each separately, linking them together when you've mastered each part. In Calisthenic V, after the arm strokes have been mastered: link this movement with the legs by hopping on the foot opposite the side of the arm strike. Hop twice on the ball of the left foot, one hop for the forehand punch, one for the following backhand move. Hop then to the other foot, as *the other hand swings into its forehand move,* then a second hop along with the backhand. Without a hitch in the timing you now hop back to the ball of the other foot, and so on. Don't be discouraged if the rhythm confuses you at first. Once you've mastered it you will own it. You can stop right here because you've already added an excellent ex-ercise to your repertoire if you merely hop and punch. Adjusting weight and frequency, you can go for 20- to 30-or-more-minute sequences, or do them heavier and faster as short intervals or por-

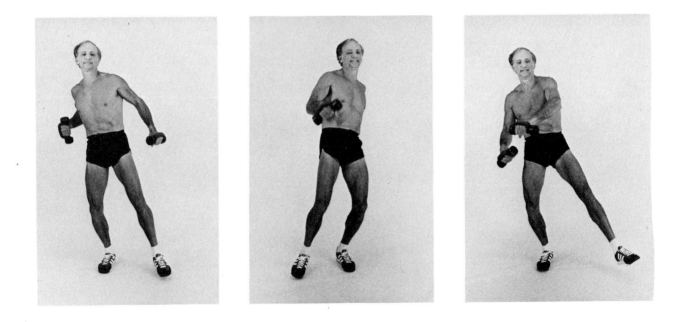

tions of medleys. The third component is a fringe benefit. It makes for a more choreographed feeling and squanders a few more calories.

Leaving everything you've learned as is, insert *four kicks*. Each kick is synchronized with a swing — so that each foot kicks twice, when the *arms on the same side* are punching twice. In effect, simultaneously you punch with your right hand, hop with your left foot, while kicking with your right foot. The hop and kick are done twice during the combined forehand and backhand swing; and the whole procedure repeats with the other side. It sounds impossible, but it's not. You'll tend to omit the hops at first, but some hard concentration will wrap it all into one movement. Initially, when confusion reigns, return to the simpler hop-and-punch variation, experimenting with the kick addition for brief moments. When you've mastered the entire ensemble, you may incorporate it into dance as well as shadowboxing. Add weight and speed when you're up to it and use the heavy-light technique to shift the emphasis from strength to speed and back, keeping your heart-lung operation fairly constant. (110–130 punches and hops per minute)

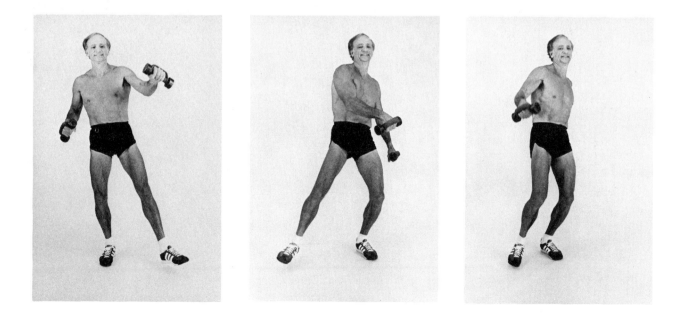

XVII. Diagonal Arm-Leg Thrusts

This is a multiple muscle mover, and difficult even without weights. In fact, try it first without weights to gain the sense of balance the move requires and a solid respect for the sheer energy it takes to fuel it. You've doubtless seen variations on the theme during tap-dance routines. It's like traveling furiously on a treadmill with exaggerated moves of arms and legs, paired diagonally as in pump 'n' run on the move. The "exaggeration" is produced by the fact that you must go slower if you expect to last beyond the first panting minute. The payoff comes, of course, in the additional strength-power route — the additional workload dumped on the legs. Hand-weights become the added touch once you've "steadied out" at an appropriate heart rate for those 3 or more minutes that give the move aerobic usefulness.

Nordic skiers will find this exercise helpful, as it increases their ability to climb those long uphill trails. Its inherent difficulty may cause you to grant it short shrift, but try to keep it in your repertoire. Nothing can raise your pulse faster. Needless to say, it belongs to any dance-move repertoire. (80–120 thrusts per minute)

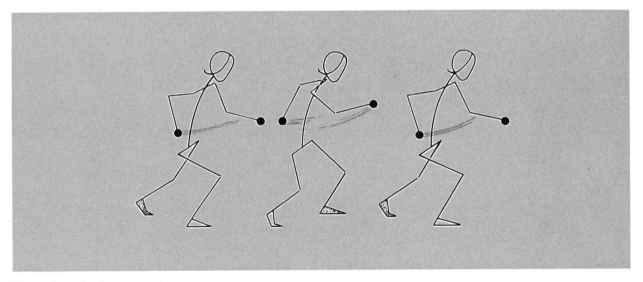

Diagonal arm-leg thrusts

XVIII. Shrug Wiggle

Use a very heavy weight, perhaps 2 to 4 times as heavy as what's comfortable in your pump 'n' run. A fairly fast tempo may be necessary to get you to target pulse because there's virtually no limb motion of the short- or long-lever variety. Stand erect with the weights hanging at arm's length, touching the outsides of your mid-thighs. Place your feet at shoulder width. The shoulders seesaw, each alternately elevating and lowering. The hips do the same, the knee on the "down" side bending slightly. The more exaggerated the better because that ultimately will stretch the range of motion of the joints and give maximal play to the muscles involved. Shoulders and hips coordinate the only two ways they can. Either elevate both simultaneously or drop one while elevating the other. Do prolonged sequences both ways. This may *not* be the warm-up exercise for you if you have serious back problems, but it will help you shake the typical uncomplicated morning backache in the flicker of an eyelash. The exercise effectively shows how muscles aside from the limbs can generate plenty of cardiorespiratory response. Remember, there's no evidence that your heart prefers one muscular stimulus over another. You could shrug wiggle to target pulse with a shoulder tendinitis, a tennis elbow, a heel spur, and a runner's knee! (90–120 wiggles per minute)

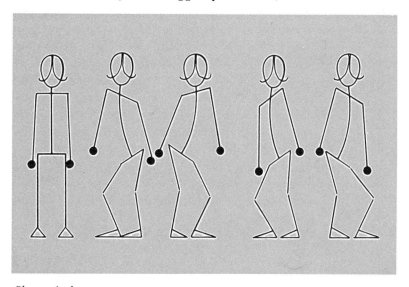

Shrug wiggle

XIX. Single Dumbbell Swing

This exercise is borrowed from standard dumbbell exercise charts. We shore it up mechanically and increase its overall effect by turning it into an aerobic exercise. Experiment will quickly dictate the weight you can manage — but remember *always* to err on the light side.

Grasp the weight handle with both hands. Make a comfortable connection somehow; a modified golf grip works for some, as many handles aren't long enough to accommodate two fists simultaneously without some sort of overlap. Soft cotton gloves can help lessen annoying friction when all those fingers are scrunched together. The feet are planted wide apart and the arms hang downward, elbows extended, the weight in front. The knees are flexed, and the weight is brought downward between the legs as far back as it will go until the arms touch the inside of the thighs. Then the weight is swung upward in an arc to the overhead position. Try to maximize the range of flexion to extension, a kind of curling and upward release of the curved spring your body becomes in the execution of this move. Try to remain relatively stiff-elbowed, but a few degrees of flexion is tolerable and may keep you at it longer.

My guess is that early and continued practice of this exercise would significantly reduce the number of herniated discs. *Don't use it to cure the one you've already popped* without official sanction from a cautious orthopedist. I've often tried to figure which muscles this exercise *doesn't* call into play. Including the facial grimaces it's apt to evoke, there aren't many. Juggle frequency and weight to achieve target pulse and hang in there, gradually increasing the duration of continuous execution. I employ it frequently as a 10-minute-interval warm-up for running. It is also good for stretching painfully stiff muscles. Establish a comfortable breathing rhythm. Depending upon the weight and pace you select and the state of your conditioning, you may elect to breathe once per cycle, i.e., inhaling on the up arc, exhaling on the down; or twice per cycle—

both in and out with each change in the direction of the weight. (30–50 cycles per minute)

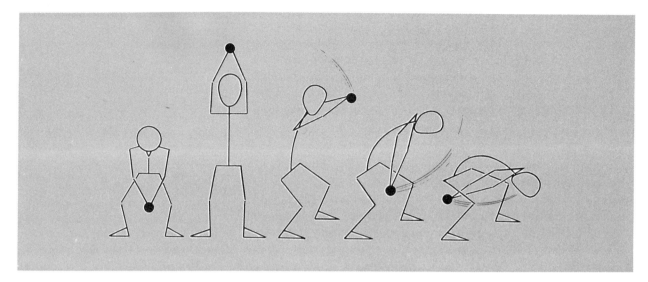

Single dumbbell swing

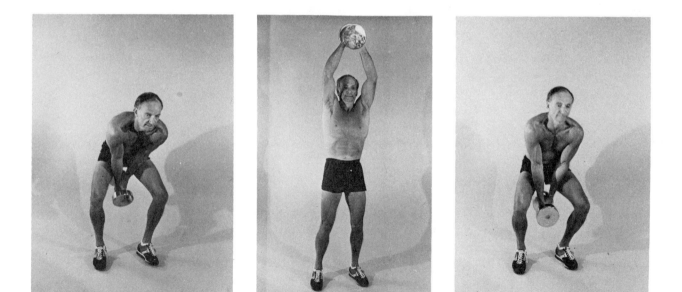

XX. Jumps

Jumping of any sort represents the most unabashed rebellion against gravity. All running contains a vertical component, albeit slight, and all sports that involve moving about invoke the antigravity potential of the massive quads. Jumping with handweights counteracts this weakness in the runner's muscular equipment without abandoning the aerobic core of the exercise. Any program can be enhanced by jumping. Here are a few suggestions:

A. Jumping curls. Just as the name suggests, you merely jump with both feet, one jump on the "up" swing of the curl of one weight, one as you lower that weight. At a tempo of 150 by metronome you will, at one minute's end, have left the floor 150 times and completed 150 curls. As always, select weight and frequency by their combined effect on pulse rate.

> **Improving jumping work with Heavyhands**
>
> Very few people I know have continued rope jumping as their staple aerobic shtick. Boredom may be a problem, but also it's a fact that rope jumpers become relatively more efficient after much practice. Since the frequency of jumping doesn't figure much in determining the workload, there's not much you can do to increase your jumping work except to go Heavyhands, which makes it a new ball game. Great control and only the sky limits the workload once the hands join the act.

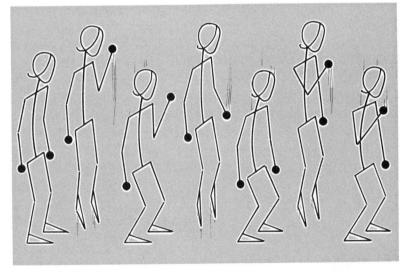

Jumping curls

B. Jumping long-short levers. This one is good for a short fast-light interval. Elbows relaxed, jump as in the above exercise, but using a lighter weight, move the hands about 180 degrees—up above the head and then down, and as far behind as is comfortable—using the same 2:1 hop-to-hand ratio as with the curls.

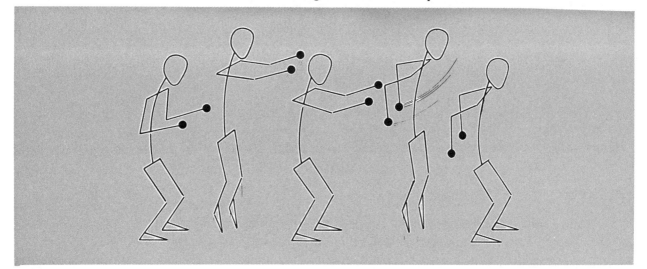

Jumping long-short levers

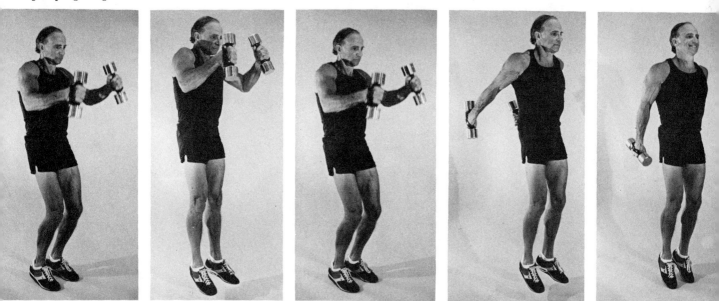

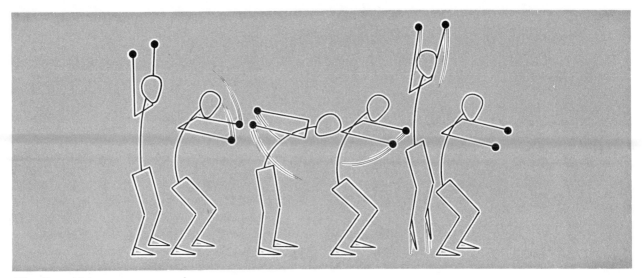

Ski-poling with jumps

C. Ski-Poling with interspersed jump or jumps. This exercise is like Calisthenic VIII, and like B above, except there's more knee bending and the added jump. (30–50 cycles with jumps per minute)

D. Lateral flings with jumps. In another variation of long-lever uppers with jumping, merely jump each time the weights are

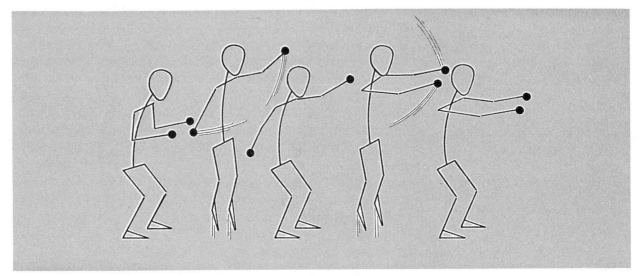

Lateral flings and jumps

brought together at mid-chest, and again as they are flung outward to full extension. Overdoing these jumps could make your calves very sore, so go easy until the muscles grow accustomed to the stress, then extend to longer intervals. With any evidence of pain *in any joint* — hip, knee, ankle — or in the feet, stop the exercise, returning to it *only if and when* that discomfort has disappeared. (140–180 jumps — that is, 70–90 flings per minute)

Lateral fling variation

Try this variation of lateral fling with jumping, using about half the weight you'd use in *that* exercise. Instead of bringing the hands together in the midline, cross them alternately, passing one hand over, then under, the other. The alternation merely keeps the muscle activity symmetrical. This is a range of motion extension and demonstrates nicely how increasing that element can substitute for larger handweight. This extension calls many of the rotator cuff muscles of the shoulder into play and will surely cause soreness if you do much your first try. It's a perfect exercise for tennis, working all of the muscle elements that make for speed-power in both forehand and backhand: the lateral deltoid, pectorals, trapezius, infraspinatus, etc. And the jumping-vertical strength element is what it takes to make some of those near impossible "gets." You will confirm the work involved by noting that with half the weights of the conventional lateral thrust you achieve a similar steady pulse rate. These exercises, together with double ski-poling in place or on the move, bring formidable training to the typically disused shoulder joint and its muscle attachments. A former victim of recurrent shoulder bursitis, I've not suffered a moment of discomfort since loading up on these movements. The weights should be small enough to keep the exercise light and lively.

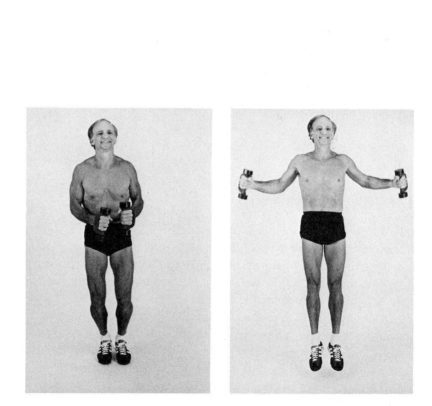

E. Jump twists. Deceptively easy, this exercise makes a good short interval by itself or in a dance sequence and brings a useful torsion component to jumping moves. The weights, held close together and parallel, are swung with only a slight bend in the elbow, back and forth across the front of the body at about waist level. The feet, meanwhile, close together, swivel during the jumps toward the *side opposite* the direction in which the hands are traveling. (Frequency to taste)

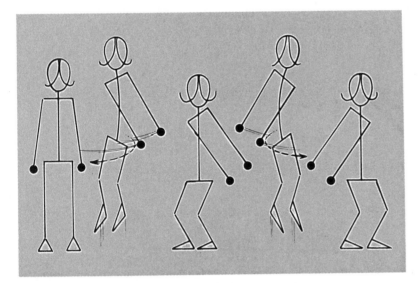

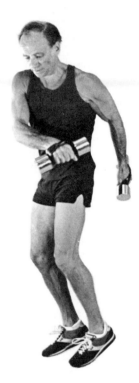

Jump twists

F. Biceps and triceps with jumps and bending. Involving a variation on Calisthenic No. XI, the trick here is consciously to use as many muscle groups as possible. It works equally well in the heavy-slow or light-fast mode. At slower frequency exaggerate the forward bend, the knee bends, and the height of the jump. The sequence goes: forward curl with jump, forward bend at waist, hands swing backward to full extension with a second jump, forward curl and jump, and so on. Twenty minutes of this in your hotel room on a business trip will undo most of the physiologic disadvantages of travel.

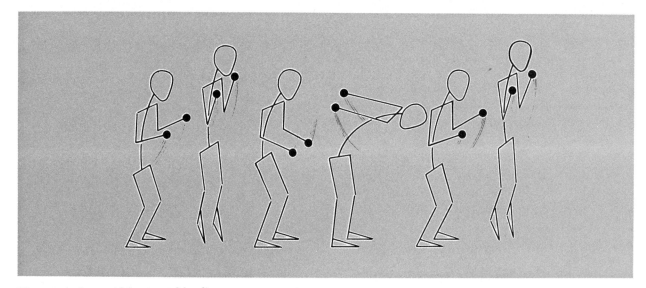

Biceps and triceps with jumps and bending

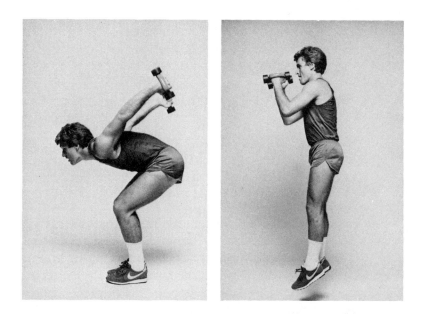

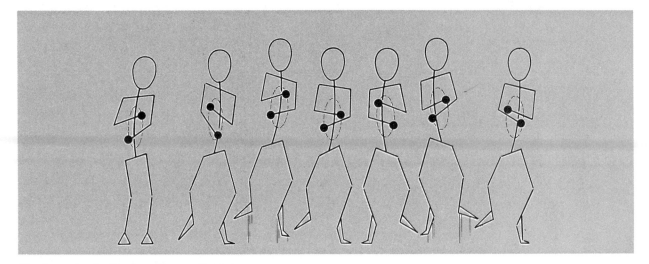

Hand over hand with alternating one-foot hops

G. Hand over hand with alternating one-foot hops. In this dependable staple, you execute a hand over hand as described in Calisthenic XIII, meanwhile hopping onto the ball of each foot 2, 3, or 4 or more times consecutively before shifting. (130–180 hops per minute)

You now have sampled more than enough Heavyhands calisthenic moves. You will, in time, come to know which ones, and at which weights and tempos, are best for you. Some you may really enjoy. Others may not be your cup of tea. Don't worry. Not one of them is indispensable. But try not to exclude any until you've given it a fair shake.

MEDLEYS

Having gotten the feel of Heavyhands calisthenics, you are aready to mix a few of them. We do this for several reasons. Combination exercises that involve both relatively trained and untrained groups of muscles may tire you quickly at first. That's to be expected: you're mixing muscle-heart duets that produce high oxygen pulses with others that produce rather low ones. That imbalance won't last long, you may be sure. At first, your untrained upper torso will speed your pulse too much, too quickly, at relatively small workloads. The more varied your upper-body work, the more quickly you will achieve higher oxygen consumption by those muscles. By spreading the work around with calisthenic mixes or medleys, you avoid overfatigue and possible injury of these untrained muscles. And medleys tend to neutralize boredom and add fluency and a sense of expertise to your workouts. Here are some suggestions as to how to hook the movement sequences together for best results.

1. Alternate hard and easy moves. That tends to steady out your pulse and breathing more effectively than if, for instance, you add a difficult series of long levers end to end.

2. Listen to your body. Any sense of localized discomfort in a particular muscle or joint that persists more than a few seconds is a signal to switch to a movement remote from that one. Frequently, the pain is a momentary spasm and you will soon be able to return to the exercise without discomfort. Of course the more moves you learn, the more expendable any one of them becomes.

3. During your calisthenic medleys, work toward longer intervals with each movement. Too frequent switching prevents the development of strength-endurance in the movement. Short strength or speed drills are fine and can be inserted occasionally to increase the workloads.

4. Think about your range of motion. As training proceeds, increase it, which should leave you not only stronger, but more supple and less prone to stiffness and injury.

5. Use slow-heavy, fast-light variations in your medleys. You can change tempo either when you change movement or during the course of any one movement. These changes bring an agility and versatility to your exercise and prevent the hypnotic effects of a single tempo. Heavyhands is thinking exercise rather than robotlike repetition. The point here is that any of these various choices cannot be wrong so long as you're neither loafing nor overdoing it. Keep your pulse rate reasonably steady at target.

6. When you are learning a new movement, practice it for a while as a solo interval, both fast and slow, so as not to dilute the movement fluency you've already established in your medley.

7. Exercise to music, unless you simply don't like it. A Heavyhands calisthenic medley can be seen as a dance, and excerise time passes more swiftly with musical accompaniment. Music may lessen

Medleys

With adequate training any of the preceding calisthenics can be done for 30 minutes straight, but that would increase the likelihood of overuse injury and it certainly would be boring. A better strategy is to mix a number of them together in your exercise. This mix is called a medley. Medleys lessen the risk of injury and, by calling into play various muscles and "muscle-duets," promote a higher level of general fitness.

the tendency to perceive yourself as toiling — even when you're hard at it.

8. Almost always ease into your exercise with pump 'n' run as a warm-up. Warming up incidentally is really just that. One literally raises the temperature of the muscle fibers so that the chemistry of contraction happens more efficiently.

STRETCHING

Most Heavyhanders will not require special stretching routines because many of the calisthenic moves and some of those employed with Heavyhands walking and running will *themselves* tend to abolish spasm and promote suppleness.

The diversity of the movements probably helps. I believe that complex movements involving strength and endurance of all of the major muscle groups is the key. Trading some speed for a great deal more strength probably reduces fatigue and therefore spasm.

I do suggest a few moves that can erase stray kinks that are associated with Heavyhands. They are novel in that they serve both to warm up *and* stretch and are performable at *target pulse*. This trio can be used prior to workouts, interspersed in calisthenic medleys or used as separate aerobic "stretch intervals."

1. The first is a variation of Calisthenics XII—side bends—using relatively light weight, it is performed at high frequency, 200–300 per minute. The upper limbs are stretched at dead-hang, and the pulse is generated by the muscles of the trunk.

2. Simply bend forward at the waist with the knees locked, and follow by a return to the erect stance. Meanwhile the shoulders seesaw rapidly, each weighted hand alternately approaching the floor in front. Two movements happen concurrently: the trunk bends forward and back 60 to 70 times per minute; the shoulders seesaw 250 to 300 times per minute. The arms and hamstrings stretch while the trunk works.

3. Merely bend forward and backward at the waist. The weights swing loosely forward from extended arms during the backbend; then down through and backward in a pendular movement while the upper torso is bending forward. At the proper tempo, when the weights are right, this too, will get you to target pulse. The

Static and dynamic stretching

Static stretching consists of extending one or more joints and holding that position so that the muscles and ligaments around the joint are motionlessly stretched. Dynamic stretching extends the muscles and ligaments while the limbs are in motion. Generally speaking, static stretching is considered *more* beneficial.

To stretch or not to stretch

Heavyhands exercise requires little if any stretching. By dividing workloads over many muscles the stress on any muscle group — particularly with beginners — is relatively small. Further, as the Heavyhander trains, muscles and ligaments around the joints are progressively strengthened. Finally, many Heavyhand exercises inherently contain stretching movements.

Stretch caveat

There is growing evidence that too much static stretching *before* a workout may not be wise. Researchers at Temple University found that increasing the temperature of muscle fibers makes stretching more effective. They suggested that 5 or 10 minutes of light but progressively intense exercise *before* stretching would increase its safety and efficiency.

---

knees are locked during the front bend, consciously stretching the hamstrings. Sixty *complete* cycles per minute is a good average tempo.

The trick here is to slip in and out of these movements, going from one to another, or to insert the trio into any Heavyhands exercise when stiffness or spasm in an extermity occurs. Some people enjoy these moves. Others, frankly, never touch them.

As your training proceeds you will quickly determine how much and what sort of stretching, if any, you need. Sometimes a new move or added workload will produce a bit of spasm that will work itself out without any special attention. Static stretching, if you enjoy it and don't overdo it, can't hurt you. There are always excellent articles in *Runners World* and whole books devoted to the subject for those who are interested. But for most people engaged in Heavyhands, stretching will be a matter of choice, not necessity.

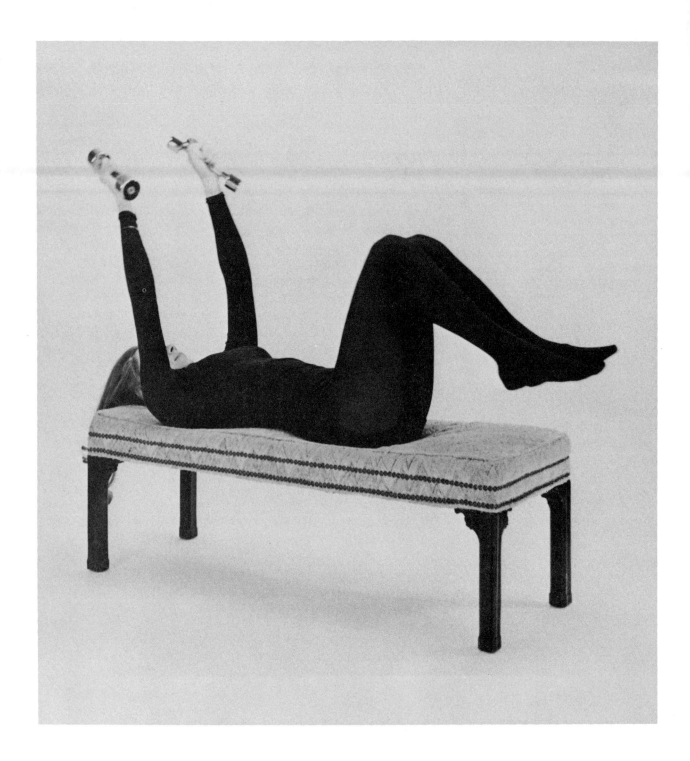

7

Bellyaerobics and Back-aerobics: Heavyhands for Abdomen and Back

THE BELLY IS something like the weather: everyone talks about it but few of us do much about it. Yet I know people who exercise *only* for their middles. I presume they do this in deference to their wardrobes or some other cosmetic concern. Belly fat is granted a special kind of unattractiveness. And if you are blessed with a flat abdomen you're dubbed slim and, some think, fit. Is the tendency for fat to accumulate at our midsections just a nasty trick of fate? Despite all the concern with our waistlines, the fact is, at any beach, those pairs of rectangles, the "washboard," that form the "abdominals" (rectus muscles) are seldom plainly visible. Does that mean that even vain folks neglect their bellies? Not exactly. Although spot reduction is mythical, the sit-up remains alive and well. I know old ladies who do 10 sit-ups daily even when grounded by the flu. A young man I once saw was so preoccupied with his waistline that he did thousands of sit-ups each day, incidentally remaining quite plump despite his ardor.

There is no question but that fat gathers where the action is least. Fat is measured by the bulk of skinfold, and if you find a skinfold thickness of 3 millimeters, which stands for zero fat, you can be sure you're examining a leg or an arm. There's not much chance of testing the theory that lots of reps chase fat until we learn to bend at our middle the same way and as *often* as we bend elbows, knees, and other joints.

We are not only paunchy, but our middles are flagrantly lacking in strength, speed-power, and endurance. It's easy to see why. Unless you're the catcher on an aerialist team or a gymnast, or shovel something all day, it's difficult to come by a fit middle outside of regular, intelligent exercise.

Implicit Heavyhand exercises for the belly

While the abdomen and back, like all muscles, need *explicit* exercise, inherent in many Heavyhand exercise is plenty of good *implicit* work. Double ski-poling, side bends, shadowboxing, and dance — any exercise in fact which includes bends at the waist — will provide a challenge for belly and back muscles.

IS THERE HOPE?

The belly is the first and last "depository" of excess poundage. If it is important to you, there are really only three ways of making a magnificent belly:

1. being fatless enough so that your abdominals show;
2. making belly muscles as strong and speedy as we want our limb muscles to be; or
3. making aerobic use of the abdominal muscles.

Many of the Heavyhands calisthenics implicitly exercise the abdomen. Double ski-poling does it, as do side bends performed vigorously and any of the other moves that involve bending. Dancing and shadowboxing are excellent, abdominally speaking, if you emphasize bending.

But I have discovered that abdominals, like biceps or "lats" or "pecs," require explicit work, too. That is, not only work that involves them as accessories, but work that invokes their most specific actions. Even neglecting these explicit moves for months at a time, I never grew a paunch. I simply wasn't adding fat anywhere. But after my first 5 minutes of overenthusiastic belly work I was sore enough that, for a week, even clearing my throat was painful. Exercising the abdomen is not easy and most of us can't manage "belly bends" fast enough or long enough to "steady out" at target pulse. But here are some moves that, if developed gradually, will be worth 5 minutes of your workouts.

The "Fold"

This is my favorite abdominal exercise. Some of my pupils swear *by* it now, but their first attempts had them swearing *at* it. It's a very unusual move; I've never seen a reasonable facsimile anywhere. Relatively small weights can produce large workloads.

It begins with you flat on your back, preferably on a padded bench, your head close to the bench's end, your arms extended horizontally beyond the bench. The floor will do, but put a pillow under your lower back. You are in the horizontal version of standing with your arms extended overhead. Use small weights or even none at all at first. With the initial move, pull your arms — elbows almost, though not rigidly, locked — upward over your head and toward your feet, while the legs, knees slightly bent, move upward, as in the standard leg raises. At some point then, your arms *pass* your legs, moving outside your knees, of course. There should be a peculiar sense of unwarranted difficulty because the upper and lower extremities seem to — and do, in fact — oppose each other in their respective travel. That's why small weights do admirably. The range of motion is dictated by the strength of your shoulder girdle, particularly the pectoral muscles and latissimus dorsi and your abdominal wall and hip flexors, and by the size of the weights. When relatively light weights are used, the range of motion can be

---

Safety first

Very, very few people have strong belly or back muscles (a major defect of our present exercise systems); therefore it is extremely important to approach these exercises cautiously. Until you have begun to develop these muscles, use light weights, go slow, and don't focus on the muscles for very long consecutive periods.

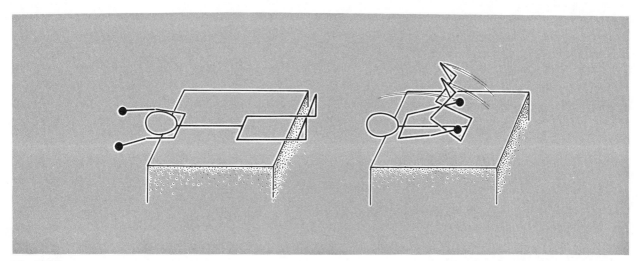

The "fold"

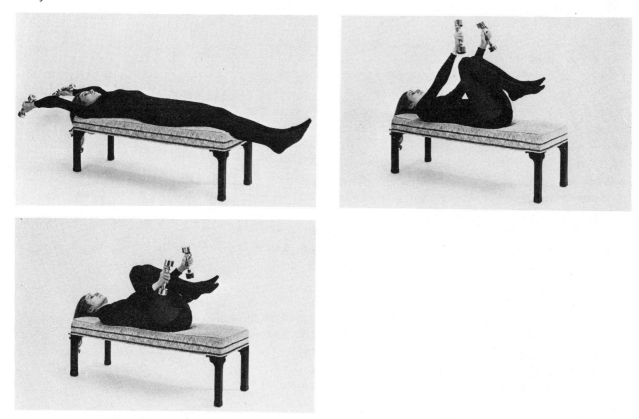

quite extensive, the hands approaching the bench on their downward arc, the knees above, even beyond, the exerciser's face. With heavy weights the limbs may barely cross.

The exercise requires patient experiment and practice to gain a place in a Heavyhands medley. Naturally, the heavier the handweights, the more resistance the legs encounter (you read it correctly) in their movement toward your head. I go heavy-slow or fast-light depending on how the spirit moves me. You'll feel an additional tension in those long muscles of the lower back that often remain weak and vulnerable in people whose limb muscles are extraordinarily developed. It is probably redundant to add that your handweights must be held palms facing each other to prevent a collision between knees and weights. This is another example of a movement mixture that you'll likely begin with a grudging few awkward repetitions. A few months of devoted practice may find your total workload capability upped several hundred percent or even more!

Why one and one don't always equal two. I believe these enormous increases are related to the combined nature of the exercise. If muscle group A is combined in simultaneous movement with group B, the increased effort is not always simply a matter of the *addition* of workload A to workload B. A separate and additional factor involves the inhibiting effect A has on B, and vice versa, whens they are combined. The "fold" presents a vivid example. An ordinary leg raise feels effortless to me. With a few pounds of hand-held weights moving toward the lifted feet, the latter seem suddenly leaden! This principle is involved in many Heavyhands combinations. The effect of one muscle group's movement on another may also make things easier. In double ski-poling, for instance, the dipping knees help the arms swing upward.

How to do it — very slowly. Here's the way to build a 5-minute or longer "fold" interval for your Heavyhands strategy. First of all select a weight that you can use comfortably for a minute at 30 to 50 cycles per minute. That could be close to your pump 'n' walk weights, but it is best to err on the side of caution.

Limit yourself to a minute the first day, practicing the movement without concern for your pulse rate. Longer work is sure to leave

> **Elementary, but paradoxical, physics while "folding"**
>
> The more weight you hold in your hands, the more resistance your legs meet as they move toward your head. The resistance your legs encounter is transferred to your abdominal muscles.

you with a sore belly the next morning. In a day or two you can add another minute, but only after a "relief" or rest interval of from ½ to 2 minutes. As your abdominals become used to the movement, increase the cycle speed gradually — thereby upping the intensity of the exercise. Then gradually decrease the rest periods until you can work for 2 minutes straight. Once you can manage 2 minutes without any discomfort the following day, add another minute, again after a rest period. As before, gradually decrease the rest period until you can "fold" for 3 minutes, and so on. Do not begin to monitor your pulse until you reach a 5-minute session.

Once you're working at the 5-minute level, check your pulse. If you're not at target, gradually increase your speed. Once you're at 5 minutes and at the proper pulse, you will find yourself easily able to go longer periods. Work on increasing your range of motion, i.e., cross your limbs more when folding. Last of all, begin to add weight. Angling my bench strategically, I can watch TV while "folding" and could really conduct an entire aerobic session with two sore feet if the need arose.

Belly Curls on a Bench

Sit on the short end of a longish bench, preferably upholstered or softened by a thick quilt or pad. Your feet are flat on the floor, only a few inches apart. Grasp a pair of dumbbells which lie on the floor just to the *outside* of the feet. If you own them, use dumbbells that are heavier than any you would consider for pump 'n' run. At the start position, your arms extend downward to the dumbbells, your biceps just touching the outside of your mid-thighs, your knees together. Your spine is curved into a *C*, your neck flexed so that your nose juts toward a point just beyond your knees. Now lift everything upward and backward so that your back flattens against the bench; the weights lift through about a 120-degree arc, stopping at the end of a curl that finds your elbows planted beside you on the bench. Don't worry about straight knees. Flexing them a bit will tend to spare your back undue strain. If you work with the right poundage, you can achieve heart rates that would astound most joggers. Use it as an extended interval when your feet hurt or when you want to work an improbable combination of biceps, abdominals, and trapezius muscles.

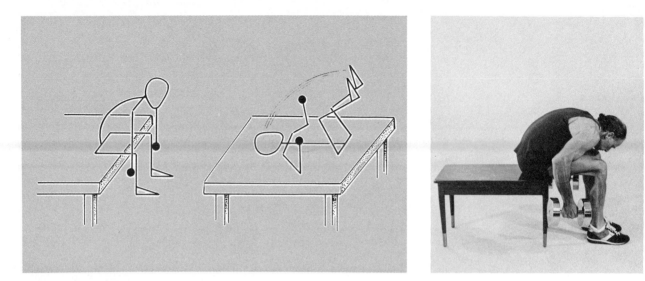

Belly curls on a bench

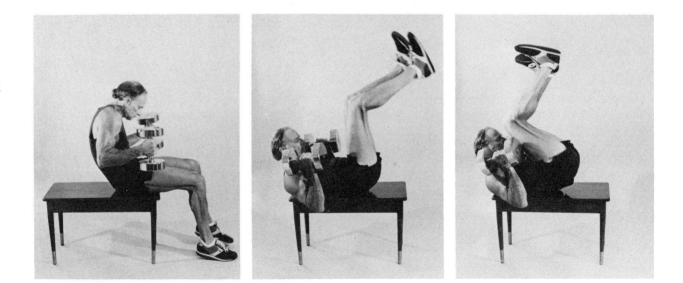

The Shovel

Less explicitly abdominal, this exercise works several of those vulnerable underused spots in our musculature and includes a large abdominal component. Get an ordinary shovel or spade and merely go through the shoveling motion, doing it a number of times, then shifting hands and doing it from the other side, like a switch hitter. Imagine you're shoveling something into a bin a couple of feet higher than your head, and keep your elbows mostly extended. You end up doing a lot of work with your long-lever deltoids along with your "girdle" muscles and the powerful hip extensors that make up the buttocks. You can get to pulse by shoveling fast or, if that's not comfortable, by adding a weight to the business end of the shovel. You can do that by taping a barbell plate of 2 to 10 pounds securely to the shovel bed. I have some screw-on adjustable dumbbells whose ends I detach and screw onto a bolt I've put through the shovel bed so that I can use varied weights for this one. I often shovel for 20 consecutive minutes with appropriate pulse or I include it in a montage of Heavyhands calisthenics. There's nothing quite like it for bringing the basics — strength, endurance, and speed-power — to the trunk and abdomen. It's good and hard enough to make most exercise seem easy by comparison.

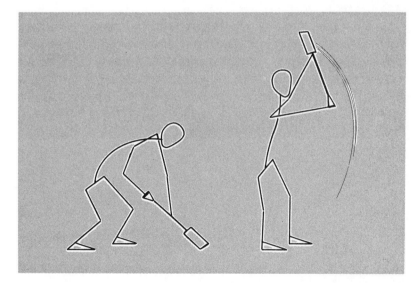

The shovel

When you shovel to the left your left hand grasps the shaft near the shovel, your right hand the shovel's handle. As you straighten up with the load, toss it high, and try to bring the arm — whose hand grasps the shovel handle's end (your right hand as you shovel to the left) — up to the horizontal. There is an aura of practicality about this exercise. Emphasizing in your program for a week or two will make you unwittingly seek reasons to bend and straighten — it feels so easy without the shovel. If you don't have a shovel, simply duplicate the motion with a relatively heavy dumbbell.

The shovel is both a belly and back exercise. I included it here because it makes a transitional exercise between the above two relatively pure belly aerobics and the exercises we'll discuss next.

THE IMPORTANCE OF ABDOMINAL EXERCISE

I encourage most Heavyhanders to emphasize abdominal work. Aside from a certain feeling of resilience that goes with extra conditioning of the middle, a strong belly wall serves as a solid central base for limb exercise, like the hub of a wheel that supports the activity around it. And your sports activities will be enhanced by abdominal specialization. The stomach muscles, along with those of the low back, need tuning and strength to tolerate the twisting, shearing forces that are part of many athletic moves.

BACKAEROBICS

Neglect of the upper torso is similar to the problems that besiege the human back. In July 1980, the editors of *Time* ran a cover story on "That Aching Back!" The article revealed some dismaying statistics: 75 million Americans are afflicted with back disorders; 93 million work days are lost yearly; 5 billion dollars are spent each year for back tests and treatment in the United States, and the figure is climbing. In Sweden back trouble is the biggest single cause of lost work!

Erect posture is generally blamed for the usual varieties of back

Buttaerobics!

The large muscle mass of the human bottom should not be excluded from Heavyhands exercise. These hip extensors brought us, literally, to our erect posture during the evolution of our species. They are badly neglected in most conventional exercise. Working the glutei in high-repetition format will pay off in maintaining back and leg suppleness in sports and in facilitating the miscellaneous body-flexions of everyday life. The hip-shoulder hops illustrated here are a bit unusual in that one side repeats *several times* before switching to the other. As you can see, they can be performed in place *or* during walking medleys. In both variations remember to accentuate the hop, which will really do your hamstrings proud. Next-day derriere soreness may locate the explicit action of these movements. The lateral-thrusting variation works a little better in place. I must admit I prefer the in-place variation generally, wherein the "hop" comes both in the forward and backward movements. With appropriate weights and frequencies these are excellent aerobically and well suited to interval cycles. You merely sandwich a "relief" between the switches from one leg to the other (see Chapter 16 on intervals). Use Buttaerobics to complement double ski-poling and other jackknifing Heavyhands.

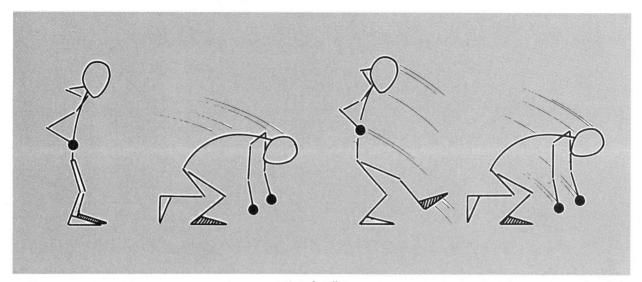

"in place"

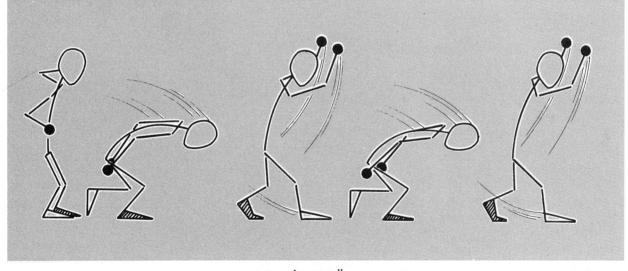

"on the move"

miseries, which are often lumped together as the lumbago-sciatica syndrome. But the fact that four-footed animals suffer similarly spoils that theory.

From the anatomist's view the spinal column is an absolute work of art, and back woes are more attributable to poor development of back function than to defects in our spinal structure.

I think we suffer from a culturally sponsored phobia of back injury. We are taught to protect the back by lifting correctly — the knees bent, the back as vertical as possible, the weight held as close to the body as we can keep it. An aura of caution becomes a semi-conscious warning to be wary when it comes to use of the back. Stories of sudden excruciating pain with long, sometimes endless aftermaths are too familiar.

Few sports demand rhythmic back motion, and endurance exercises raise the heart's workload *without* involving the back. Finally we are loath to do anything that might risk back problems. As a result of this gingerly treatment few adults have either a very strong back or one that hasn't suffered discomfort at one time or another. Some studies indicate that more than 90 percent of adults over fifty show X-ray evidence of disc degeneration and 60 percent of those have painful symptoms.

In short, the human back has become a potential Achilles' heel because use of its muscles has been intentionally avoided. Although exercise is invoked as a preventative by some back specialists, most of the exercises prescribed are of the limbering-stretch variety.

PROTECTING THE BACK BY USING IT

Heavyhands takes a different approach to the care of the back. I call it counterphobic — a word psychiatrists use to describe behavior that runs directly in the face of a conscious fear. Learning to fly to overcome a fear of flying is a well-known example.

I came upon backaerobics accidentally. Heavyhands double ski-poling (see Chapters 6 and 8) was designed to strengthen the shoulder muscles, the latissimus, the trapezius muscles and the pectorals. But it also involved a jackknifing movement of the trunk, and this had a remarkable and salutory effect on my aching back. This, in turn, lead to the development of more explicit back exercises: the short-lever jackknife and "reach" variations of pump 'n' walk.

Fitness and the bad back syndrome

1. Upright posture tends to lead to disuse of back muscles in all but a few people.

2. Typical workloads of work and play don't train trunk muscles.

3. Abdominal muscles become flaccid, fatty, and surrounded by fat; the abdominal cavity, poorly supported, becomes less protective of the spine.

4. The spine becomes increasingly susceptible to overload.

5. Injury occurs. Muscle fibers are torn, leading to painful spasm, which in turn leads to inhibition — which results in more disuse and atrophy of muscles.

6. Tolerable workloads diminish progressively and inhibition increases; relaxant drugs and rest are prescribed, superseding activity; back muscles become flaccid or spastic; and the victim of back trouble becomes more confused and depressed over how much exercise — or even movement — is possible.

7. Cardiopulmonary training may be out of the question because every limb motion poses a threat to the weak, nonsupple back.

Back, belly, and mind

There is a curious, permanent stamp that often accompanies a bad back. It becomes a continual harsh reminder to play it safe or suffer. Always sniffing about for mind-body connections, however obscure, I sometimes think I detect a parallel in the lack of fluidity in the *thinking* of chronic back victims. Intuitive jumps seem to become as *verboten* as do the corresponding body moves. The law of cognitive dissonance half explains: we try to retain body-mind unity even when it's harmful to us.

The back-belly girdle effect

Our orthopedic colleagues implore us to keep our middles in shape, to strengthen our abdominals, and to stretch out our backs and hamstrings. Belly- and backaerobics go further. The same sense of lightness that happens to high-repetition-trained limbs begins to inhabit that problem-laden middle of our anatomies. With an aerobically fit middle you feel supple, strong, tireless. The expression "tone up" is an utter *turnoff* for me where it comes to "middle" management. It implies a just-passable treatment of a series of muscle groups that need much more of those fitness elements of which they are traditionally deprived: strength, endurance, speed, power, varied and increased range of motion.

For years severe back discomfort had forced me into a protective ritual each morning — I rolled out of bed onto my knees and onto the floor. But as I began backaerobics, first with a minute or two, later with much more, of these new exercises, my back problems — for the first time in over twenty years — disappeared completely!

Backaerobics are called that because they introduce the high-repetition, heart-priming format to the back muscles. While most of us don't need much strength-endurance of the back muscles either to earn our bread or for our leisure activities, I believe that the long muscles of the spine, and other trunk muscles, can be developed — and protected — adequately only by the same sort of rhythmic movement that builds aerobically competent limb musculature.

The exercises that follow are clearly heretical. The weights, often held at arm's length, are at such a distance from the spine as to produce considerable mechanical strain. The bent knees lessen the strain somewhat, but the back continues to receive its fair share of the work.

Jackknifing

The exercise is the same as pump 'n' walk, except you bend the trunk forward during the first two steps and return to an upright posture during the next two steps. Initially, you will probably only bend your trunk forward about 45 degrees. Later, as you become more adept, try to increase the bend to 90 degrees so that the trunk, at its most forward position, is horizontal, parallel to the ground. Maintain the usual curling or pumping motion of the arms as you bend and straighten.

Use smaller-than-usual weights while learning. After a brief period of adaptation you will be able to handle almost the same load with this as you do walking. What begins as a chore for your lower back will become a hearty aerobic assist, and a promoter of strength and a suppleness where, sadly, few have it. Insert just a few of these jackknifes into your walk when it occurs to you, gradually increasing the number of reps in succession. Watch for the low-back cramp that may signal strain. At its subtlest and earliest signs, shift back to erect walking. At first a few seconds of jackknifing is a nice embellishment that will immediately raise your pulse. Because the back muscles are so underused, progress will be rapid,

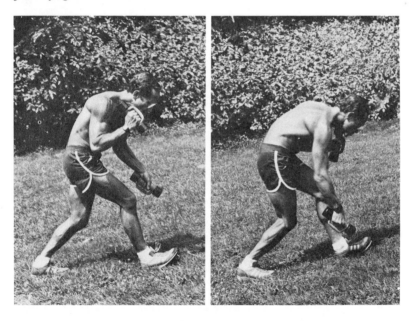

Jackknifing

large, and extended; and you will be able to continue as long as you wish. Once you've mastered this exercise, you can increase the workload by increasing the weights or speed or by exaggerating your leg lifts. I like to jackknife going up hills, lifting my thighs high and leaning into the slope.

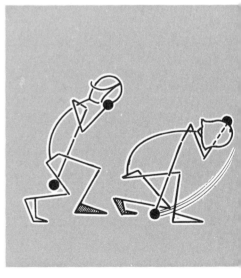

The "reach"

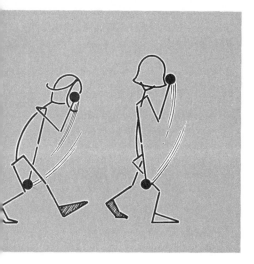

Jackknifing may at first seem awkward. That's quite all right. Don't abandon it. If it embarrasses you — or if any of these exercises do — practice it inside and alone when privacy is possible. One day you'll use these exercises unabashedly. Remember, fifteen years ago, the jogger was an unusual (and some thought comic) sight.

The "Reach"

This is the most difficult version of pump 'n' walk. Like the jackknife, you bend forward on the first two counts, straighten on the next two, but instead of dropping or uncurling the arms, you literally reach very low during the first two steps of the cycle and come up higher with the curl on steps three and four. As you get better with this, other subtle movements develop naturally. You'll find yourself striding somewhat pigeon-toed, especially when the weights are on the heavy side for you. Your hips and upper body will twist slightly to help you reach, while the head swivels toward the side of the curling arm.

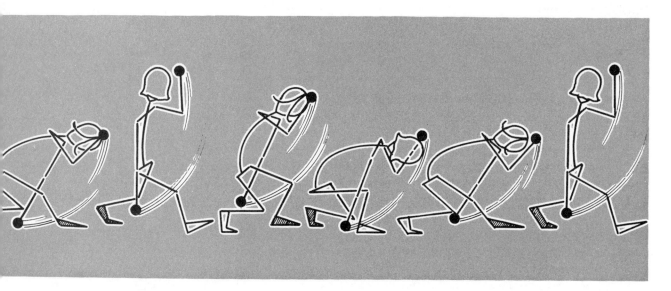

THE BENEFITS

I believe that adding jackknifing movements to Heavyhands could prevent many of the common and agonizing back syndromes, and, practiced with good judgment, could "cure" some of the "chronic backs." The butterfly stroke in swimming with its dolphin kick may produce similar benefits, but Heavyhands enjoys additional factors of graded increases in workload and greater range of motion.

Most of the Heavyhands walking variations that you will find in the next chapter include a good proportion of the jackknifing moves of either the short- or long-lever variety. The aerobic output is greater than that produced by upright exercise. It is hard to imagine the work a back can perform. I have double ski-poled with weights that totaled 23 percent of my body weight, for 4,200 arm cycles (16,800 small paces) in two hours. At the end of such exercise, my back is absolutely supple — a far cry from those years when my movements were cautious or painful and when I was often bedridden for days at a time.

If you have a back problem it's important that your doctor give any exercise an okay. Not all back disorders respond to this exercise equally. *Always* use small weights to start with; going through the movements *without* weights is a good way of checking out your back's initial response.

Backs are complicated structures and back disorders are not simple. Backaches frequently involve psychic factors, and back-problem personalities have even been described. Although I can't pretend to have all the answers to a problem that continues to defy the best orthopedic, physiatric, osteopathic, psychiatric, and chiropractic thinking, I would suggest Heavyhands backaerobics for these reasons:

1. While the aerobic capacity of the upper torso has been neglected, the trunk, including the back and abdominal muscles, *has not even been considered* from the aerobic standpoint.

2. These muscles are not different structurally from the muscles of the limbs, so there is no obvious reason for granting them short shrift in endurance exercise.

3. Our experiments show that the trunk is quite trainable, capable of great endurance and strength.

4. All muscles may be injured if given tasks that exceed their capability. Weak muscles are statistically, then, more susceptible to

---

Passive and aggressive care of the back

PASSIVE CARE OF THE BACK
1. Lift with knees bent — let the legs do the lifting.
2. Keep the back vertical while lifting.
3. Keep the weight close to the body's vertical axis.
4. Use stretching exercises to lessen spasm and increase suppleness.
5. Do a number of bent-knee sit-ups daily.
6. Sleep on a hard mattress: add a bed-board if necessary.
7. Be careful!

AGGRESSIVE CARE OF THE BACK
1. Exercise back and abdominal muscles, hip flexors and extensors (ski-poling; jackknifing; doing the reach, the shovel, the fold, the single dumbbell swing).
2. Gradually add strength, speed, power, range of motion, and endurance components to trunk workloads.
3. Augment these with limb "assists" to keep in target pulse range.
4. Continue to add as many movements as you can through calisthenics and free forms of Heavyhands (shadowboxing and dancing). Include twisting, torsion movements to work the muscles through many angles of contraction.
5. Enjoy your back!

injury. We tend to avoid reinjury by progressive inhibition of movement, which further weakens the muscle, inviting new injuries. In a classic vicious circle, each successive injury leads to more inhibition, atrophy, weakness, and greater risk of injury.

5. Stretching techniques — the only exercises usually applied to the back — are not especially strengthening.

6. Strength-endurance training of the trunk muscles results in the same changes that produce greater working capacity and reduced risk of injury in the muscles of the limbs.

7. Only after the spinal and abdominal muscles receive their share of endurance-training can we properly evaluate current theories as to the cause of back disorders, e.g., erect posture, obesity, sedentary existence.

8. By the nature of the Heavyhands backaerobics you become a *bold* rather than a *defensive* manager of your back. In double ski-poling and in short-lever jackknifing and the reach and shovel, the weights travel at some distance from the body's vertical axis. This creates the mechanical "disadvantage" that will strengthen. My friend and colleague Dr. Richard Kalla tells me that aside from injuries resulting from accidents, he rarely if ever saw a coal miner with a back disorder during the days when digging was largely accomplished manually. When we consider the biomechanics of shoveling, we see that the experienced shoveler lifts and moves significant weights at extended arm's length from the spine, which coils and straightens again and again. This is persuasive evidence that erect posture may not be the sole culprit in back disorder, but, instead, that moving the back as little as possible to protect it may produce dangerous muscular deterioration.

Everyone can enjoy the physical advantages of hard labor! A 5-minute Heavyhands backaerobic interval can provide, depending upon the work intensity, the equivalent of several months of the back usage typical of a sedentary life. It is also likely that the abdomen protects the spinal column by its ability to absorb the shifting stresses that occur during exertion.

THE INEVITABLE WARNING

Our life-styles, including our work and play patterns, leave all but a few of us with weak backs. Any attempt to strengthen runs the

Back caveat

If you're a back victim, don't be so whipped to enthusiasm by this spiel that you shove off impulsively toward a Pain-Free-Back Nirvana. It would be absolutely folly to try to undo by an explosion of zeal what healing time and medicine may have been unable to accomplish. The key word is *gradual*. Decide upon a rate of progress, divide it by three, then ease ever so cautiously into that. Once into it, keep the faith.

risk of injuring. Don't start backaerobics when you're hurting —
and always remember to *proceed gradually:* gradual additions of
weight, tempo, range of motion, and duration. The rewards for
patience will pay off handsomely. Complement your backaerobics
with bellyaerobics. When doing short-lever jackknifes, "reach"
walking or double ski-poling, let your thighs and back tell you when
to shift the workload betwen back bending and knee flexion. When
your back stiffens or aches use more knee flexion, less back, and
vice versa. Soon you will find yourself able to handle a 3-minute
interval, or, if you choose, a 3-hour marathon.

You're bound to experience some "healthy" soreness at first.
Your back muscles — accustomed to their disuse — will naturally
rebel a bit. But backaerobics will become favorites for most, combined as they are with tremendous limb work and appropriate heart
action.

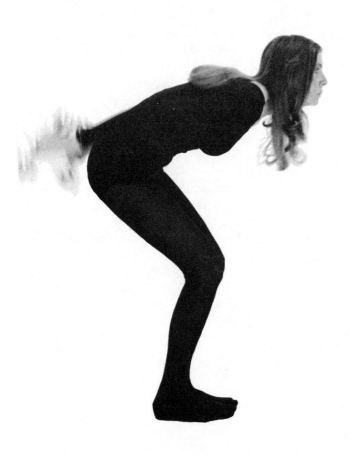

Some folks will view your public backaerobics as odd exercising antics. But as the number of healthy backs increase they're apt to join you. The psychological advantage of a strong, healthy back can't be fully appreciated by those who haven't suffered with a bad one. I often think that improper "care" of the back is a good parallel to what we call neurosis. Backs and personalities deprived of the joy of *active* growth can become real liabilities.

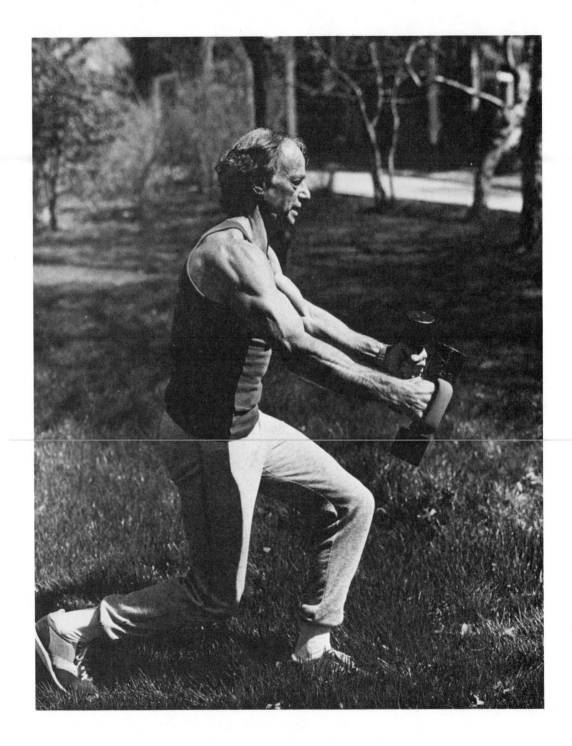

8

Heavyhands Walking

A GROWING NUMBER of knowledgeable people believe that walking is destined to become *the* exercise of the 1980s. The most enthusiastic advocates of walking are the physiologists and doctors who see running as too injurious. Walking has a very low rate of orthopedic complications. I personally would not settle for the fitness levels I could attain with just plain walking. Why? Remember, all exercise can be understood as a product of intensity times duration. Given a husky pair of legs and healthy central oxygen-transport apparatus, almost anyone can walk an hour a day or more. And it's true that it's better to invest that hour than not. But what about the intensity or rate of work we produce while walking? There are some great walkers to be sure. A few can hit a 7- to 8-minute-mile pace, fast enough to spark envy in many runners. Walking tends to become onerous at speeds of about 200 meters per minute (8 minutes per mile). At that point, the walker feels like breaking into a jog. But the vast majority of habitual walkers never reach that point. My hunch is that most people don't walk faster than a 20-minute-mile pace.

WALKING WORKLOADS

If we figure roughly 100 calories used per mile, the average walker drops 300 calories per hour, since he covers 3 miles in that amount of time. That corresponds to 5 calories per minute. It could be 600 calories over the same distance and time if you weighed 300 pounds, because the work done is proportional to the body mass moved. Incidentally, that still would be a poor strategy for losing calories fast!

Israeli researchers have now shown that significant conditioning can occur in young men willing to walk three miles or so several times a week with a few sealed bags of water in a backpack. Why not? Increase the workload and conditioning increases willy-nilly.

HEAVYHANDS AND WALKING WORKLOAD

More to the point, walking on the level at 140 steps per minute (about a 14-minute-mile pace), my pulse, which had been 70 at the

---

High-calorie miles

A hundred calories per mile is a rule of thumb for "legs-alone" walking. Heavyhands calls for a whole new set of rules for determining calories per mile. If you know your MET load, your body weight, and wear a watch, our charts will enable you to calculate oxygen consumption per minute, and thus calories. If you cover a mile in 15 minutes at 15 METs and weigh 154 pounds (70 kilos), the answer is about 275 calories per mile. It takes less than 13 of those miles to incinerate a pound of fat — not the usual 35 of the walkers and runners. Incidentally, knowing your steadied-out calorie pulse (see the Appendix) is all it takes to compute Heavyhands calories per mile. Fifteen cal per minute at 4 mph walking speed will cost 900 calories per hour, or 225 calories per mile.

WORKLOAD INCREASES WITH PUMP 'N' WALK

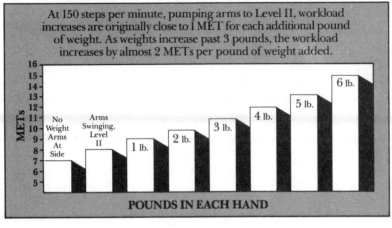

At 150 steps per minute, pumping arms to Level II, workload increases are originally close to 1 MET for each additional pound of weight. As weights increase past 3 pounds, the workload increases by almost 2 METs per pound of weight added.

start, rose to 90. When my pulse had returned to 70, I began walking, carrying but not pumping 7-pound weights. Moving at the same pace and stride length, my pulse hit 100. In a third interval, I pump 'n' walked and my pulse rose a cool 60 beats to 130.

The experiments were an attempt to learn how these three variations would affect my heart rate. Our admittedly rough calculations suggested I was doing conservatively twice as much work with pump 'n' walk than I was walking unencumbered. Such an experiment isn't useful with subjects untrained at Heavyhands. Arm work for the untrained literally drives the pulse "off the chart."

A well-trained competitive walker would probably equal my pace with a pulse as slow or slower than my 90. But if he were to carry or pump weights he would doubtless find his heart rate higher than mine, especially during the pumping trial. And if I continued walking and pumping for, say, 8 minutes, my pulse would continue, steadied out at 130, while the competitive walker with untrained arms probably would not be able to finish.

It boils down to this: walking for most people is a very limited exercise. The price one pays for a low injury rate is a low level of conditioning. Adding upper-extremity work, however, makes walking a new ball game. Depending upon their load, the arms' activity in pump 'n' walk can amount to a hefty slice of the total work. Exceptionally well trained Heavyhanders can actually bring their arms to *outperform* their legs.

Heavyhands hill work

The pumping action of Heavyhands walking, depending upon how fast, how high, at and how heavy the weight, makes any slope feel steeper because your oxygen transport is being more heavily taxed. Respect hills: a 6-percent slope adds about 30 percent to your oxygen requirement. With added weights the labor involved fairly jumps. You'll often find yourself above "anaerobic threshold" suddenly, gulping air when moments before you were steadied out. Hill training, pursued with cautious diligence, will lift you to new aerobic heights.

But such heroics are unnecessary. A 120-pound woman pump 'n' walking with 3-pounders can reach a work level that loses 5 or more calories from legs alone, plus 3 or more calories per minute from arm work. These are modest figures. Heavyhanders have lost 10 to 20 or more calories per minute pump 'n' walking with negligible risk of injury.

If you add up benefits of a year's worth of pump 'n' walk compared to conventional walking, the numbers are pretty convincing. Aside from producing a higher grade of conditioning, a couple of 3-pounders over 624 miles — a reasonable distance for a year walking 4 hours a week — would shed at least 10 pounds of body fat, arm work alone!

Although outsized strength is not an essential for pump 'n' walk, strength *does* make a difference. Pumping 6-pound weights over that 624 miles would burn some 150,00 calories per year — over twenty pounds of fat — arms alone. And of course the greater the hand-held weight, the greater the leg's work, because inevitably they must support it all. So any addition to what the hands are doing pays off below as well. The legs must stride against the added burden, toughening ligaments, tendons, and joint structures as well as muscles. We now know that our bones mineralize — adding strengthening calcium and other elements — when we work our limbs harder. One X-ray, showing the porous thigh bones of those who for some reason quit walking, would convince you of the prime necessity for muscular work to maintain our skeletal structure.

STRENGTH VERSUS SPEED

As in all Heavyhands techniques, one enjoys the option of going slow-heavy for strength or fast-light for speed. Muscle bulk is definitely related to strength, but strength is *not strictly* limited by the size of the muscles. Large-muscled men will naturally be capable of using heavier weights than petite women. But by focusing on the speed-power axis, women can produce enormous exercise intensities and some believe they may have greater "staying" capacity than men. Finally, I do believe that this form of walking is the answer to most of the concerns raised by some obstetricians about the bad effects of running on the pelvic floor of childbearing women. Walking trades speed for "legato"; a welcome nonjarring of the body as the feet meet unyielding earth, nontraumatically.

RUNNING VERSUS WALKING

Do runners walk? Yes, of course, but seldom for exercise. And the reverse holds true. Walkers seldom run. The trade-off is neat and explicit. Walkers can follow their footloose inclinations for a lifetime with small chance of injury beyond an early heel blister from badly chosen shoes, or fallen arches in those whose arches were destined to drop sooner or later. Over three-quarters of the runners who train heavily will develop one or more injuries severe enough to halt their exercise, sometimes recurrently, sometimes permanently. Both runners and walkers gamble. Runners bet against the odds that favor injury. Walkers settle for a level of fitness that probably falls short of what doctors prescribe.

Heavyhands walking bridges the gap: more work with less injury risk. When you train in Heavyhands technique, *both* walk and run can be retained as part of your repertoire of exercises. Endurance-strength training of the upper extremities makes the difference.

Heavier weights can be handled in Heavyhands walking than in running work. The planted feet make it possible, as does the slower pace and the shorter stride. The range of arm motion is usually greater; the slower moving, more stable stride allows for more deliberate, thoroughgoing arm movements. As I shall describe presently, the walker's base allows a wider variety of complex arm and trunk movements.

With adequate arm training the options for the walker's strategy are endless. Juggling pace, stride length, and handweight, one can construct walking medleys en route, shifting on impulse from one combination to another — always remaining at target pulse. By imaginatively using these variables in your exercise, you can move the workload upward and downward as the spirit moves you. You can push feet, rest arms, reverse that, bring in long levers, do more things with legs generally than mechanics of running will allow.

Terrain know-how

Heavyhands walking is an excellent way to acquire body savvy. You already know, for example, that downhill walking feels easier when unencumbered. But pumping weights to Level III is hard work even when descending. The arms don't reap gravity's advantage: indeed the hands must pull against the added drag. It's a bizarre sensation at first because you've been conditioned to relax on the downside of a hill.

Heavyhands and cold weather

I used to be one of those people who sort of shrunk into himself during cold weather. I made fetishes of warm gloves, constantly scouting about for better ones. All that has changed. I now see winter as an excellent season for training — a time when I can exercise hard, air-cooled.

Pump 'n' Walk

To review: in this diagonal stride-curl combination, hold your weights with your knuckles out, your palms facing your thighs. Remember to keep your elbows pretty close to your sides in this basic form. With Heavyhands walking, the curl, regardless of the

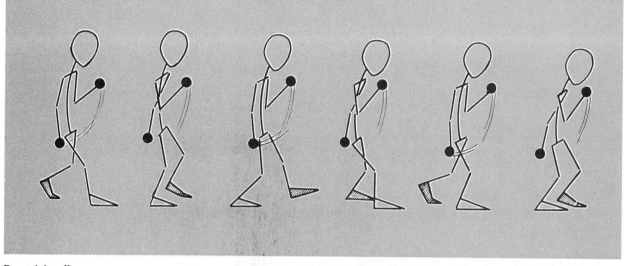

Pump 'n' walk

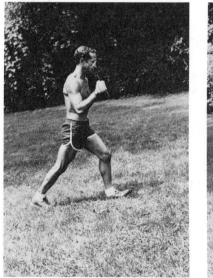
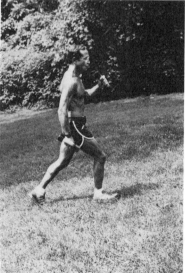

weight you decide upon, should move through a larger (higher) arc than you'd use while jogging with weights.

Measuring as carefully as I can, I have found that my walking curls rise and fall an average of 3 to 4 more inches than they do during a jog. It's easy to see why. The slower pace gives you time to really jerk the weight upward with a cheerful vengeance. To avoid occasionally bumping yourself, tilt the plane of the curl *outward* as it rises. Experiment with it. None of us is the structural clone of anyone else. Minute differences in the complex lever systems involved — inborn and acquired — make for delicate nuances. If something isn't right, you will automatically adjust it.

Avoiding the pain that comes from overuse, you're looking for comfortable ways of being outrageously *inefficient*. Walking in the Heavyhands manner isn't the efficient way of getting from point A to B.

Vary what you must to get to target. If your arms are aching (increased lactic acid, usually), go slower, lighter, or both until you're able to continue for several minutes comfortably. Muscle ache en route often responds nicely to a walk-stretch tactic. Just let your arms hang loosely in full extension. Bending forward slightly, continue to walk at an undiminished pace. When the ache leaves, begin curling again. Gradually the relief intervals will shorten and become necessary less often. If you're winded of course you'll need to cut the load. Again, go slower and/or lighter. If you need to use tiny weights in order to remain at target, do precisely that. At this stage in the game you're not able to imagine what will come easy for you a year hence. You couldn't play a succession of tough chords after your first piano lesson either — it's a good analogy to the acquisition of strength and endurance. Be patient and confident. The inescapable laws that guide your body function are working for you. All you need is time and practice.

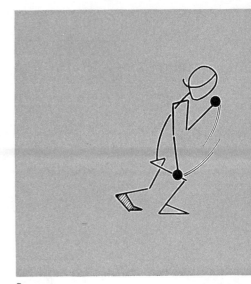

Swagger

Swagger

This is the first and least radical departure from the basic move. Swaggering is a dancelike addition to walk. The head swivels slightly to the curling side. The raised weight isn't simply allowed to fall: it is resolutely pulled downward. In swagger a peculiar torsion of the body helps swing the weight-hand upward. Perhaps you've watched the almost comical movements of the race-walker; the

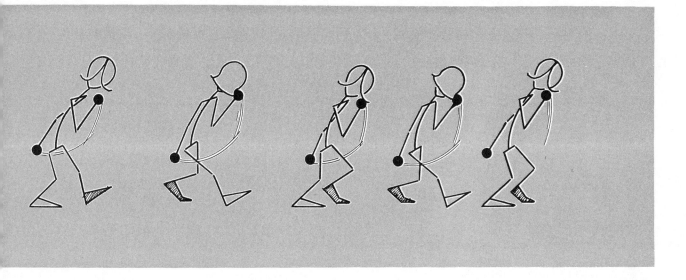

characteristic wiggle. In Heavyhands walk, the hip motion is come by naturally. The swagger provides opportunity to increase the strength-endurance of trunk muscles and the smaller accessory muscles that surround the shoulder joint.

Jackknifing   See Chapter 7.

Reaching   See Chapter 7.

WALKING PULSES

One day I determined the pulse increase for these exercises, starting each with a pulse of 60 and walking for 3 minutes at a stride frequency of 150 steps per minute.

	STARTING PULSE	ENDING PULSE	PULSE DIFFERENCES
Walk (no weights)	60	70	10
Walk (with weights at sides)	60	90	30
Swagger	60	125	65
Jackknife	60	150	90

The numbers are presented to give you an idea of the work possible when additional muscle groups are added to the simple act of walking.

Of course your pulse rates will differ from mine for a host of reasons — body-weight difference, weights, upper torso, training, age, amount of body fat, efficiency, and so on. The differences don't matter. The point is almost anyone using Heavyhands walking can produce big, useful workloads. Many strong practitioners of the "reach" will be able to achieve MET levels of 20 or more for prolonged intervals. That means their body will do 20 times the work it does at rest.

Double Ski-Poling

Given the choice of a *single exercise* here's the one that gets my nod. Double ski-poling has, I think, most of the attributes of the ideal exercise. Here's why:

1. It produces workloads large enough to bring the central oxygen transport mechanism to high intensity with sufficient duration.

2. It mobilizes the largest mass of skeletal muscle.

3. It is performable by almost anyone.

4. It has an open-ended quality that permits growth, yet offers maximum control of the workload components: strength, speed-power, muscle-heart endurance.

5. It develops agility and grace.

6. It increases flexibility.

7. The injury rate is very low — much work with little risk.

8. It provides a kind of a fitness package that covers the broadest range of activities of the work and play of everyday life.

9. It creates the lowest subjective sense of effort in relation to the workload.

10. There is a low dropout rate; complex enough to challenge but not so difficult as to discourage — most rewarding by objective and subjective measures.

11. It's convenient: good indoors and out.

12. It emphasizes those muscles and functions least used ordinarily and therefore most in need and most trainable.

I have already mentioned the high oxygen-consumption rate of cross-country skiers. Exaggerating their movements, Heavyhands

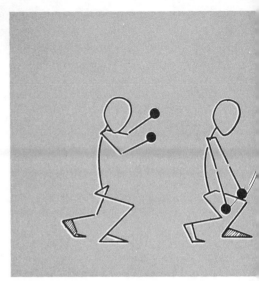

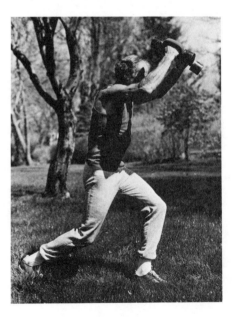

Double ski-poling — knee flexion

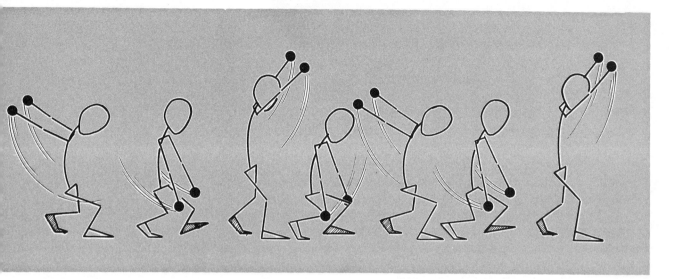

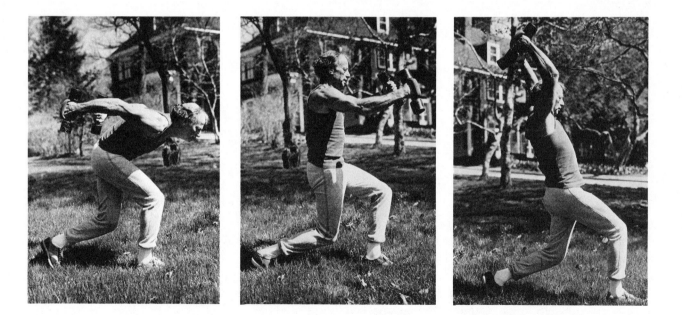

double ski-poling creates a continuous high-intensity exercise which mobilizes as much as 80 to 90 percent of the muscle mass.

Double ski-poling is the same exercise described in Chapter 6, except, of course, here it is done on the move.

The arm-leg coordination for this double ski-poling exercise is similar to pump 'n' walk with jackknifing. Both are four-step cycles. The arms, extended almost overhead, sweep down, through, and back (see picture) with steps 1 and 2; returning forward and to the nearly overhead position on steps 3 and 4. The trunk bends forward during the first two steps, and straightens during the third and fourth. As in the jackknife, the closer you come to a 90-degree bend — with the trunk at its farthest position parallel to the ground — the more effective the exercise. At the first sign of back discomfort, cease bending the trunk. You can compensate for the loss of workload and maintain your pulse by exaggerating and deepening the bend of your knees as you walk. Light weights should be used initially. At 30 to 50 cycles per minute, plenty of work is performed with any payload since the weights may travel a total of 6 to 8 feet during each cycle. Eventually your shoulder musculature will be able to manage the same weights you use in pump 'n' walk.

While breathing should be free and spontaneous, I find myself breathing comfortably once per cycle, inhaling deeply on the up-stroke, exhaling hard as the weights are pulled sharply, not dropped, in the downstroke.

Aside from the general benefits, already enumerated, of double ski-poling, there are specific benefits to particular parts of the body which are worth listing.

1. *Knee flexion:* Having assumed a semicrouch during the lowering and raising of the arms, the thighs' quadriceps muscles are given continuous strength, speed-power work. These movements build the *vertical lift* so frequently lacking in runners. I believe extensive Heavyhands double ski-poling could reduce the all-too-frequent incidence of runner's knee (chondromalacia patella). Treatment of this condition often consists of strengthening the quadriceps through weight training. Perhaps prevention would be the best cure.

2. *Trunk flexion and extension:* Like knee bending, this movement is common to double ski-poling and jackknifing. The collective mass

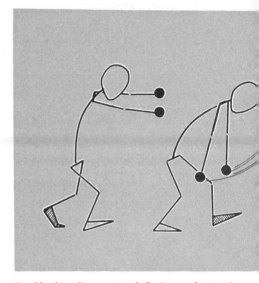

Double ski-poling — trunk flexion and extension

Warning: double ski-poling for women

Because of the smaller ratio of shoulder to hip width, women must be more careful at first to angle the weights *outward* during the downstroke to avoid bumping themselves. A good way to ensure safety from the beginning is consciously to draw diverging lines with the weights as they streak through your field of vision. By using these "after images" you can construct and fix a pattern that will carry you through hundreds of thousands of reps without a scrape or bruise to your outer thighs. The diverging downstroke is, of course, plain sensible for the male double ski-poler as well.

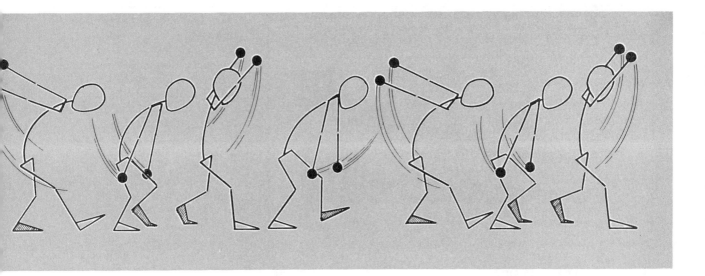

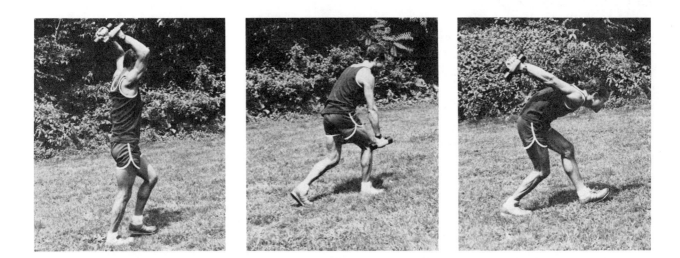

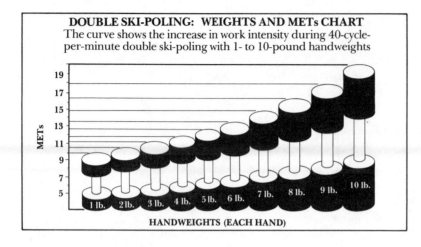

DOUBLE SKI-POLING: WEIGHTS AND METs CHART
The curve shows the increase in work intensity during 40-cycle-per-minute double ski-poling with 1- to 10-pound handweights

of the trunk and abdominal muscles, the great hip extensors represented by the gluteus and upper hamstrings work continuously. In brief, if your belly, back, hips, or fanny need work, this is the exercise that will do the job.

3. *Shoulder girdle:* The anterior and posterior deltoids, trapezeii, pectorals, and latissimus are directly involved in the poling movement.

Repetitive motion of all these muscles with open-ended possibilities to increase speed, strength, and endurance occur in no exercise or sport. The possible increases in workloads are truly exponential simply because these muscle groups are so specifically underused in our lives.

4. *The back:* As elaborated on in the last chapter, this exercise will do wonders for your lower back. But, remember, if you've had recurrent back problems, seek medical advice before beginning. Even the healthiest backs will experience some initial spasm and ache because of the overwork of the unused low-back muscles. Shift to erect exercise when that happens. Adding continuously a little more to each workout, it won't be long before you can perform miles of double ski-poling at comfortable workloads that are mind-boggling.

Double Ski-Poling, Three- and Five-Step Variations

I have thought, and some colleagues agree, that a four-step double ski-pole pattern may not suit all physiques because even-numbered

One the back side of double ski-poling

One way to improve your double ski-poling is to yank the weights high in back at the end of the backswing. I can't think offhand of another movement that asks that much of the shoulder joint. It's a bonus extension to trapezius and triceps muscles, as mild next-day soreness will announce after your first try. That extension, incidentally, is mechanically wise because it occurs just when your nose leads your knees by a few inches — so it makes for balance. Abandon that option, however, on significantly steep downhills lest you find yourself somersaulting.

Climbing *à la* double ski-poling

When moderately advanced, you'll find yourself surprisingly able to negotiate rather steep inclines double ski-poling. I often find myself paradoxically resting "into" a hill after a brisk anaerobic interval. There's a curious, pleasant intimacy with terra firma when chin, knees, and weights swoop into the down phase. On cold winter nights when the footing's good, I prepare this way for snow. A backpack makes the struggle even more delightful.

stride-cycles leave each leg repeating the same movements each time. Purists are concerned, perhaps with reason, that this could disturb the body's symmetry. I've probably double ski-poled hundreds of miles doing the four-step and I've heard of no problems thus far from others. But the three- and five-step versions

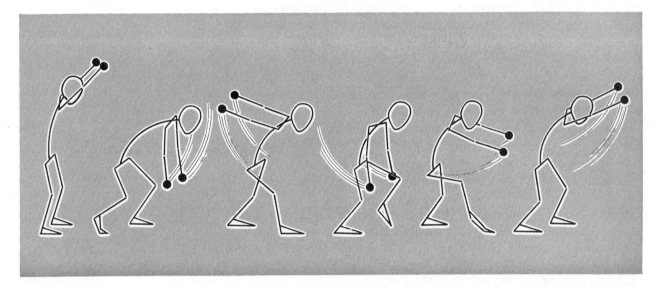

Double ski-poling

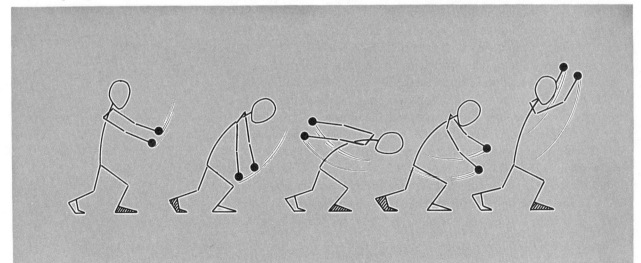

will avoid movement asymmetries and they are fun to switch to now and again. Some prefer them outright and never return to four-step double ski-poling.

Level III "High pump 'n' Walk"

We described this in Chapter 4. For the serious Heavyhander who favors walking, high pumps can add an incredible increment to exercise intensity even when using *small* weights. For example, by measuring oxygen uptake in the laboratory we found that a 150-per-minute stepping pace, pumping 3 pounds to Level III (3-foot lifts), achieved 15 METs or better, despite the short stride and a walking pace of just 3 miles an hour (20-minute mile). The energy required jumps from about 6 calories per minute, conventional walking, to about 18 calories per minute when performed by a 154-pound (70-kilo) person! This exercise, continued for many minutes, is by no means easy. But such poundages are well within the reach of almost any healthy, diligent Heavyhander of either sex.

Stretch-Strength-Striding (SSS) with High Pumps

Here's a movement that will add strength and suppleness to your underpinning without neglecting any major muscle group that mobilizes the shoulder joint. It's a chance to bring heavier weight than you typically use to Level III because the tempo is, of necessity, slow. The drawings come close to being self-explanatory, I think, but there are a few details to be kept in mind. Performed properly I believe it will tend to protect against the knee problems encountered by some runners. While the striding foot is landing flat, the back foot is on its toes. The stride should be long enough so that a slight pulling sensation is felt at the upper inner thigh and groin of the back leg. Some next-day soreness may occur at the inner thigh just about the knee (the vastus medialis muscle). As the back foot kicks off for the next stride, the front leg straightens — its foot moving from the flat to the toe position. The visible and felt effect is bouncy and fluid, the back leg's knee coming within a few inches of the ground. A diagonal arm-leg pattern is probably best. Don't do much the first time or you're sure to be hobbled next day. Add it gradually during your walking medleys. Use small weights until you've mastered it.

My stride at SSS is about 32 inches, so at 100 strides per minute I cover about 3 miles per hour. Walking unencumbered, a 20-

---

Double ski-poling on the move: weights and METs

The relationship between the size of handweights and work is not, strictly speaking, proportional in Heavyhands. For example, going from 1- to 5-pounders at 40 complete cycles each minute, one moves up about 3 METs; the next 5 pounds take a greater toll — an additional 6 METs, approximately. This is true of all Heavyhands exercise — as you add pounds the work increases faster per added increment of weight. The reason for this "curvilinear" relationship between added pounds and work is that both arms and legs are forced to share each increase — hands are "heavied" and the body weight is effectively increased beyond what the added amount would anticipate using simple arithmetic.

Anyway, double ski-poling on the move at 40 cycles would produce this curve which plots METs against handweight. (See page 138.)

minute-mile pace is worth about 5 METs. Depending upon the handweights used, I have seen some people reach 18 to 20 METs at that pace doing SSS! At paces faster than 100 strides per minute, it becomes difficult to include the toe lifts of the front foot. The quads are strengthened two ways: as they contract in their elongated condition when the striding leg is bent (so called *negative work*); and when the bent leg straightens the quads contract concentrically, i.e., while shortening.

SSS will mollify your taut hamstrings and facilitate forward bending with the knees straight. The muscles of the buttocks and calf are strengthened, too. With somewhat lighter weights I add two variations: (1) a slight conscious hyperextension of the back (backward lean) during the stride; (2) a lean toward the side of the "down" hand. Try alternating SSS with double ski-poling for several minutes during your workouts.

This move will appeal to strength athletes — the lifters, shot putters, and footballers whose oxygen transport will "move up" on SSS with high pumps. Competitive runners will find this exercise quickly makes them more proficient on the hills.

Stretch-Strength-Striding to Level III in Place

Good for indoor Heavyhands generally, this exercise has a subtly different effect from the on-the-move form. The striding leg is

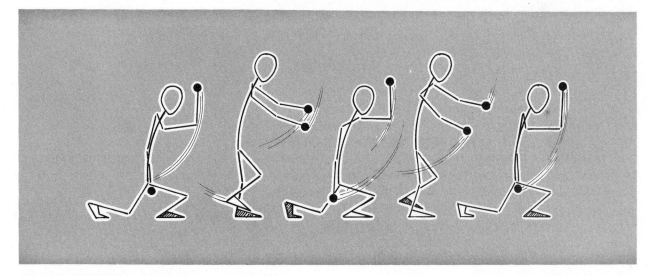

Stretch-strength-stride to Level III

returned to its starting position on the second count, whereupon the other leg repeats. The arms simply switch as in the on-the-move version — moving with every stride and return. Five minutes of practice is enough to make you expert and to gain your respect for the unexpected workload involved. Difficult enough that a slow tempo brings you to pulse, it's a good bet for TV viewing.

The Killers

Here are two additional moves inspired by watching Eric Heiden's electrifying performance at the 1980 Lake Placid Winter Olympics, where he took five gold medals. Not likely to produce Eric's 29-inch thigh in the casual exerciser, these moves do mimic the speed skater's body while adding as much upper-torso work as you can manage. They are designed for roadwork, but will serve equally well in any calisthenic medley, in dance sequences, or as a 5-minute warm-up for conventional running.

A. Pump 'n' duck walk. This is a diagonal move as with pump 'n' walk. The knees are deeply bent so that the forward striding thigh is almost parallel to the ground. The weights are lifted quite high — the arms are semiflexed, somewhere between the curl and the nearly overhead position used in alternate ski-poling. The pace

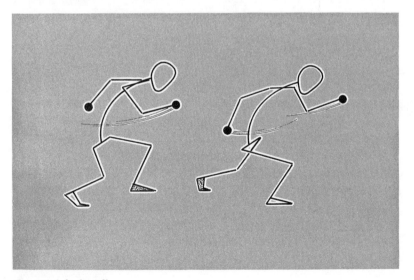

Pump 'n' duck walk

must be kept slow. This is a good example of a strength-builder engineered for progressively longer intervals that is excellent aerobically. You will need to keep the handweights modest.

B. Heavyhands duck waddle. Prompting an astonishing assortment of contractions from head to toe and promoting any and all of the fitness components along with a large measure of skill, this is a very difficult exercise. Going heavy to light you can lumber along or fairly scurry. Either extreme will produce maximum heart-lung action. For this movement you curl into a low crouch, your chin above your flexed knees. The weights are held at dead-hang. As you waddle forward, your shoulders seesaw so that the downside weight passes close to the ground as the foot on that side strikes flat on its sole. The back foot rests on its toe at the moment before shoving off. You will probably experience soreness in your legs after first trying it. This may occur in the back and front large muscle groups of either thigh or calf. If too sore, skip a day or two. This exercise will also strengthen the great hip extensors that you sit on, so some buttocks soreness is likely also.

These two exercises are so difficult and represent such an awesome workload that you can afford to bide your time, slowly adding

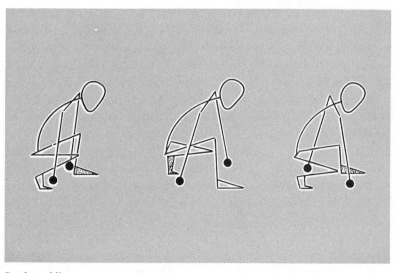

Duck waddle

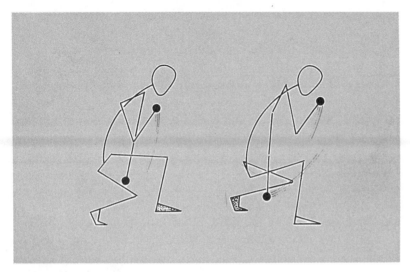

Duck waddle with heavy curls

small increments of handweight, range of motion, or frequency. They are very strength oriented, so if you're less enamored of that component, you needn't bother with them.

If, on the other hand, your state of conditioning and your gluttony for punishment are outsized, you can make them even tougher. Use lateral raises from the waddle position. Here the long-lever arm is lifted from the side while the same-side leg steps. Alternately you can throw in a few curls along with the seesawing shoulders, the curl of course executed by the downside arm, which in this instance acts with the diagonal foot as in pump 'n' run on the move. When you think of acquiring facility, power, even grace with these concoctions, plan a time frame that spans months or even years to be realistic. When you are able to lateral raise and waddle carrying weights that amount to 20 to 25 percent of your body weight at 90 to 100 steps per minute for 10 minutes, you will enjoy the aerobic capacity of an expert Nordic skier, the strength of a gymnast, and the balance of a tightrope walker.

OTHER LONG-LEVERED WALKS

You can insert all sorts of moves to make interesting medleys of your Heavyhands walking. With lighter weights, lateral pulls and raises can be added to any of the above moves, along with alternate ski-poling. You will soon discover about how far and fast you can go with a particular move yet stay out of oxygen debt. Don't prove your mettle through pain. The "train, don't strain," admonition is equally applicable to the Heavyhander and the practitioner of other aerobics. Switching from one muscle group to another helps enormously; or using intervals when you merely stop the arm action, let the weights hand loose and low, and wait for your body's chemical miracles to recycle themselves, then start again. That way you'll complete your workout pleasantly tired, not overly wilted and sore.

Sometimes well-trained legs produce too slow a pulse at a pace that the arms can't sustain — and the target pulse isn't reached. A loaded backpack can fill in admirably until increased pace or arm strength-endurance become sufficient to pick up your pulse. This technique amounts to a strength-loaded walk — the backpack burdens the legs so that the arm work become a smaller percentage of the total work expended.

Walking rehabilitation

A surgical procedure may be likened to an injury. Postoperative bedrest is itself deconditioning. The exerciser's blood volume may drop 15 percent and cardiopulmonary fitness drops rapidly. General anesthetics may have some psychic and physiologic effects that inhibit activity temporarily. The incision's soreness may discourage movements depending upon its location and the extent of the surgery. A good friend and colleague found himself able to resume Heavyhands walking medleys a week after a hernia repair. Within two weeks of his surgery, he was, in fact, exceeding his best prior workload intensities and durations! The wider distribution of the muscle work again seems to make reconditioning go faster and smoother.

ADVANTAGES OF HEAVYHANDS WALK

1. For tired or tattered runners. Supposing a runner true to his or her sport for years ends up with a beautiful heart-lung apparatus and a pair of legs so blighted by injury that the effort is painful too much of the time. Ordinary walking, more bearable, doesn't cut the aerobic mustard. Settling for the walker's pace, this runner will decondition. Enlisting the arms, he or she is saved.

My good friend Irwin Cohen of New York City is a perfect case in point. Irwin had been a top-flight heavyweight weight lifter, who turned to running. Dropping from a hulking 235 pounds, Irwin was as assiduous a runner as he had been a strength athlete. For years he was a familiar face at races in the area, ran the New York Marathon each year until an Achilles tendon tore clean through. Consultants told him he'd not run again. A colleague of mine told Irwin about my interest in exercise and Heavyhands. A few telephone conversations and a couple of meetings in New York followed. Irwin's determination, spirit, and knowledge in the field of exercise made him a perfect candidate for Heavyhands. He now combines the best of his previous worlds as an exerciser. He walks at a 12- to 13-minute-mile pace pumping 10-pounders, for as much as 8 miles or more — as many as 20,000 consecutive arm curls, while walking at this most respectable clip! He feels fitter and stronger than ever at a very young forty-six. All this after a short year of training. Needless to say, his workloads will continue to spiral upward for a long time. When inclement weather scotches a walk, he works out with Heavyhands calisthenics indoors.

2. For nonrunners. Some people will not run. They didn't do it much as children and they're even less eager to do so as adults. They can't be proselytized to its advantages, however tempting the pitch. A host of structural realities may make this a wise choice. Obesity or big bones and muscles may cause them to lumber gracelessly, and be prone to bad knees and painful feet. If they're inclined to be competitive, their poor times discourage them. Trying harder can be dangerous. Some, concerned about fitness, turn to swimming, where they are less blatantly penalized by their dimensions. These people often make good Heavyhanders. Not sleek for speed, their size lends itself to exploiting the strength axis.

3. Women. Women may be especially attracted to walking. In his book on walking, Bill Gale mentions Ellen Minkow, who held the boy's state record for the one-mile walk, both indoors and outdoors. As a college freshman she later won the indoor mile, competing with college men. Apparently body build is less crucial to race walking than it is to running. Doubtless this has to do with the vertical vector, which is reduced by the requirement to keep one foot on the ground at all times. Women have leg strength that is comparable to that of men; any increase in walking pace with handweights added would produce respectable workloads. The more solid base provided by walking allows the female Heavyhander to concentrate on the neglected upper torso. Women also find the hip and knee action of walking more comfortable than do many men. As relaxed walkers they are efficient walkers; energy savings can be invested in arm and trunk work — boosting their total work intensities significantly.

4. For runners. I see no reason why walking and running should not be compatible. In Heavyhands they become complementary. Heavyhands walking pushes strength in the four extremities at the very least. "Strength" walking can fill in when the foot strike of running is painful. Some running coaches believe arm strength is a definite advantage and advocate weight lifting. What runners

Aerobic stretching

I think this is really a new species of stretch. Physiologists have compared the benefits of static stretching — holding a position for 30 seconds or so — with the dynamic variety which includes a bit of "bouncing" to extend the stretching. Most experts favor the static variety. I consider SSS (strength-stretch-strides), with or without back and side leans, double ski-poling, pump 'n' jackknifing, and the reach to be excellent both aerobically and for the purpose of stretching. When your back and/or hamstrings are taut, it's a good idea to use these for extended intervals of 10 to 15 minutes or even your entire workout.

High pump Heavyhands walking and mitochondrial density

Mitochondria are the tiny intra-cellular energy plants that are said to increase both in number and size in well-trained muscle fibers. Trained athletes, especially the endurance type, might be said to enjoy increased total *mitochondrial* density dramatically. Lots of large mitochondria makes the heart-lung-blood vessel-blood delivery system a great deal more efficient, much as a high concentration of customers makes a given milk route efficient. The delivery truck doesn't need many more horsepower to deliver more milk along the identical route. When you pump weights fast and high (level 3 or even 4), you are probably building mitochondrial energy "transducers" in muscles that seldom are more than modestly endowed with them — i.e., lats, traps, delts, pecs, to nickname a few of the major upper torso groups, as well as a slew of those little-used leg muscles like abductors and adductors of the hip. A good delivery system plus plenty of users (mitochondria) spells ultimate effectiveness in oxygen transport.

clearly require is not outsized strength or muscle size; strength-endurance, produced by large numbers of repetitions with moderate weights, makes more sense. Runners such as Herb Lindsay, who perform well despite sizable upper bodies, must be considered exceptional. These athletes may consume more oxygen at a given pace than runners of slighter build. Runners should walk heavy and run light — typical running weights being 70 percent or less of those selected for walking. Juggling weight and pace is a matter of intuition, trial and error. The workload totals, as reflected by the working pulse rates, will, in most instances, be quite close. What happens in practice is that the Heavyhands walk facilitates the lighter run, which in turn facilitates unencumbered running. While this is happening, the exerciser is fitter than he would be if he ran exclusively.

5. For gravity-dodging exercisers. I refer to those whose aerobic exercise doesn't deal with the full effect of gravity. In swimming and biking, excellent exercises both, the body weight is supported: by the swimmer's buoyancy in water; by the bike itself for the cyclist. That doesn't preclude vigorous heart or muscle work and training effect. But many of the antigravity or postural muscles are neglected. My friend Dr. Fred Marks is a perfect example. In his early fifties, Fred, a pediatrician, is expert at swimming and biking, spending an average of 4 to 7 hours weekly working at them. Fred acknowledged, however, a tendency to tire early when walking, a bothersome ache in the hollow of his back, and some recurrent ankle problems. Given his state of fitness, when I showed him two or three Heavyhands movements, he took to them instantly. When we spoke a couple of weeks later, he had already noticed lessening of his symptoms.

Fred is far better off than most exercise specialists, because he combines swimming and biking. Biking specialists don't enjoy the great strength-endurance of the upper torso that Fred gains from hard swimming. And swimmer's legs are relatively neglected, especially in the crawl stroke. I cite Fred's case because it demonstrates neatly that "good" exercise may not always train the muscles that implement the activity of everyday life.

Incidentally, competition swimmers, those who swim 15,000 to 20,000 meters daily, frequently suffer swimmer's shoulder and back problems. The former presumably stems from grooved overuse;

the latter from the peculiar "hyperextension" of the back that is characteristic of the expert free-styler in training. Heavyhands offers prompt antidotes for these hazards.

6. Those whose livelihood is derived from muscular work. Ballet dancers practice for grueling hours. The work is extraordinarily demanding but seldom produces high degrees of aerobic power as compared with endurance athletes. A ballet dancer who wants a level of fitness beyond what his occupation confers needs something to increase oxygen consumption without jeopardizing the body. Something that would strengthen without threatening the suppleness that is essential for the dancer. Walking Heavyhands would provide an answer — large workload; small risk of injury; strengthened muscles and ligaments around the joint: all useful adjuncts to the dancer's occupational requirements. Dancers quickly make a dance of walking, bringing every variation I've suggested and many, many more.

How about ballplayers, steelworkers, hod carriers, cellists, pugilists, and wrestlers, acrobats, animal trainers, homemakers, referees, window washers, miners, mechanics, movers, stock boys, and hundreds of others whose muscle generates income? For people whose work life calls for strength and endurance, multifaceted, high-level fitness pays a dividend: energy with which to do the job well, with plenty left over to cover an active leisure.

7. Body types and Heavyhands walking. Running suits the narrow-shouldered, sinewy-legged physique well. If speed over distance is what you're after, a large-muscled upper body is not an asset. Even the great sprinters, though well muscled, are not behemoths. Beyond some point the drag of great bulk begins to overtax the oxygen-transport system. For each of us there is probably some optimal amount of muscle: enough to do the job without creating problems. For genetically wide-shouldered and large-chested body types who want aerobic conditioning, walking with weights is superior to running. Their body weight precludes speed. But their size and strength can produce higher workloads without speed. For most of us, whose legs are already strong enough, "strength walking" helps the upper torso develop into a better proportioned match.

For anyone dubious about running, walking is a safe, solid bet. Heavyhands walking, in fact, demonstrates that for each and every body type there is an optimal combination of components — hand-weight, speed, and range of motion — for achieving the highest exercise workload.

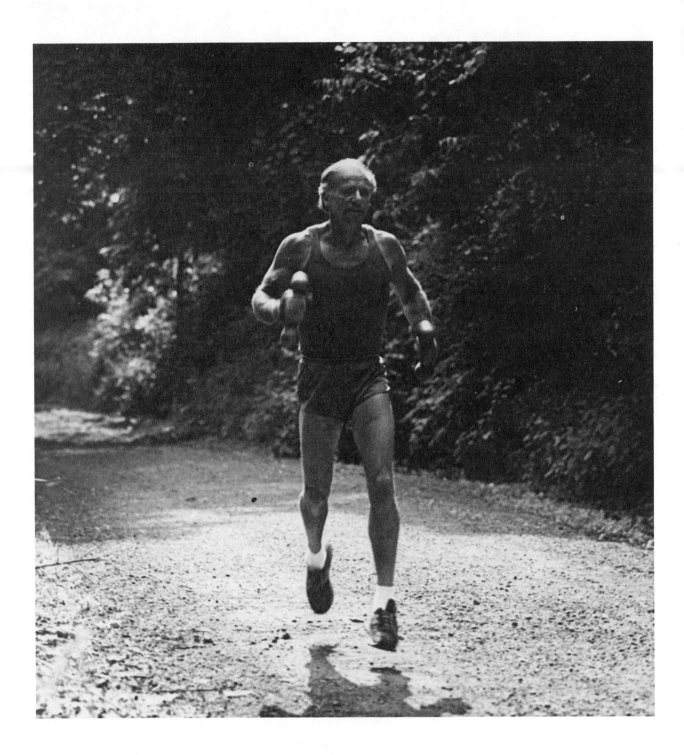

Heavyhands Running and Heavyhands f)r the Runner

THIS CHAPTER IS for four groups of runners:

1. exercise runners, those for whom running is seen as an acceptable way of keeping fit;
2. competitive runners who may seek to improve their times;
3. injured runners of either variety; and
4. eclectics — those for whom running is one of many exercises.

EXERCISE RUNNERS

Those who run simply for fitness generally run at moderate paces. Most of them will probably find whole-body aerobics and its greater total work capacity a beneficial addition. Dozens of the ones I've worked with certainly have. Some fitness runners add weight training or strength calisthenics like push-ups, chin-ups, or sit-up drills. Unfortunately, these movements do not enhance the oxygen-transport system. When all is said and done, these exercisers must depend solely upon their running to increase their aerobic power. Running alone for these people simply doesn't generate optimum workloads.

Combining running with strength work, such as push-ups, chin-ups, or weight training, isn't logical. Arm strength can easily be added *within* the aerobic mode to increase heart-lung efficiency and arm-muscle endurance simultaneously. Leg strength and endurance increase during the body's natural development, and while their emphasis in aerobics is understandable, we typically neglect the upper torso's remarkable potential as an aerobic driver. Recent research tells us there is nothing special about the leg muscles. Starting with small weights and adding speed, range of motion, and endurance, the arms can readily be trained to duplicate the legs' aerobic power. We are merely following the legs' example. If greater strength be necessary, the Heavyhander merely adds a selection of heavier lifts to expedite matters. Not hours and hours of heavy weight training unless we need the awesome one-shot strength and the bulk that goes with that.

This group, the runners who are primarily exercisers, may contribute the largest number to the Heavyhands movement, once they discover the fallacy of excluding the upper torso and trunk from strength-endurance work.

COMPETITIVE RUNNERS

There is reason to expect your running can be improved through Heavyhands training. Some of my notions are theoretical, because Heavyhands is too new for me to have collected enough data to be certain. So I'll run through the logic for what it's worth.

1. Lots of studies show that the upper extremities are a real help to the runner. Subjects on treadmills whose hands have been immobilized run more inefficiently, for example. The upper extremities of great sprinters are powerfully muscled. As noted before, many coaches advocate weight and circuit training to strengthen arms and thus improve times and diminish upper-body fatigue.

2. High-repetition work involving light to moderate weights is not apt to produce sufficient new muscle mass to impede the runner significantly.

3. Hand-held weight is ultimately supported by the lower extremities. The muscle, joint, and ligaments of the legs are strengthened in their adaptation to the added resistance.

4. Pump 'n' run and other Heavyhands exercises strengthen those other parts of the leg that remain relatively weak despite a lot of conventional running. For example, pump 'n' run strengthens the muscles of the thigh-front that receive insufficient work in level running. This development strengthens the "vertical lift" that is part of all running and that aids in climbing hills. And any strengthening effect will reduce the risk of injury.

5. Heavyhands calisthenic routines, shadowboxing, and dance provide aerobic strategies for the abdominal and trunk muscles, explicitly neglected in the mechanics of running. In typical running training, these muscles are given short shrift — quite outside the aerobic mode.

6. Initially the additon of handweights may dismay the elite runner since his pace will inevitably slow. But the arms' oxygen consumption capability will increase rapidly — so that total workloads will increase correspondingly. We are not sure how much these increases will affect the elite runners' heart-leg duets. But his overall oxygen transport will be improved and that theoretically should enhance his running.

Let me add a practical note from personal experience. Over the past four years I have reduced my yearly running to 100 miles

Ordinary running and Heavyhands running

I think running is a sport more than an exercise. Every athlete interested in winning is willing to sacrifice something, and runners sacrifice a good bit of their musculature in order to concentrate on their heart-leg duet. Indeed, running is so specialized that only part of the leg and certain fitness factors receive emphasis. Everything else is "relaxed" to reduce unnecessary oxygen utilization by body parts that don't figure directly in increasing the pace. If the conventional runner requires strength and flexibility of other muscle groups, he or she must acquire them during separate "satellite" exercise sessions. The Heavyhander, training at his game, is simultaneously preparing for other games, including running.

Heavyhands exercises and running speed

The addition of double ski-poling on the move and strength-stretch-strides appear to have had most resounding effect upon my fast running. Liberal use of these exercises also seems to have cured the painful left hamstring that had inhibited my attempts at fast running for four years. And running slowly didn't challenge my oxygen transport sufficiently. Now equipped with healthy thighs, I fully expect to do a 5.5-minute mile or better before I'm done, on zero miles of unencumbered running per year.

Weights and pace

I run a comfortable 10-minute-per-mile pace pumping 10-pounders within a few inches of Level II, at about 150 paces per minute. At the same pace and reaching a similar pulse rate I run the mile in 9 minutes when I switch to 8-pounders. As I drop to even lower weights, the slowing effect is less; at 2 pounds it's almost imperceptible. In novice Heavyhanders those same 2-pounders make a terrific difference. Oddly enough, in experienced marathoners the pace-slowing effect and heart rate increase with handweights may be enormous. One explanation is that some runners have arm VO_2Maxes as small as 58 percent of their legs, while the average in untrained healthy subjects tends to cluster at about 70 percent.

Horizontal-vertical Heavyhands running

On long jogs use weights that you can handle comfortably to Level II at least. Use a "vertical"-oriented, short-striding bobbing jog, landing on the balls of your feet with pumps to Level II. Then switch to a longer stride, Level I pumps, landing on your heels. Repeat the cycle en route ad lib. Don't forget to begin and finish with some stretch-strength-stride and/or double ski-poling. That will warm you up and cool you down aerobically and keep you supple.

while training steadily with Heavyhands. My times, which had plateaued before that, then began to improve. I can only attribute this to my increased oxygen-consumption rates and to increased leg strength resulting from an assortment of Heavyhands exercise.

INJURED RUNNERS

To what form of exercise can the injured runner turn? This is an important question because there are injuries that either preclude running outright or hamper or dampen its "joy." For aficionados, few alternate aerobic forms seem satisfactory. Usually the workload is insufficient or the technique, as in swimming, is for some reason unacceptable. I know of seasoned runners who trained seriously for two decades or more then simply quit following an injury. Nothing seems to fill the void. A few walk, but don't reach paces that could begin to restore them to their earlier level of conditioning. Some make the rounds of specialists hoping for a newly discovered treatment. Slightly embittered, a few continue to follow their sport from the sidelines, enjoying vicariously. When running had been motivated mostly by the *need for exercise,* most injured runners can be reconditioned.

The Heavyhands repertoire must be combed for elements that won't impinge on the injured parts. In Achilles tendon injuries, for example, jumps and moves that involve landing on the balls of the feet must be excluded. A high percentage of injured runners can use many of the calisthenics and Heavyhands walking. Given a doctor's okay, these movements can often be continued while running injuries heal. With high degrees of arm endurance, arms-alone exercise can prevent massive deconditioning. Some Heavyhanders can produce prolonged workloads well in excess of those required to run 10-minute miles. Injuries involving the feet and ankles do not interfere with movements like double ski-poling and Heavyhands walking. The very moves that tend to strengthen and *prevent* injury will *maintain* the fitness of the athlete in the *event of injury.* A number of athletes, initiated to Heavyhands when injured, have continued this form of training after their recovery was complete.

ECLECTIC EXERCISERS

Heavyhands, as I noted before, has been very good for my own running. In the past five years my annual mileages have dropped from a high of about 1,200 miles to less than 100. Most of my unencumbered running happens on vacations. During this period my running time for the mile has diminished from 12 minutes to 6.5 minutes — and is still improving — and I am fifty-seven. My best gains, significantly, came after I began to train with Heavyhands. Most garden-variety runners, who run 20 to 25 miles a week, quickly reach a maximum pace at which they continue for years. My experience suggests that the Heavyhands eclectic, the exerciser who prefers not to become overspecialized, will sacrifice nothing in his running. A number of Heavyhands disciples have described similar findings. Sharing their exercise time between running and Heavyhands has not diluted their running excellence. They enjoy the best possible of exertional worlds. Neither intensity nor duration need be reduced. Sometimes they're increased significantly. Exercise becomes more interesting, more open, more adventuresome. That triad may make quitting more remote.

HEAVYHANDS MEDLEYS FOR RUNNERS

Many of the movements we described in the chapter on Heavyhands walking can be included with minor changes in running medleys. You will want to use lighter weights because being airborne is more taxing than the supported walking stride. For interval work you can vary the workloads from hard pump 'n' run to easy pump 'n' walk. On the other hand, walking at a 150 pace will feel more difficult and will usually evoke more pulse rate response than jogging at 150 strides per minute. If you've selected the proper weights, you may literally be able to rest while you pump 'n' jog.

Paying careful attention to your body you will learn to include segments of double ski-poling at the first hint of leg stiffness, especially of the hamstring group. With relatively light weights double ski-poling can be performed while running. Remember the downstroke should incline slightly outward to avoid the collision of weight and leg. With practice, and a tempo somewhere between

---

Heavyhands for runners who plateau out

The typical course of a running career goes like this: in a year or less of *serious* training, say 4 hours or more per week, speed and oxygen consumption stablizes, regardless of the runner's age. I've known many new runners in their middle years who never could manage multiples of 10-minute miles *comfortably*, if at all. That means their maximum steady states were probably less than 35cc of oxygen per kilo of body weight. Jogging with small weights to Level II, within 3 months, their steady VO_2's often rose to 40–45, in a few cases even higher. Their arms literally had lifted their oxygen transport a healthy notch higher, and with it, of course, their calorie loss per minute of exercise. A few years ago, such increases in work intensity in vintage exercisers were unheard of. Even more exciting are the instances in which running times improve after the addition of Heavyhands training effects. The mechanism is as yet uncertain.

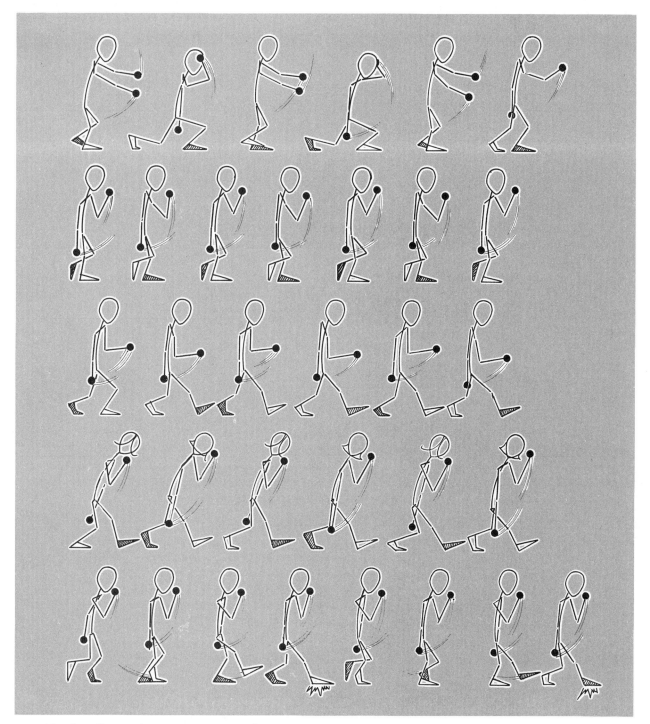

Heavyhands medleys on the move

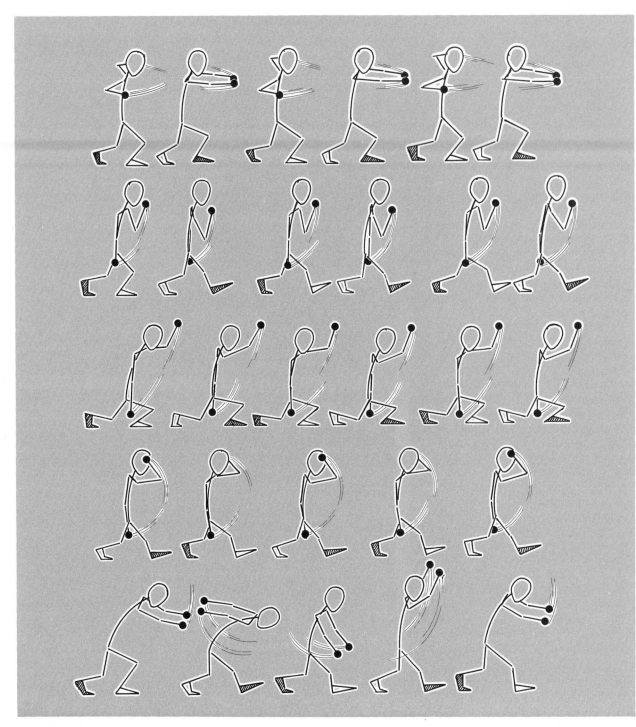

Heavyhands medleys on the move

On-the-move medleys

We've drawn ten movements to choose from and depicted them in sequence. Needless to say you needn't do them all. More than likely you'll settle in to a few favorites and even though you change every few minutes over a 30 or more minute session, you may only use three or four of this group. I'd suggest starting and finishing *every* session with either stretch-strength-strides (SSS) or double ski-poling (DSP). That way you are likely to return home more supple than when you set out. And, en route, any kind of tightening of the thighs should lead you to substitute SSS or DSP for their dynamic stretch quality that will head off overuse spasm. So a typical medley on road or track might scan like this:

SSS	3 min.
Pump 'n' jog — Level II	6 min.
Pump 'n' walk —	
Level III	5 min.
DSP	5 min.
Reach	3 min.
Pump 'n' jog — Level I	4 min.
DSP	4 min.
	30 minutes

Use weights that get you to target at the suggested frequencies. Adjust, of course, if your numbers don't agree with my suggestions. They are only approximations and will vary with the individual and with the level of arm and leg conditioning at a given point in training. Medleys can be more interesting when you vary the sequences and the emphasis and when you intersperse them with long sessions devoted to a single movement.

30 and 50 complete cycles per minute, you will find yourself exhaling with each hard downstroke. Comfortably into your target range, your respiratory rate is quite negotiable, since pulmonary ventilation will happen nicely at a variety of breathing rates. That applies incidentally to many Heavyhands moves — either on the road, track, or in your living room. Synchronizing a certain phase of the movement with your breathing can create a pleasant rhythmic pattern, even though you may be breathing slightly faster than you need. Soon you will do that automatically with every variation.

In running double ski-poling you may enjoy switching between the jackknife and knee-bending variations often. That adds interest, avoids injury, and will iron out any residual soreness from something you did yesterday.

When pump running, I like to vary my foot strike, moving from the balls of the feet to my heels. Also, shifting the workload upward and downward often produces a subtle kind of interval effect while your pulse holds steady. That shift is accomplished, as mentioned in Chapter 8, by varying stride length, stride frequency, the extent of arm curls or raises, and the addition of trunk movements and knee flexion.

FAST PUMP 'N' JOG

With small weights, 1 or 2 pounds will be sufficient for all but advanced Heavyhanders — jog at 150 strides per minute. Your strides will be small, of course. Pumping to Level III is so demanding that with *unweighted hands* you will be working at 10 METs — the equivalent of running at a 10-minute pace! At a 200-steps-per-minute pace most subjects I've tested have hit the 14- to 16-MET level. Many who had not been able to attain a 10-minute-mile running pace found themselves able to do that and better after a few weeks of this exercise. At Level III, tempo 200, I've not seen anyone yet who could exceed 5-pound handweights!

KEEP ON RUNNING

The ranks of runners may be thinning, in part a natural falling off from the high numbers that reflected a first blush of national enthusiasm. Perhaps the addition of Heavyhands will help keep more runners aboard without jeopardizing the art of running in any way. Heavyhands can shore up a runner's strategy by:

1. building strength into the running workload;
2. bringing multiple muscle groups to full aerobic status;
3. increasing total oxygen-consumption rate for a given running pace;
4. strengthening, en route, those muscle groups that tend to receive little work during conventional running;
5. making running workouts more interesting;
6. including flexibility work within the exercise proper;
7. adding fitness components that may augment other activities of work and play;
8. making the runner less dependent upon weather and less apt to suffer seasonal deconditioning;
9. widening the runner's training and athletic horizons; and
10. lessening the risk of injury.

Most of my students have been and continue to be runners. None that I know of has abandoned running. Interesting physiological changes occur in runners who take up Heavyhands seriously. At first the weights seem to discourage. The pace slows and the heart rate quickens — a rather bad combination for any athlete. But the immense gains made by the pumping arms quickly overtake the legs' performance which has very nearly plateaued in those who've logged respectable mileage. A small percentage of high-intensity interval running is often enough to preserve the runner's best times while the endurance component is kept alive and well through a variety of "LSD" — long, slow, distance work — using Heavyhands combinations. At the end of a few short months of training, the pulse rate during pump 'n' run and other combination exercise will have dropped surprisingly — in proportion to the arms' new work capacity.

Most runners who get into Heavyhands enjoy the new upper torso–trunk strength endurance. I recall reading a statement selling the virtues of running that suggested no one ever died of weak arms. I'd be afraid to bet on that one. Early last winter after a heavy snowfall, we had several deaths within a few hours from snow shoveling. I seriously doubt we've had that many bona fide total deaths from running here since *Aerobics* was published over a de-

---

Great race!

A few hours before I wrote this I joined ten to twelve thousand others in the annual 10 K Great Race in Pittsburgh. It was my first race. I hadn't run an interrupted mile with or without weights in over a year. I decided to pump 'n' run with 5-pounders. Most would have properly thought my attempt to be foolhardy if not downright stupid. I finished the race — averaging a 9:20 pace; calculated my oxygen consumption to be equivalent to that of a 215-pound runner moving at the same pace; had no post-race soreness anywhere; and never exceeded a 155 pulse rate. But I learned something interesting. Over the hilly course many runners passed me on the *downhills* and I passed quite a few *going up*. Explanation: the pump 'n' runner doesn't get much relief on the downhills because the arms actually work *harder*. On the uphills the Heavyhander takes advantage of his powerful thigh fronts — the quads derived from "poling," SSS, and Heavyhand work on the level. Heavyhands has a place in the training of runners.

Running better as a Heavyhander

Am I being presumptuous when I predict that Heavyhands will one day figure prominently in the training of runners? I realize the idea goes against the grain of the specificity doctrine: that one should train as nearly as possible at the activity one expects to perform. Heavyhands work enhances what the runner's training does, only more so. It adds these advantages:

1. Aerobic flexibility
2. Endurance strength to the muscles running studiously neglects
3. Speed-strength — little weights at fast tempos
4. The prevention of overuse injury; irons out mild hurts
5. Good cardiopulmonary training when bad weather precludes running
6. Increase in the vertical strength that runners conspicuously lack
7. Guarantee of cardiopulmonary training even when injuries prevent running

---

cade ago. Arm excellence is too useful and so quickly available that there's small point in not having it, whatever your first exercise love happens to be.

HEAVYHANDS RACES

By the time you read this, hundreds, perhaps thousands, will have run 5–10K races pumping Heavyhands, and more than a few will have pumped stride-for-stride in full-length marathons. What's nice about Heavyhands race running is that clock time becomes less important and *competition* — considering the many added by variables such as stride-pump frequency, range-of-motion, and hand-weight — simply ludicrous!

DANCE FOR RUNNERS

Why do I recommend Heavyhand dance for runners?

1. It provides the chance to train, to music, muscles that *help* the runner, but which are *not trained* by the act of running.
2. It is a relative diversion from the gruelling business of logging big weekly mileage.
3. The dancer can studiously work back and hamstring flexibility into his routine.
4. Its MET level will rival, if not exceed, what he achieves on road or track.
5. It's a splendid conditioner for days when bad weather, bulging schedule, or travel make running out of the question.
6. The inclusion of grace as an attribute of running might well be catalyzed by dancing. Grace should help a runner manage a given pace more efficiently.
7. Dance might reduce the need for stretch, which could both save time and spend calories.

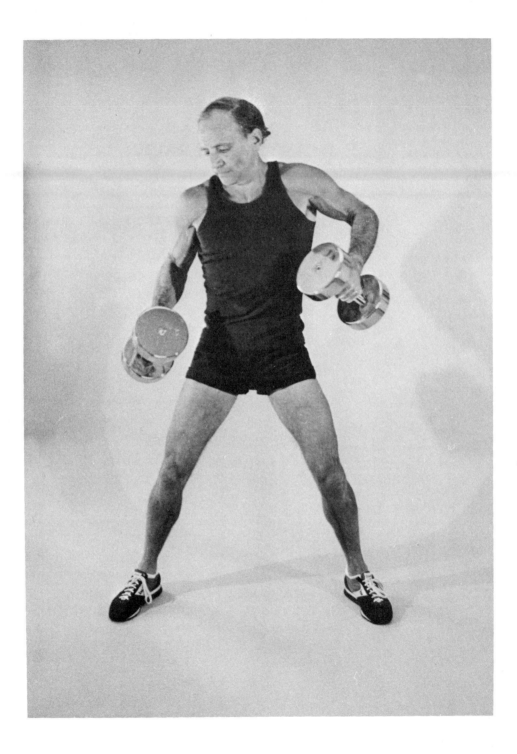

10

Heavyhands for Lifters and Body Builders: The Strength Specialists

Bitty weights for behemoths

Why are strength athletes, who can bench press 400 pounds repeatedly, unable to move their hands as fast and long as a trained Heavyhander? The answer lies in the muscle chemistry that relates energy. Lifters may scoff at using 1- to 3-pounders to turn a respectable pulse, but it's the road to speed, endurance, *and* strength.

THIS GROUP OF ATHLETES and exercisers will provide the world of exercise physiology with some exciting data over the next few years. The musclemen and more recently some very capable strength-trained women generally consume oxygen at modest rates. Typical lifting amounts to heroic work performed over a short time. In order to produce greater muscle mass their exercise consists of few repetitions (6 to 20 generally). These short bursts of strength don't rev the oxygen-transport system sufficiently; neither central (heart-lungs) nor peripheral elements (skeletal muscles) are trained to sustain large workloads over extended time. To make matters appear worse, relative VO_2Maxes are low, especially in massively muscled men, since their modest consumption of oxygen is divided by their large weight. A body like Arnold Schwarzenegger's, weighing, say, 100 kilos (220 pounds) would have to consume 7.5 liters of oxygen to equal the levels achieved by many elite runners. And I've never read of a level that high even from the best and biggest endurance-trained athlete.

MUSCLE BULK AND OXYGEN

There comes a point beyond which muscle bulk lowers the body's oxygen-using efficiency. But, one wonders what would happen if strength athletes would train for muscle endurance? What sort of workloads could they produce with moderate weights moved thousands of times? Trained with Heavyhands, the large-muscled strength athletes will consume enormous amounts of oxygen but their relative VO_2Maxes will probably never exceed the top levels produced by champion cross-country skiers. The important question is whether their heart output could keep up with the demands of their outsized musculature.

Heavyhands training in strength athletes might help decide which determines the limit of human work capacity — the heart-lung complex or the skeletal muscles. To hazard a guess: heart-lung mechanisms may be the limiting factor for the iron pumpers; skeletal muscle chemistry may limit the speed-endurance-oriented athlete.

TIME, WEIGHT, AND WORKLOAD

Many top-flight body builders train for twenty or more hours weekly. Reduced to actual work time, these hours shrink because heavy-weight work requires long rest intervals. It is clear that far less time is neded to maximize strength than most devote to it. The body builders train longer than the competitive lifters, partly, I suspect, to keep skinfold fat to a minimum. Despite the huge weights used, the total workload involved is relatively small, which in turn means few calories used.

Despite these problems with weight training, Heavyhands-trained strength athletes will soon produce the largest workloads ever seen. By that I mean that strength-endurance in some optimal combination, involving large percentages of the musculature in simultaneous activity, will produce a larger amount of physical work within a given time segment than has ever been done before.

Lifting as sport and exercise involves big numbers. Lifting big weights is the aim. To that end, few repetitions became the best prescription for both enormous strength and matching muscle mass. With that, the potential for strength training as a producer of *great and extended workloads* has been lost.

But strength athletes who adopt Heavyhands techniques are in a good position to build both endurance and work intensity. What they lack in speed can be more than compensated for by the terrific weights they can manage. Since their strength need not be sacrificed, Heavyhands brings stamina of both central (heart-lungs) and peripheral (muscle systems) components to the oxygen-transport mechanism. Once conditioned, strength-oriented Heavyhanders can probably reduce their strength training time without sacrificing muscular bulk or definition. Indeed, a high-repetition, moderate-weight Heavyhands strategy may produce the best muscle definition. Two factors will contribute to that. Prolonged high-intensity work chases calories and thus incinerates skinfold fat most effectively. And Heavyhands strategy using a large variety of movement will activate muscles largely neglected in conventional strength programs.

Strength-muscle and strength-endurance-muscle

While Heavyhands produces more modest increases in muscle bulk than programs oriented toward "pure strength," the story doesn't end there. Someday I hope to compare the work capacity of units of muscle mass added through each method. Also I'd like to develop a simple scheme for judging how much new muscle is optimal for a given life-style. I *can* say unequivocally that new muscle acquired through broad-based Heavyhands training will produce enormous total workload capabilities (METs times minutes) as well as surprising levels of brute strength.

Heavyhands and strength

Good evidence exists that muscle bulk is not the only route to strength. I believe Heavyhands will make a significant addition to that body of knowledge. I can't, of course, claim that Heavyhanders are the strongest specimens. But experience will show that *gram for gram,* a piece of Heavyhands-produced muscle is stronger and can *outwork* by a huge margin that produced by any other kind of training.

Large muscles needn't be excessive

I read recently of a young oarsman weighing 100 kilos (220 pounds) whose VO$_2$Max was 71.2. That means he could consume 7120cc of oxygen in a single minute of maximum work! That level would inspire envy in most of the lankiest roadrunners. Rowing is incidentally a good example of combined exercise. The young man's lung bellows pumped a whopping 288 liters of air while that gargantuan oxygen uptake was recorded — twice what many world-class endurance athletes can manage.

Lifting for Heavyhanders

Some heavy lifting will not interfere with Heavyhands training. The proportion of Heavyhands to pure strength work should be freely negotiable. If skinfold fat loss is a major concern, Heavyhands has no rival. And even when strength is your highest priority, the mixture of Heavyhands with strength work will maximize the benefit per unit time of the latter.

Lifting, strength, and Heavyhands

I can't prove it yet but I do believe that 2 hours per week of power repeats like punch 'n' dip, and lateral thrusts with jumps, will edge a lifter's strength upward a bit while boosting his cardiopulmonary values startlingly.

THE APPROPRIATE HEAVYHANDS EXERCISES

The entire range of Heavyhands exercise is well suited to complement a strength program. The first priority should be heart-lung conditioning, the element most often lacking. Heavyhands calisthenics, Heavyhands walking and running, and Heavyhands dance and shadowboxing all will produce sufficient heart work to do the job. Strength athletes who have not attempted aerobic exercise may find the continuous format strange at first.

Heavyhands walking and running, including light-fast work, is of special value. Sessions should quickly grow to 30 minutes in length, especially in young exercisers, Sessions of 1 to 3 hours at reduced intensity may be added to lose skinfold fat. Heavyhands dance, which develops grace, agility, and balance will use calories faster than any activity a typical strength athlete encounters. Generally the best gains will come from intensifying the staple 30-minute sessions. Weight trainers may wish to add movements such as those that push the weights overhead. But I find these "presses" clumsy for the most part, inhibiting during ambulatory exercise, and generally unnecessary. The muscles involved are trainable by an assortment of other movements; pushing things overhead may be one of the chores with lowest natural incidence among activities of everyday life!

Though lifters already deal with gravity superbly, Heavyhands should improve that factor as well. Plenty of *jumps* from among Heavyhands calisthenics gives a springy nuance to the lifter's solid base. But Heavyhands walking may be a wise investment before going to the airborne moves of jog and run. I encourage strength athletes to do extensive walking medleys: *swagger* for style, grace, and relaxation; *jackknifing curls, duck walks* and *waddles* to add endurance and balance to their great leg strength.

OTHER WEIGHT PROGRAMS

Recently a form of strength, training called circuit training has enjoyed growing popularity stemming from the hope that it would provide an answer to the weight lifter's aerobic deficiency. It consists of a series of strength exercises performed consecutively with 15- to 30-second rest periods between each. Unfortunately, a number of studies suggest that only insignificant increases in oxygen consumption rates occur with intensive and prolonged circuit training.

Many who would never consider weight training are addicted to push-ups. But push-ups are weight-training movements. The triceps muscle functions whether it's pushing weights skyward or raising its host's prone body. And the oxygen-transport system responds with equal indifference to either exercise. I recall as a young man doing push-ups. When I tried it recently I found myself easily able to double my best previous total. The push-up, however firmly ensconced in our culture, is not generally aerobically fueled, uses only a few of the many muscles that need work, doesn't develop great strength, may push the blood pressure higher than its value warrants, and produces precious little in the way of muscle endurance. Yet I heard a man the other day mumble something about giving up running and going back to push-ups. Easier is seldom better.

HOW MUCH MUSCLE AND HOW MUCH STRENGTH

Few repetitions with heavy poundage produces maximal strength. Aside from competition in body building or weight lifting are there logical limits to the need for strength? Pure strength is developed at enormous cost in time and at the expense of the other components of fitness. I have watched twenty-year-olds, strong enough to bench-press 350 pounds, attempt to "bag punch" with 10-pound weights at 100-per-minute frequency. Inevitably they reach pulse rates of 180 or better within a minute and many can't continue the movement for an entire minute. Muscle tissue is muscle tissue. A few minutes daily deducted from their ritual "sets" of curls, presses, and pullovers would quickly convert their muscle enzyme capabilities from one-shot to the sustained performance and give their hearts a steadied-out ride in the bargain.

Isometrics

We tend to dichotomize too much. Small wonder fads swell and recede in the self-help area: it's *either* calorie or carbohydrate counting; *either* rest or work a sore muscle. Similarly, we label exercise either isotonic or isometric, depending upon whether the muscles involved contract and relax rhythmically or remain in fixed contraction for a prolonged period. Actually, there's probably some of each mixed into every movement. Push-ups, for instance, are clearly both. Recent studies show that isometrics may be more beneficial than had been previously thought. Dr. Paul S. Fardy, writing in *The Physician and Sportsmedicine*, summarizing the state of the art, tells us that healthy hearts take well to isometrics; even people with coronary artery disease, he says, so long as the crucial left ventricle's function hasn't been compromised significantly. You'll need your doctor to answer that one.

Work capability and strength

Many don't really understand the fundamental difference. Some believe strength and work capability to be synonymous. While big muscles almost always suggest outsized *strength*, they are often poor predictors of *work* capability. Work means steady energy output measured over minutes, even hours. Strength implies heroic output measurable in just a few seconds. Work should conjure things like heart-pump strength and oxygen transport efficiency. Strength associates to power lifters, work to triathletes. In body terms, strength and work call upon two separate chemical-physiologic systems. Heavyhands combines the two in strength endurance, by repeating high-resistance movements enough times to allow them to qualify as *work*. And, while strength has always gotten high billing for its theatrics, work is the stuff that makes civilizations tick.

Exercise	Strategy (1 Yr)	Strength	VO$_2$Max	Muscle Endurance
Weightlifting	210 minutes per week 6 to 15 reps per set	great increase	little change	little change
Jogging/ Running	30 minutes, 5 to 7 times per week at target pulse	little change	increase of 15–25%	great increase, limited largely to legs
Heavyhands	30 minutes, 5 to 7 times per week varied Heavyhands repertoire	moderate to large increase	increase greater than 25% common	great increase in large number of muscle groups

THREE EXERCISE METHODS COMPARED FOR STRENGTH, VO$_2$MAX, AND MUSCLE ENDURANCE

The addition of a single pound to each of a Heavyhander's hands is a big event at higher poundages. I am not sure that pure strength as well as the more health-oriented endurance-strength can't be achieved outside the conventional weight lifters' 6- to 10-rep strategies. I know people whose strength ranks them in the ninetieth or above percentile of our population who have never touched a heavy weight. Muscle mass may be necessary for special kinds of strength, but strength-endurance may be increased with imperceptible additions of muscle mass.

I often wonder what reactions would occur in a group of strength athletes once given a taste of high repetition (500–20,000) exercises with moderate resistance. How would they then view their bodies' generous proportions? When Heavyhands gains wider acceptance and the workloads of Heavyhands-trained strength athletes are evaluated, we'll know more about how much muscle is *enough*.

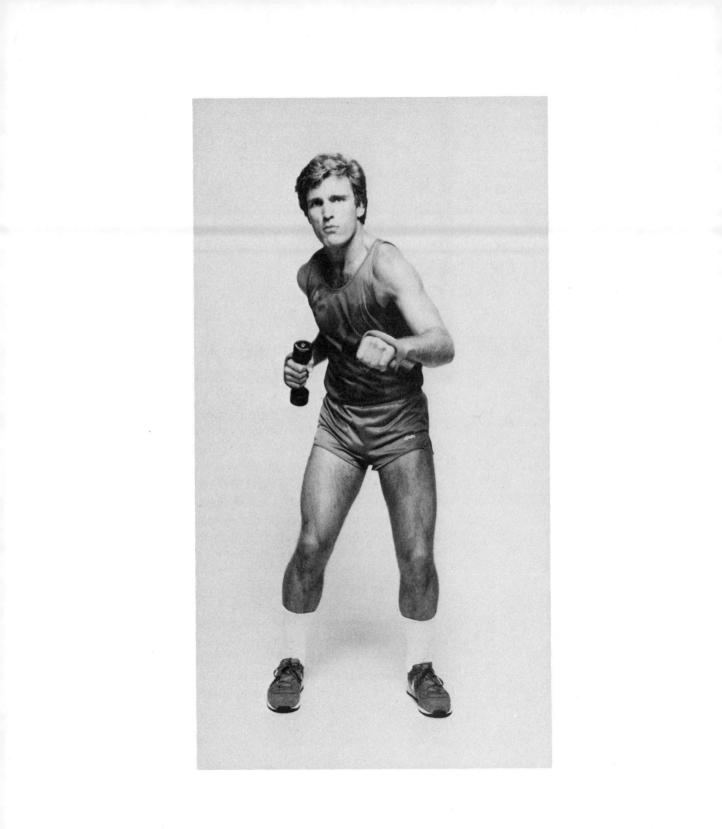

11

Shadow-boxing

I'M DEFINITELY PARTIAL to this exercise. It has all of the big components I keep prattling about. Anyone can do it, and like dance, it is something that gets better with conscientious practice. I am saddened by some women's reluctance to shadowbox, but their aversion tends to balance out the shyness many men feel with dance. Shadowboxing is like dance but is more structured, so it belongs between dance and fixed forms of Heavyhands. Shadowboxing performed with zeal turns rope jumping into an also-ran.

HOW MANY ROUNDS CAN YOU GO?

One day four years ago, just for fun I began shadowboxing on my patio. Using a couple of 3-pounders, I hopped about bobbing and weaving, feinting and thrusting vigorously. Three minutes of this had my pulse tripping along at 170 beats per minute, and I was yearning for the bell! So I rested a minute "between rounds," counted my pulse, and went after my imaginary opponent for another 3 minutes of sweaty flailing. Soon I was cut down to size by my own ambition; round five found me laboring, arm-weary, throwing fewer punches, even ducking with somewhat wilted enthusiasm. Whoever he was, my opposition was wearing me down at a frightening rate! For a few days I practiced this encumbered routine thinking in terms of its exercise potential, calculating likely oxygen-consumption rates by extrapolating from pulse rate and laboratory experience. By more realistic pacing I was able to quit the rest minute and found myself moving along nicely at 60- to 70-percent oxygen-consumption rate for 20 to 30 minutes at a time. On my toes a good bit of the total time, I ran into slight, expectable calf soreness but that vanished quickly. I now shadowbox Heavy-hands style when I feel I need a pick-me-up at the speed-power level. It's comic relief after heavy work with long levers and 5 to 10 minutes as a warm-up for anything, including running, is perfect because you're so very much in control.

Shadowboxing can be done while watching television because you actually needn't lift your feet from the floor for long periods. I now spar for as long as 2 hours with 5-pounders to make up for lost exercise time; and when traveling, that 10 pounds beats any

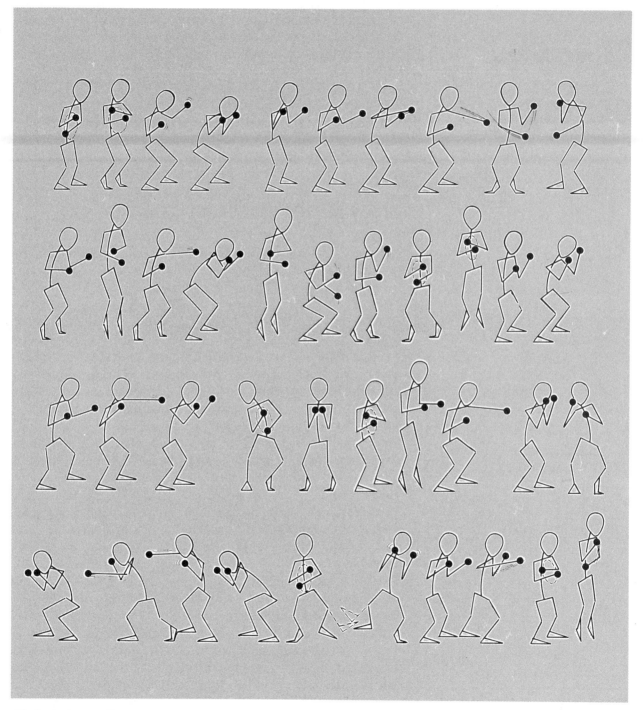

Shadowboxing sample

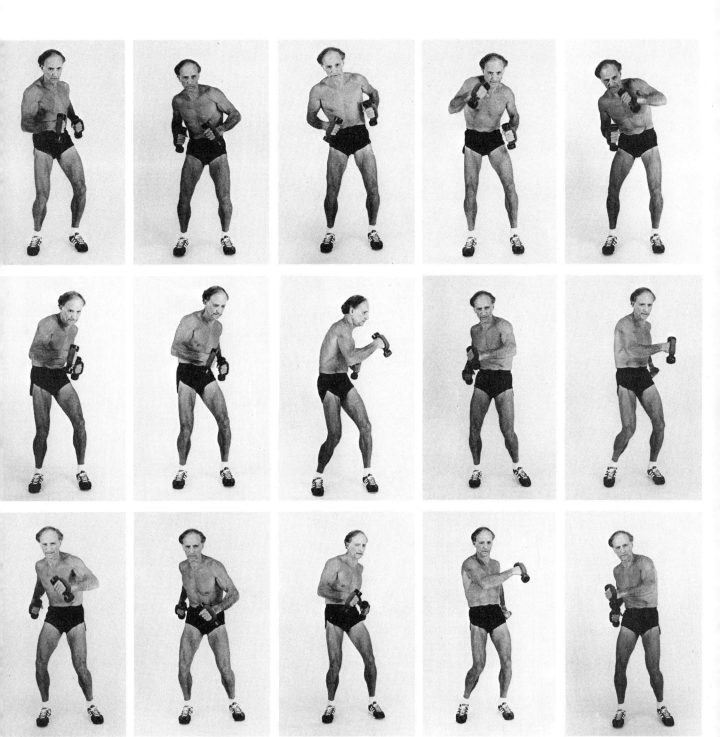

exercise device I could stuff into my luggage. I would be willing to challenge any exercise with Heavyhands shadowboxing *alone* on a point-by-point checklist covering everything from the physiologic measurables to psychic imponderables. And, as the saying goes, I'll make book on it.

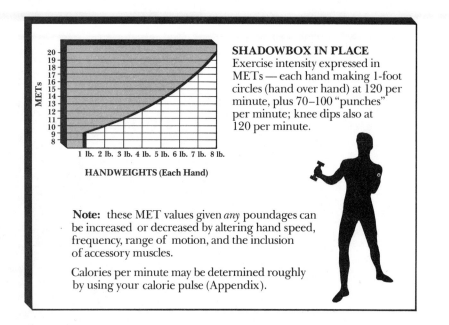

SHADOWBOX IN PLACE
Exercise intensity expressed in METs — each hand making 1-foot circles (hand over hand) at 120 per minute, plus 70–100 "punches" per minute; knee dips also at 120 per minute.

Note: these MET values given *any* poundages can be increased or decreased by altering hand speed, frequency, range of motion, and the inclusion of accessory muscles.

Calories per minute may be determined roughly by using your calorie pulse (Appendix).

(Graph labels: METs on vertical axis from 8 to 20; HANDWEIGHTS (Each Hand) on horizontal axis: 1 lb. 2 lb. 3 lb. 4 lb. 5 lb. 6 lb. 7 lb. 8 lb.)

If a single picture is worth a thousand words, a single demonstration could just be worth a tomeful of them. I can't really teach you to shadowbox Heavyhands style. My best bet is to get you going in a way that at least guarantees the physiologist's requirements. Regardless of your vaunted notions of your own strength, start with the smallest weight you can find. One-pounders are already big weights, especially if you're a typical tyro and have not been punching at something lifelong. If you happen to be very strong in your upper body, you can compensate for the weight by the number of shots you fire and the speed-power dimension. If moving all limbs steadily at a brisk tempo with 1-pounders fails to bring you *beyond* target pulse within 3 minutes, you either have third-degree heart block and should fetch your physician *now,* or you don't understand what I mean by "brisk" (90 or 120 moves per minute).

SOME HAND AND FOOT BASICS

Remember hand over hand, Calisthenic XIII? Use it here. Considered bad form in the ring because it squanders energy, it's very good as an exercise for the very same reason. The orbiting hands release their punching fusillade intermittently. Short or long bursts. Combinations like the old one-two, a jab with the lead hand and a cross or hook with the other as follow-up. Or a succession of jabs. With a flurry of rights and lefts, throwing iron at a devastating frequency, your hands alone can control pulse. When arm-weary, do what the pros often do: drop your hands and dance out of your opponent's reach. Bring your arms back into play by "bag punching," Calisthenic V.

As you become stronger, the number and power of your punches will increase. Finally you can increase weights. It might help to do strength drills: a few extra minutes of heavy work intermittently to begin acclimating yourself to your next "glove" size. You will note certain muscle changes that cannot accrue from other exercise. The trapezius muscles and the complex of anterior deltoid and chest muscles — the pectorals — will get special work. You should at first experience the reassuring slight discomfort of morning-after soreness.

FOOT MOVES ARE KEY

Sore elbows

Don't overdo the number of consecutive jabs you throw until you're sure you're up to it. Overambitious repetitions, thrown hard, are apt to be rewarded by something resembling tennis elbow, or worse.

Early in the "fight" game you will run out of upper-torso gas and will need your legs to keep up your oxygen use and pulse rate. Watching boxing on television will give you some of the feeling of footwork. Knees should be semiflexed and bouncy, not rigid. Awkward feeling at first, as the involved muscle tones, trains, and gains facility, grace follows. And you should consciously try to add a bit of grace to any Heavyhands moves.

I feel comfortable at a 120 metronome pace, which means that my footwork follows that frequency. That's a convenient tempo because it incidentally corresponds roughly to the beat of much popular music. And when I Heavyhands shadowbox, I nearly always use music. Much of your foot activity will depend upon how your hands are getting on. Along with quick hand over hand, try a half-dozen quick little steps, backward and forward. Or try wheeling sharply around 90 degrees, even 180 degrees, spinning on the front toe and resuming punching promptly. Use your imagination. Imagine yourself in different defensive-offensive situations. It's good for your body and won't hurt your image.

USING THE WHOLE BODY

Involve your trunk muscles. As you dip your knees abruptly to duck, bend sharply at the waist and come up fast with hard left-right combinations. Do it again. And again. Jab five times quickly with your lead. Throw a haymaker. Waggle back and forth at your waist, avoiding pretended onslaught. Listen to the music. Duck back from the jab coming at you, or bend quickly forward and to the side from the waist, to let would-be blows slide past your moving head.

Shadowboxing needn't be purely that. I now include some jumps that push oxygen transport, when I'm working with weights that are on the heavy side. I especially favor the jump with lateral flings. Its a beautiful long lever that works the antigravity muscles both above and below. Don't be afraid to work up to 3 to 5 minutes or more of this, spliced into a shadowboxing workout. Remain flexibile — insert any or all of the calisthenic moves when they occur to you.

Shadowbox on days when you feel lively and don't want to use heavy weights. Shadowbox during Heavyhands walks.

PUNCHING PROBLEMS

Some beginners find the punches difficult. The tendency is to abort the punch prematurely, pulling it back before complete extension,

In place

If you have a sore leg, are not fond of jumping, or feel you can't do it, here's a way to condition 500 muscles at your target pulse without either foot leaving the ground! Just what the doctor ordered for TV watching. Stand with your feet planted at shoulder width, somewhat pigeon-toed. Throw all of your punch combinations and/or keep hand over handing while you knee dip rapidly. Reverse the direction of your hand over handing and it will soon become equally comfortable both ways and there is considerable biomechanical advantage. Also exaggerate lateral knee movements, bends at the waist, and hip action, without letting up on your hooks underneath and "over the top." Try it with feet very close together. That challenges the postural musculature more and will give you the balance of a downhill slalomer. Some physiologists would bet against an averaged-sized individual spending 20 or more calories a minute without moving their feet.

Intervals

One reason I like to work walking medleys on a short course like my backyard is that I can have several pairs of weights available. Even though it means lots of laps, I keep my pumping action going at the turns. I can intersperse 5 to 10 minutes of shadowboxing, using half my walking handweight anytime I feel the urge and end up with a satisfying 30-minute stint that has enlisted 95 percent of my musculature in wide-ranging activity.

Power

In shadowboxing you come to understand the intimate relationship between muscle power and aerobic work. The object is to generate heat by getting your weighted hands to many high-velocity "shots" per minute. Training proceeds as these increase. Weights are added only when you're satisfied with your hand speed and punch frequency.

Special effects

As in dance, an active imagination coupled with cheery aggressiveness make for pleasurable, productive workouts. The defensive moves repeated exaggeratedly are probably as good for middle conditioning as anything you can do. The jerky quality of shadowboxing sets it off from the smooth changes characteristic of dance. Both are good and necessary ingredients for your Heavyhands strategy — a bit of toughness and a bit of grace.

Aerobic control

With practice, your heart's response to shadowboxing will be exquisitely tuned and controlled. Backing off can be managed in subtle reductions of hand velocity, hop-shuffle frequency, and the duration of flurry combinations. It can be engineered like interval work, in which high-intensity levels are interspersed irregularly with lower-intensity segments.

which makes it an awkward, tight, restricted, chopping motion. The punches are really throws made with relaxed grace but with plenty of steam. Don't sacrifice this element in favor of heavier weights and correspondingly cumbersome motion. You can *always* add poundage.

Quite consciously bring the muscles that surround the shoulder joint into play. You can work the trapezius muscles, pecs, lats, and deltoids. They will make punching feel easier — because the load is being distributed — will prolong your pleasure, and diminish lactic-produced arm ache. Also bring knees and hips into each thrust so that the whole body literally gets into the act.

The addition of a pound of iron to each hand with this exercise must be considered a major event. To go from 2- to 3-pounders without sacrificing frequency is to increase upper-body workload by 50 percent. That means it really can't be done effectively and safely. Cut back in frequency to help accommodate the tremendous increment in resistance. Another tactic is to use weights 50 to 80 percent heavier, but for shorter, more deliberate periods — just to enhance ballistic strength.

Shadowboxing may come to blend spontaneously with Heavy-hands dance, which is introduced in the next chapter. But even without that you should feel somewhat like a dancer as you shuffle and hop about. Remember the way strength and grace are connected. Time will pass very rapidly, incidentally, while boxing or dancing, in part because improvisation distracts from the onerousness of the exercise. I hope you come to love this exercise. If you do, it will love you in return!

Here's a wake-up exercise I often do with 1-pound weights, within a minute of rising in the morning. I hop on my *left foot,* throwing a hard right hook at the same time. Then I shift, hopping on my right with a simultaneous left hook. Next I do two hops, two hooks, on each side, then add one each time for 20 or 30 units of hops and punches. Going to 30 units amounts to 930 hooks and hops — done in little more than 5 minutes.

Don't start with 30!

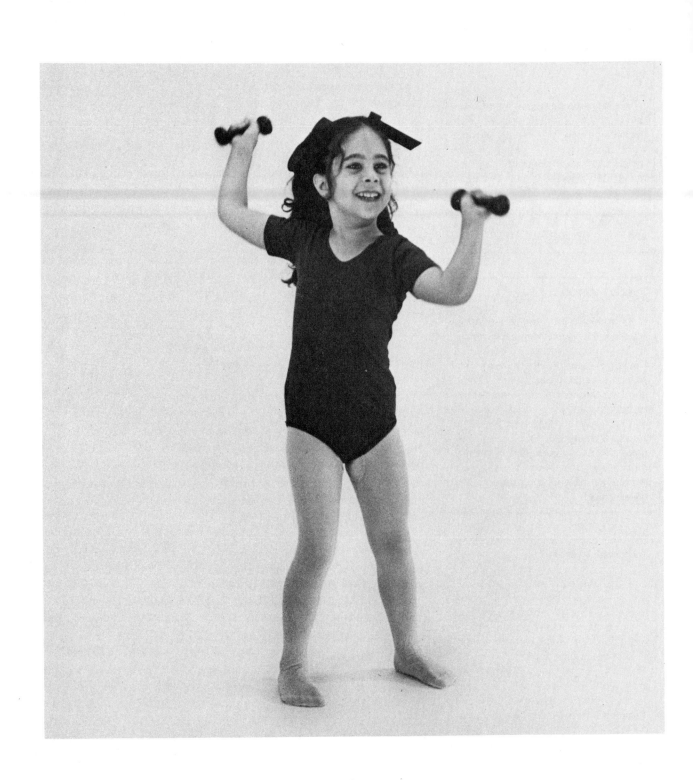

12

Heavyhands Dancing

Who's for Heavyhands dance?

Strangely enough, we'd like to attract from the whole range of the people-spectrum: from those quite expert at dance to those who shrink from the very notion. Expert dancers can immediately place it in the service of acquiring super fitness. The shyer ones, and that includes many of us, have more to gain; beyond physical training there's the unrivaled bonus effect spelled in terms of a new sort of confidence.

HEAVYHANDS DANCING IS an extension of the already popular aerobic dancing inaugurated by Jacki Sorensen. Dancing is an absolute natural for aerobic exercise, using music and rhythmic movement to bridge the gap between hard physical labor and play. Heavyhands dancing evolves naturally from the notion that the hands and arms are well equipped to take the lead in exercise.

Music tends to make us tap our feet. Interestingly enough, after a few weeks of Heavyhands dance, I found myself responding through my shoulders, arms, and fingertips. While a poor match for the legs' superior brute strength, the arms are more mobile and capable of complicated, swift, prolonged activity at workloads, as we've indicated, that can rival the legs' best effort.

Dance is different from other exercises, and has its own specific and peculiar advantages. Overall self-confidence may be deeply rooted in how well our bodies function; motor skills may dramatically alter the self-image that makes us more at ease socially; and very few exercises combine grace and skill the way dance does. Music's percussive component is a metronome dictating the tempo and regularity of the movement. Its melodic line says something else. It has "direction," moves toward an end point, and can parallel many typical emotional states. In a word, it craves interpretation.

WHAT IS HEAVYHANDS DANCE?

Heavyhands dance, along with shadowboxing, is free-form exercise. Rather than following staid movement patterns, the dancer obeys spontaneous sequences of movement impulses. The hands rather than the legs lead the action. The free-floating arms execute in huge arcs of movement at higher velocities than the legs can muster. The Heavyhands dancer, intent upon graceful performance as well as the elements of fitness, achieves high levels of oxygen transport along with the impromptu movement. As in other types of dance there can be fixed movement patterns, but the option to improvise remains open. In the four-limbed variety of dance the integration of the limbs is more complex and kaleidoscopic than in any form of exercise. The fitness possibilities are limitless; the highest workloads are available with dance. The Heavyhands dancer's control, part of the art, becomes a physiological advantage.

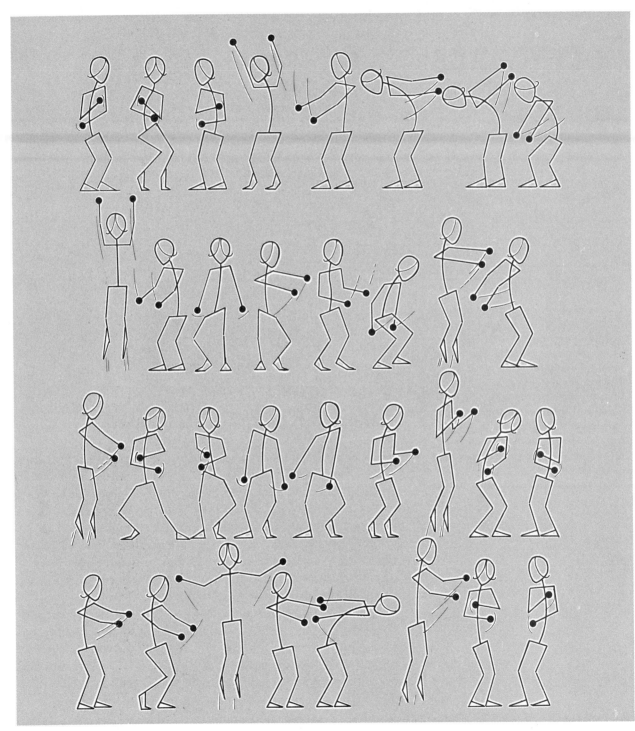

Dance routine example

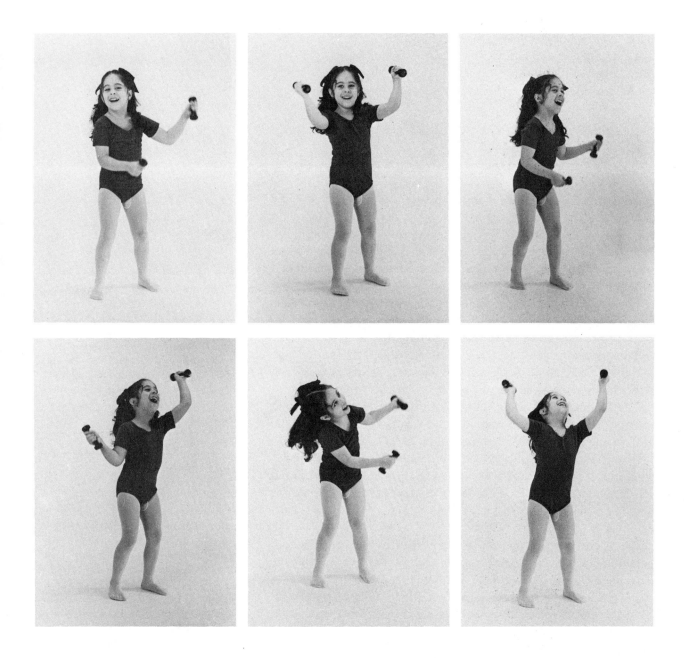

Within the confines of any muscial tempo endlessly flexible manipulation of the workload is possible. The various forms of Heavyhands exercise, ambulatory, calisthenics, and shadowboxing, are readily included into Heavyhands dance routines.

ADVANTAGES OF
HEAVYHANDS DANCE AS EXERCISE

Heavyhands dance differs from the conventional forms in some important ways. The ordinary aerobic dance class tends to motorize everyone to an identical MET level; i.e., in step with the music everyone may hit 6 to 8 METs, a physiological fact that continues session after session. In order to accommodate the deconditioned member of the group the pace is kept modest. This makes good sense socially, for no one is left out. A few struggle beyond their target heart rates and a number of healthy young people find the going too easy to constitute a real challenge. The addition of variable handweights along with the possibilities in tempo and range of motion make it easy for individual dancers to work at their own target heart rates while remaining "in synch" with the group.

Free-form exercise is less apt to bore than the more stereotyped forms of aerobics. Injuries are less frequent, simply because the movement pattern shifts frequently enough to avoid overuse injury.

Heavyhands dance is a bad-weather beater. Never to be considered a mild substitute for real exercise, dance can make a trained Heavyhander shed calories in 20-calorie-per-minute bunches as long as the music lasts. You can't decondition if you dance conscientiously — and you'll have fun!

Dance has been recognized for centuries as a natural antidepressant. The dancer, locked into the music and intent upon the movements, is drawn away from the immediate concerns of everyday life. The entire personality, one might say, is consumed in the stimulus and with the challenge presented by the need to match the music's mood to movement. Four-limbed exercise presents a novel and diverting problem to the game participant of dance. The addition of hands to dance, aside from the obvious physiological advantages, may stimulate unexplored thinking-imaging patterns. And by the way, dance becomes the best, most vigorous form of

---

Injury and dance

Some mild hurts of the legs, like shin splints or sore feet, can occur with dance. Going virtually flat-footed, you can kneedip, sway, bend, involve the arms and shoulders in a higher percentage of the total work, without extending your injury and without deconditioning.

Heavyhands dancing and intelligence

Freewheeling pleasure begets grace and vice versa. Ordinary smarts aren't always a help in gaining the feel for dance. It's often as though one must divest oneself of everyday intelligence. Freedom and intelligence match up uniquely in dance, which is why we're so apt to be polarized on the subject: either you "catch on," so to speak, or you tend to sever yourself from the temptation to dance. The ironic rub is that we never know how close we are to "catching on."

Men and women and Heavyhands dance

Men and women seem to dance Heavyhands differently. Women are lighter on their feet, fancier, more "pelvic," sort of choppy with their hands. Men are more likely to shoulder or muscle through the music. After a few years of Heavyhand dancing together we may see a unisexual movement, rid of such nonsensical stereotypes.

Ballet and fitness

An exercise expert recently declared that ballet dancers may be as fit or fitter than most professional athletes. Yes and no. A recent study of some of the nation's leading dancers showed them to have VO_2Maxes that correspond to those of the best sprinters, i.e., 50 to 55. They don't come close, however, to recording the high values of endurance athletes — runners, cross-country skiers, bicyclists, swimmers. Heavyhanding might add an extra edge to the speed-strength-endurance components of gracefulness that dance itself can't always easily supply.

noncompetitive sport you can pursue indoors, and without the start-stop disadvantage of games.

Dance is an effective antidote to spasm and cramp. Back from a long run I've frequently added 10 to 20 minutes of dance to mollify the painful muscle spasm I gathered on the road or at the track. Dancing, a form of stretching in itself, doesn't require additional time devoted to static stretching.

My wife and I frequently dance together Heavyhands style. Indeed it is she who, as far as I know, invented the idea. Returning from my hospital rounds one Sunday morning I found her dancing to a Latin rhythm with a couple of 4-pounders. Wondering why I hadn't tried that before, I've never stopped trying since. The point is, and I've made it before, Heavyhands is the best exercise for togetherness involving people of unequal fitness.

Your calorie pulse (see the Appendix) is well suited to measure your energy output during the free-form Heavyhands dance and shadowboxing. Aside from direct measurement of oxygen uptake in the laboratory, the energy expended in dance would be hard to estimate. But once you've checked out your Heavyhands oxygen pulse (see page 28), you will be able to calculate calorie loss at any pulse rate you generate while dancing. Soon enough your subjective sense of effort and/or your breathing pattern will be translatable into terms of calories per minute with an accuracy of 10 percent or better.

TIPS ON HOW TO DO IT

Dancing with weighted hands will at first feel different, because we have been conditioned to respond to music primarily with our feet. But a lot is lost in that sort of specialization, and fitness is just one element. Heavyhands dancing demands coordination, which calls upon our brains to organize and choreograph *all* of us in something simultaneously stimulating, vigorous, and even meaningful.

At this point in the text you have tried more than enough movements to take your first steps, and pumps, at Heavyhands dancing. Even the simplest pump 'n' step in place is enough to put to music for beginners. After that the spirit of adventure plus the belief in the benefits of exercise will set you free.

Music does things to the psychophysiology of exercise. Once you start to dance you become instantly less aware of your body and its responses. Guided by the music and the beat you sooner or later will find parallels to piano playing: the legs managing the base rhythm, the hands carving the fast melodic trebles in the space around you.

Use your smallest weights. If you start with something even a bit unwieldy, you'll cramp some of the style and panache that makes dance fun. And since we know that any of us can get to panting anaerobics with 1-pounders, I'd recommend them for even the most muscular of behemoths. You needn't worry about target pulse at first, but I'm sure you'll get there simply by going high and fast and long-levered whenever you sense any inner slowing. If all else fails to get you to target, cautiously add small increments of weight.

Tend to concentrate on hand speed, range of motion, and endless planes of movement. Remember that just one pound of additional weight at 150–200 tempo will add 1 to 2 METs of additional workload. At average body weight, that amounts to 1 to 2 calories per minute. While not insignificant, you absolutely shouldn't worry about increasing your weights until every other fitness element has been used.

You can stay at target rate using any of the Heavyhands variations you've learned. The trick in dance is to shift unabashedly from one to another when the spirit moves you. Those "shifts" make up the nucleus of fun that people refer to when they speak of dance. Dance has precisely what jogging, biking, swimming, and walking aerobics lack — the prerogative to shift.

Think "exercise" while you're enjoying Heavyhands dance. Think range-of-motion, long- and short-lever options, muscle groups that need action and stretch. Bring in flexions and extensions of the trunk frequently. Use jumps, difficult ambulatory moves like duck walks, reaches, and ski-poling with hops to the action. Be as imaginative as you can. Avoid the hypnotic repetitiousness that may find you loafing well below target rate. Go slow and fast using a variety of weights. Improvise new movements. Using four limbs and trunk muscles, you cannot exhaust the movement possibilities within a lifetime. Learn how to rest by utilizing movements that produce smaller workloads long enough to bring you down from anaerobic excesses.

Think "regional" in terms of muscle groups. Think heart rate,

Doing what comes naturally

Heavyhands dance forces us to embellish and dramatize what should come as naturally to humans as it does to four-footed creatures; the sequencing ritual by which we presently train muscle groups one at a time sounds something like what's been said about strolling and chewing gum on separate occasions.

The music model

I keep rhapsodizing over the music-learning model as a guide to the building of a repertoire. Any child who has tackled an instrument knows that the thrill of learning lies in the discovery that what seemed impossible *to do* later becomes almost impossible *to forget*.

think skill, flexibility, gracefulness. Think halving and doubling the tempo. Include sports moves you like that need practice; music lends a grace to them which can enhance effectiveness. Think strength, speed-power-endurance.

Try all sorts of music. Anything from symphonic to rock; opera to folk; ethnic to Dixieland; easy listening to progressive jazz. Each will affect uniquely the mood and therefore the movement patterns you will spin. Don't be afraid to follow your silliest inclinations. Indeed, push toward the kind of freedom that you knew as a child, intoxicated by the absence of adult concerns. That's what dance is about, and when you've achieved it, you will keep it forever.

I must say the grind of ordinary aerobics is somewhat pallid next to Heavyhands dance. I have found it physiologically comfortable to perform "50-50 exercise" in which arms and legs contribute equally to the workload with Heavyhands dance.

HEAVYHANDS SLAP STEP

This is a simple new twist to what you've already learned. It's actually pump 'n' run in place or on the move, with a tap step added. If you've ever tap-danced you already can do it and even if you haven't you're very close to becoming an expert. The slap step increases the legs' workload a bit, adds a cheery wrinkle to pump 'n' run, and a pleasant ta-tum, ta-tum cadence to your ordinary "soft shoe" Heavyhands dance.

Standing without weights, bend your knees and lift your right foot backward slightly, then kick it forward sharply so that the ball of the foot strikes the floor on its swing forward. That's called a "brush" forward in tap language. Without stopping, bring the same foot back to the floor whence it started, slapping it down audibly on the ball of the foot.

The knee bends easily during the whole brush-forward slap procedure. The "ta-tum" sound comes from the brush and the slap, respectively. The same thing then with the other foot. Any kind of shoes will do it, even your running shoes will make a sound. Then add the pump — same side when doing the slap step in place; diagonal when on the move. If you like you can do swagger and jackknifing extensions to pump 'n' slap steps. As you get better at

---

Dance: The ultimate exercise?

Can one make a good case for dance being the ultimate exercise? Easily, I think. If one studies closely the limits of human work capability, the discouraging effects of injury upon the exercise motive, and the continuing requirement among exercisers for diversity if not fun, Heavyhands dance is the best answer. Four-limbed dance could rival any known exercise or sport for sheer workload; four-limbed dance would injure less and dance has always worked well as an antidote for boredom. As to the psychic benedictions of dance, one can only conjecture, but all those generations of dancers couldn't have been produced by pure chance.

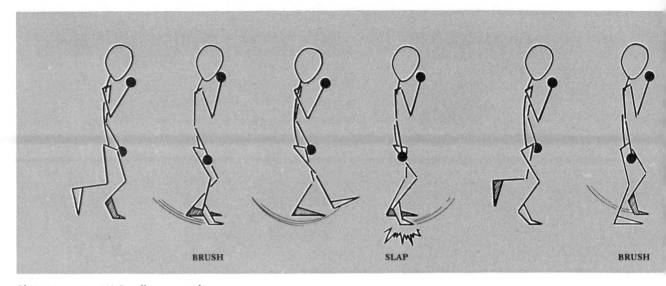

BRUSH SLAP BRUSH

Slap steps — pump 'n' walk or run style

it you'll automatically tend to speed things up. Even 200 to 250 steps per minute are possible. When it's acquired second-nature status, toss it into your pump 'n' run. I've slap-stepped running with moderate weights 3 to 5 miles many times and you probably will too. The brush-slap "ta-tum" sound makes good company on a lonely run.

HEAVYHANDS DANCE A CAPPELLA

I decided to experiment with Heavyhands dance without music when I discovered to my absolute delight that some children uneducated in matters of rhythm and tempo can dance nonetheless. Dancing without music feels different and lends itself to different strategies. Music "works" simply because the human sensory-motor mechanism is built to respond to the structure of music. But that "inner rhythm" works well even when not supplied with the "outer" structure music provides. Children demonstrate it beautifully.

Where music tends to invite repetition, a cappella Heavyhands may or may not, depending upon that elusive, momentary whim.

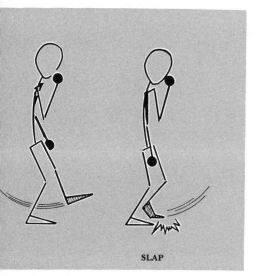

SLAP

I do believe both kinds of Heavyhands dance belong in any repertoire. After starting to experiment you'll soon find that your instincts will guide you to one or the other, based upon anything from mood to some special training effect you're after at the moment.

A cappella is especially good when your energy is high; when you feel like using very heavy weights or fast frequencies. And since frequent changes of tempo are inherent in this form of dance, the mind and muscle can make a special adventure of the impulse to change.

A cappella is good for wide ranges of motion. And even though the patterns are the most structureless of any in the Heavyhands repertoire, after short experience your heartbeat will average out at the level you wish. A cappella is a chance to let your imagination and your oxygen transpsort recombine in endless variation. To keep changing patterns, sliding from one to the next gracefully, is truly a challenge.

The pictures of my two friends doing a cappella, on page 184, are particularly interesting because this was their very first attempt. The photos were shot immediately after they'd received a two-minute instruction. It's amazing how quickly the developing human forgets the kind of spontaneity and pleasure in movement you see here. Once properly inhibited we apparently settle for simple stereotyped movement patterns that doubtless feel safer.

With appropriate weights one can go heavy-slow or fast-light and it can be so demanding that it is perfect for short-interval work. The movements can accentuate extremes of range of motion and thus enhance flexibility by working in uncharted movement territory. Once proficient at a cappella dance, your work intensity may rival that required to run 5- to 6-minute miles!

This exercise qualifies beautifully for use following injuries that make foot movements and strikes painful. Here, too, the feet may remain quite fixed during an entire session.

With small weights you are not apt to injure yourself because movements are slower on average and repetition is virtually nil. When performed optimally the movements "proper" are hardly distinguishable from the transitional movements in between. Ideally it would be one continuous chain of movements which, like a kaleidoscope, weave the body's structure into an endless series

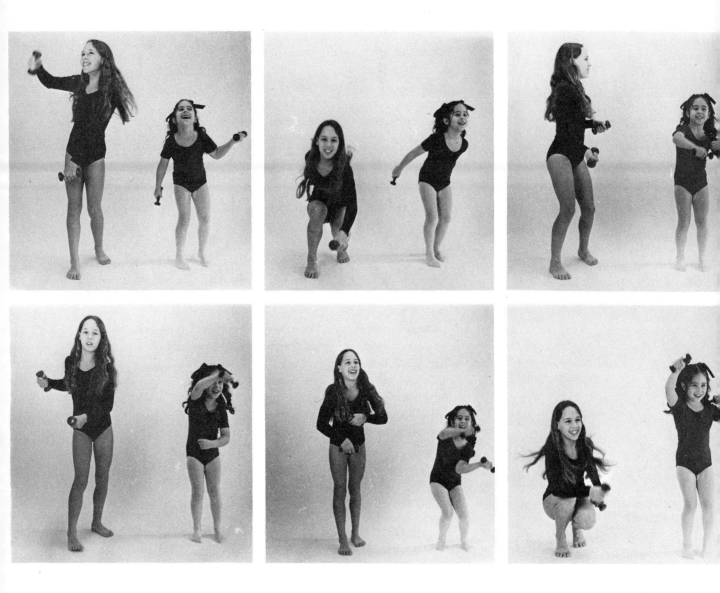

of transformations. As you practice a cappella you'll get better at it and increasing fitness will make a more aggressive performer of you.

This exercise works well in groups. Practicing alone, you come to believe you've tried everything. The group situation erases that illusion. In any event, it's a good way to experience the magic and power of nonverbal communciation while performing your constitutional.

CAVEATS

There are really not many warnings of the don't-overdo-it kind to be issued. Music is a kind of lubricant for exercise. It may massage you into such a comfortable reverie that your original motives for training may recede a bit, inadvertently. So the main warning is to avoid underdoing. The fun factor jousts with the achievement factor, when the two are brought so intimately together as in dance. Just mutter, or shout if you care to, "long lever," or "traps, lats, or deltoids," or "high pump" instead of the lyrics! Some music is naturally soporific and will lullaby you below target if you're less than determined that day. Using that kind for warm-up purposes makes good sense and you can replace it with a more spirited variety once your nervous system is aroused and ready.

Avoid too much repetition. Remember the few recycled steps you clung to with your first clumsy-anxious trials at dance? You can become so efficient with a few moves that you do them to the near exclusion of much else. Again conscious determination will rescue you. You must go at it with the dual personalities of the trainer and dancer.

If you're shy at dance and always have been, you may find the mere psychic act of labeling your dancing "exercise" helpful. If not, practice alone or with someone you can trust not to break up with laughter every time you pump 'n' step. Nothing adds to confidence like skill, and since there are not too many really skillful at Heavyhands dance as of now, you're automatically an in-on-the-ground-floor "belonger."

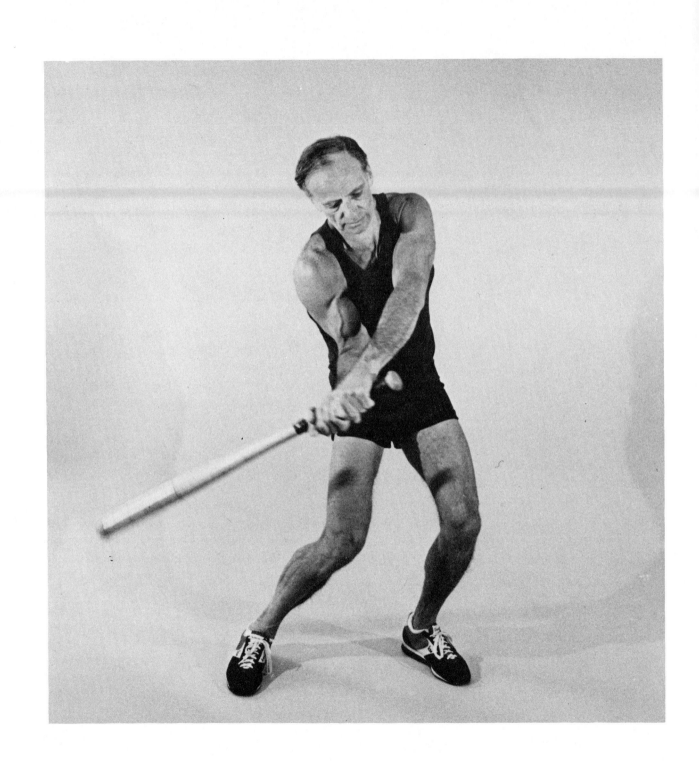

13

Heavyhands and Sports

Sports and fitness

Some people continue to believe their favorite sport can make and keep them superfit. The nature of the specialization required by a given sport makes that unlikely. Aside from long races of any sort, athletics seldom demand the MET-times-minute numbers that generate ideal fitness in a given individual. Even the diversified decathlon can be won by athletes who have achieved only modest cardiopulmonary capacity and little in the way of arm-shoulder endurance.

It is difficult to know how ultimate fitness levels would influence contemporary sport. Enhancement and fewer injuries, one would predict first off. One more guess: general acceptance of whole-body aerobics in the strength-endurance mode would probably touch off the invention of new, more challenging forms of athletics.

GENERAL AND SPECIFIC SPORTS MOVES

HEAVYHANDS MOVES can be of value in almost any sport, even if the specific moves of a given sport are excluded outright from your routine. The Heavyhands *package* prepares your body generally for sports without neglecting any of the fitness essentials. Then, too, the practice of movements particular to a sport can be programmed into your Heavyhands routine to improve your performance. A balanced, diversified Heavyhands program will make you a better match for athletic activities ranging from team sports to track and field events. While it is axiomatic in the art that one must train specifically for one's sport, it would be foolish to imply that one's sport constitutes the *best* form of training in the area of overall *fitness*. By their nature, most sports are limiting in one way or another as compared with "ideal" exercise.

Physiologists have determined the average aerobic requirement for all of the major sports in rather precise terms. So we know about what oxygen-consumption rates are required to play hockey, soccer, baseball, football, tennis, etc. at the professional level. Most sports consume oxygen at rates signficantly *lower* than those posted by Nordic skiing and marathon running. It is probable that many professional athletes don't find it necessary to increase their aerobic capacity beyond that produced by practice sessions and competition. So it is not uncommon for serious, though noncompetitive, runners to test out at levels far above those of many professional athletes.

Every sport can be analyzed into an assortment of moves that identify it, and those interspersed moves that are not specific to that sport. Your Heavyhands strategy can enhance both. And when it comes to the specific moves — the variety of swings, kicks, punches, and throws — it is doubtful that merely "playing the game" constitutes the best sort of training.

Heavyhands, with its high number of repetitions and increased resistance that make for strength, speed, and muscle endurance, provides the serious athlete with a method of improving the specifics of his sport. *Within the same time frame* he can build the aerobic power that equips him with maximum endurance; and increased strength and endurance of muscles provides extra protection against a variety of injuries.

A CAUTIONARY NOTE

If you practice swings with weights or weighted bats as preparation for competitive sports, you must "try out" your newly acquired strength *before* game time. Initially your timing will be *off* somewhat since you will tend to "overswing" using regulation equipment. You will readjust rapidly when your central nervous system learns to "integrate" the effort expended with various resistances. Real increases in muscular strength are likely within just a few days and these will be reflected in the increased speed of bats, club head, rackets, and the "muzzle velocities" of thrown projectiles of every size, weight, and shape.

Throws or swings using multiples of regulation weight should duplicate the desired move precisely. Again one should be prudent about the selection of weights. For *most* people practicing throws calculated to strengthen a pitching arm, starting with 5 pounds would invite certain disaster. A baseball weighs a little over 5 ounces. A multiple of sixteen for starters simply makes little sense. Start out with a 1-pound weight or less, either in the form of a sphere or a cast dumbbell. Throw easily first to get the "feel" and to duplicate your actual throwing motion.

When practicing throws or swings with weights, use both arms — not to develop ambidexterity, but to obtain symmetrical effects and increase cardiopulmonary output. When returning from cast iron back to horsehide or racquet, throw or swing gently until your arms, getting the message, accommodate to the regulation equipment's feathery feel.

As the seasons change, design your workouts to include whatever sports you're into. Keeping your heart in mind, go slow-heavy and fast-light as in other Heavyhands exercise. Both will contribute to your athletic prowess.

Diet, training, and sports

It is my distinct impression that a large number of professional athletes diet in order to keep their weight within manageable range for their playing season. Since repeated dieting may reduce muscle mass substantially, that strategy could jeopardize or abort athletic careers. Few professional fighters, for example, train year round and often resort to what I view as hazardous procedures devoted to making the weight — usually heroic starvation and dehydration. In sports in which only peak output intensity is required, the periodic trainer may get by. I remain dubious both regarding the individual athletes overall durability and the future of the quality of sports performance generally, so long as intermittent conditioning and dieting are considered acceptable practices. I am frankly alarmed by the published longevity statistics for American athletes. It may be ironically too often true that exercise for health and for competition are mutually exclusive propositions.

Heavyhands moves for sports

SPORT	MOVEMENTS	HEAVYHANDS EXERCISE
Baseball	Hitting and bunting; running; throwing; sliding; diving; reaching; twisting.	Pump 'n' walk and run; dance; aerobic bat swinging; HH mock throws. Calisthenics: I, V, VI, VII, VIII, IX, XII, XIV, XVI, XVIII, XX.
Basketball	Dribbling; running; jumping; shifting; body twists; shooting.	Pump 'n' walk and run; shadowbox; dance. Calisthenics: I, III, VII, X, XI, XII, XX.
Golf	Swinging; hip rotation; ankle movement.	Pump 'n' walk, including variations. Calisthenics: VII, XI, XII, XIV, XV, XVIII, XIX.
Tennis and Racquetball	Forehand and backhand strokes; hip flexion and extension; lunges; running; rapid starts and stops.	Pump 'n' run (light); pump 'n' walk (heavy); shadowbox, dance. Calisthenics: I, IV, VI, VII, X, XII, XIV, XV, XVI, XIX, XX.
Boxing	Variety of swings; feinting moves (hip flexion and extensions); hops, shuffles; pushing; "tying up" movements.	Shadowbox, dance, pump 'n' run (ligh?); pump 'n' walk (heavy). Calisthenics: I, II, III, IV, V, VI, VIII, IX, XI, XII, XIII, XVI, XVII, XX.
Volleyball	Jumps; serves; various strokes; twists; dives; lunges.	Shadowbox; dance. Calisthenics: I, III, IV, VII, XII, XVIII, XIX, XX.
Cross-Country or Nordic Skiing	Crouching, poling (double and single); gliding; turning.	Pump 'n' walk and run; special emphasis on double ski-poling and variations of pump 'n' walk; dance. Calisthenics: II, III, IV, V, VII, VIII, XI, XII, XIV, XVIII, XIX, XX.
Downhill or Alpine Skiing	Crouching; hip flexion and extension; twisting and turning.	Pump 'n' walk and run; dance. Calisthenics: II, III, V, VI, VII, VIII, IX, XII, XVIII, XIX, XX.
Bicycling	Pedaling; crouching.	Dance; pump 'n' walk and run; shadowbox. Calisthenics: I, V, VII, VIII, X, XI, XV, XVIII, XIX, XX.
Running	*Sprint:* rapid strides on balls of feet; thrusting arms.	Pump 'n' walk (heavy), including all variations; dance; shadowbox. Calisthenics: III, V, VI, VII, VIII, IX, XI, XVI, XVII, XIX, XX.
	Long Distance: Heel strike; less movement in arm carry than in sprint.	Pump 'n' run (light); pump 'n' walk (heavy); dance. Calisthenics: I, II, IV, VII, IX, X, XII, XIV, XVI, XIX, XX.
Swimming	Various strokes and kicks; body flexions associated with turns.	Pump 'n' walk and run; dance; shadowbox. Calisthenics: III, IV, V, VI, VII, XI, XII, XVII, XVIII, XIX, XX.

HEAVYHANDS EXERCISE FOR SPORTS

On page 189 is a list of some popular sports, the movement patterns characteristic of them, and selections from the Heavyhands repertoire that provide appropriate training. If you're an old hand at any of these sports, you'll of course make your own decisions.

Don't be afraid to switch around. In some instances I picked calisthenics that fit the sports moves involved. At other times, I chose moves that augment fitness where the sport is plainly lacking. Thus I included antigravity exercise in sports like swimming and biking, which neglect those abilities. The aim is to make the athlete *better* both at his sport and the larger business of living vigorously.

I did not include Heavyhands bellyaerobics. I think 5 minutes four to six times weekly should be included in *every* Heavyhands strategy regardless of how passionately one is devoted to sports.

Six or seven calisthenics can be worked together in one of a hundred different medleys that reflect the needs of your game and the condition of your body. Good exercise is more than a collection of workloads. It should draw on good judgment and the particulars of your appetite for movement at the moment. Each workout may be likened to a model of life. Each exercise montage is a blend of work and play — what's good for you and what feels good. Put these together in the right amounts and you will exercise forever.

> ### Advantages of a high VO₂Max
>
> Studies of top players in many non-racing sports show their oxygen-consumption rates to be modest. Even games like soccer, hockey, and basketball don't produce the high levels posted by endurance athletes. High VO_2 levels might prove useful in sports that don't specifically seem to require it. As we have mentioned, a high VO_2Max is almost always associated with slow resting pulse and a rapid return of the pulse following activity. Sports in which a number of sprints are called for consecutively make a quick pulse return a real advantage: a wide receiver running a series of completed pass patterns without interruption; in tennis, during especially long ralleys, going from base line to net with plenty of cross-court action; in soccer the readiness to resume at high tilt after the briefest time-outs; in boxing the minute between rounds allowing for quicker restoration after 3 minutes of hard give and take.

ADDITIONAL REWARDS

Interesting things may happen when your Heavyhands technique includes sports moves. Those with an aversion to exercise for its own sake may find this attitude changing as their workouts take on a new "practicality." Training may lose the chorelike quality that rankles some. Indeed, using sports moves in the aerobic mode may convert some people to exercise movements less wed to the specific mechanics of play. I have witnessed "players" shift allegiance to the more disciplined art of exercise. I am not antisports. But weekend athletes should remember that sports, even though they involve relatively modest workloads, when played hard are far more apt

> ### The Doctrine of Specificity
>
> As with any doctrine, practicing the specific moves by which to win at sports can reach the hazardous extreme. Money may, ironically, make things worse: Practicing the skill that earns one's *living* could produce a seemingly good excuse for not looking after the bigger issue called *life*.

Track and field

Reading through Ken Doherty's classic encyclopedic "Omnibook" devoted to the subject of road and track, I decided Heavyhands is the way to train. I put the question: locked in a small room with no more than 25 pounds of total equipment, how could one best train for that most elite of contests, the decathlon? Heavyhands won, hands down! Here are the individual events:

> 100-meter dash
> Long jump
> Shot put
> High jump
> 400-meter dash
> High hurdle
> Discus
> Pole vault
> Javelin
> 1500-meter run

I must admit the hurdles, pole vault, and high jump lose something in translation, but then with little space and lots of time one could train Heavyhanded for a marathon too, and even Decathletes don't do well in long races, ordinarily.

to injure than the higher workloads of more controlled endurance exercise. Competition motivates many sports players, but others may tire of the pain of habitual loss or find the joy of easy victory less than transporting after a while.

A growing number of elite and professional athletes, coaches, and trainers the world over have taken to Heavyhands as a main training strategy. As of this writing the list includes: tennis, hockey, boxing, cross-country and downhill skiers, baseball and softball, football, swimming, Karate and other martial arts, sprinters, long-distance runners, triathletes, power lifters, body builders, track and field specialists, and racquetball.

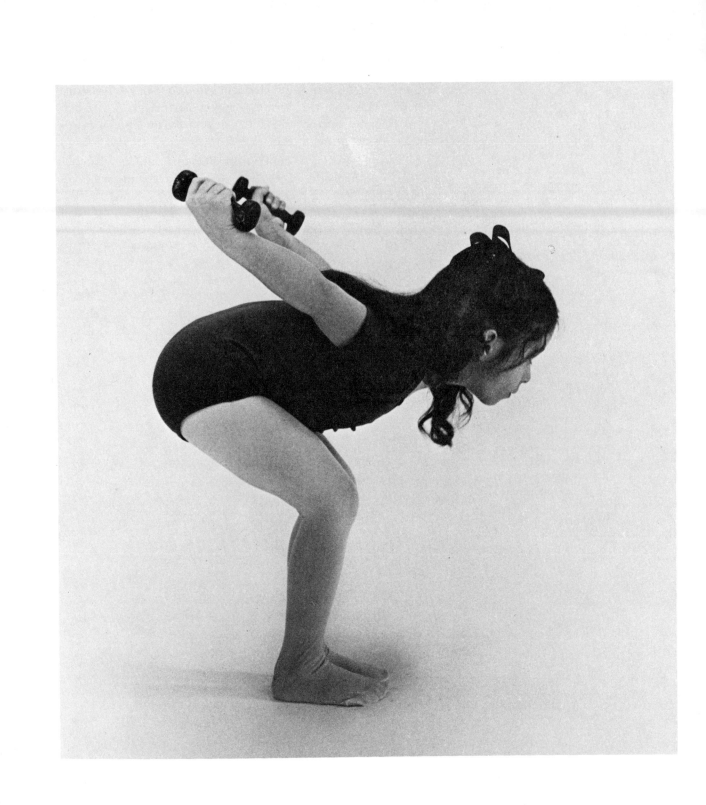

14

Heavyhands and Injuries

THE SUBJECT OF INJURY is too broad and complicated for me to deal with exhaustively here even if I were an expert, which I'm not. So what follows is a rough summary of what I've gleaned as a physician, from my reading, and from my own experience as a runner, as a swimmer, and as a Heavyhander. Millions of runners have taught us how the lower limbs respond to repeated pounding and a few things about prevention and cure of injury. I believe that a diversified program of Heavyhands will result, workload for workload, in fewer sidelining injuries, because that's been my experience as a "laboratory animal" and as a teacher of the method.

Since many Heavyhands moves don't include the actual foot strikes of running, the method enjoys some automatic protection. But even when you are running, the inevitably slower motion that results from carrying weights provides additional insurance against injury. Handweights do increase the *strain* on muscles, ligaments, and joint structures, both directly in the upper extremities and indirectly on the legs that support these extra burdens. But those weights *strengthen* and thus *protect*.

THE LEG

Generally, the leg is well equipped to endure the added burdens of Heavyhands. When one considers the enormous poundages weight lifters manage, the weights encountered with Heavyhands are tiny by comparison. This is not to say that Heavyhands work doesn't significantly increase leg strength, which is further buttressed by the endurance developed.

Risk obviously increases as one approaches extremes of weight or pace. Keeping that in mind, every Heavyhander should approach his or her exercise sessions at least vaguely aware of where he or she is with respect to the chance of injury.

THE UPPER TORSO

The upper torso may be more vulnerable. First of all, since the exercise is unique, everyone is a beginner. There are great differ-

---

Speed freaking

Some humans are speed freaks. They seek every opportunity to go fast and yet faster. It is interesting to note that fast hands are less apt to produce strains and sprains and other miseries than fast feet, especially if you get fast gradually.

Heavyhands running and injuries

You may or may not win your next 10-, 15-, or 42-kilometer race after you've become a member of the Heavyhands tribe, but I'll bet you'll injure less frequently and severely. Runners can become a lot stronger without increasing their muscle mass. And I'll warrant that those increases in strength will not reduce your speed. Many run faster.

ences among beginners, however, in terms of shoulder girdle and arm strength. Strength athletes, such as weight lifters, may be surprised at their rapid fatigue, even using weights only a small fraction of what they've been accustomed to. They may run some risk of injury because of their understandable failure to respect the stresses generated by moderate weights moved rapidly and repeatedly. Curiously, some people totally inexperienced in strength exercise are better able to tolerate the *gradual* increases that make for injury-free progress.

ACHES AND PAINS

Thus far I have not heard of one stress fracture sustained during Heavyhands training — nor a herniated disc, nor the gross tear of a single muscle. Any of those can, and probably will, happen once the ranks of Heavyhanders have grown sufficiently. My best guess, based on what I've learned during the past five years, is that the most frequent difficulties will come from sore tendons and an assortment of mild annoyances about the shoulder, elbow, and neck, especially the trapezius muscles. A bursa may become inflamed here and there, and a few of the exercises could cause a backache if improperly performed or overdone. Most of these are minor afflictions at worst, and usually will not stop the exercise. And with the relatively low leg-injury rate, exercise will almost never be halted outright. In fact, Heavyhands may produce the lowest rate of injury in relation to workload of any known exercise. In experimenting over the past five years, I have had my share of little aches and pains. Most have resulted from calculated risks taken at the brink of my own strength and endurance. None has resulted in a missed workout. Compared to running's alleged 54- to 72-percent casualty rate, the Heavyhander is heavily ensured against damage.

Sore muscles will always continue to accompany hard exercise. But the wide range of Heavyhands movement and the unusual upper-torso workloads will pay off. With Heavyhands, few sports moves and even fewer everyday chores will produce muscle or joint soreness. Even minor pulls, strains, or aches become less likely if one anticipates and gradually introduces new kinds of exertion during his daily workouts.

> **Hamstring woes and Heavyhands**
>
> I know I keep harping on the subject of sore hamstrings, but I don't suffer alone. Anyone who risks running fast is a potential victim. I love to run interval 220s uphill for kicks. Two years ago I did so at my continuing peril. If you are a victim of this, try double ski-poling and stretch-strength-strides. They may not cure you, but then you probably wouldn't be trying them if anything else had!

THE SAFEST APPROACH

The safest approach combines caution with vigor in proportions that approach neither foolhardiness nor hypochondria. Risk is greatest when trying new movements and when increasing workload. Those changes require active vigilance and willingness *to stop* the particular activity at the subtle border between slight overuse and frank hurt. Each of us learns in time, at the cost of a few errors on the wrong side of discretion; *no one*, alas, can really tell you how to avoid injury *absolutely*.

It would be wonderful to go through one's life freewheeling and hurt-free, but the way most of us are built the heart is able to fuel our skeletal muscles to the point of overuse injury. Heavyhands attempts to deal with this perilous balance by strengthening the muscles—altering their structure and function so that they can continue to receive the trained heart's bountiful supply of oxygen without jeopardy to themselves. One of Heavyhands' great advantages is its *panaerobic quality*. The workloads are not concentrated on a few muscles, but spread throughout almost the entire musculature.

THE GROUND RULES FOR HEAVYHANDS SAFETY

1. Arm and shoulder injuries are most apt to occur when moving a relatively *heavy* weight at a *faster*-than-usual velocity. One false move—one extraordinary effort—can do the damage. Unfortunately, healing is a far slower process. When you decide to increase handweight or work at a faster-than-usual tempo with your usual poundage, i.e., when you increase workload, start out with *short intervals* at the new level, extending them gradually during subsequent workouts as they prove safe.

2. Injury is also apt to occur when you employ muscle groups you haven't previously pushed during sports or work. Sudden extensions of the range of motion beyond the usual use can injure them. Your common sense, judgment, and self-awareness play a large role in protecting you.

Sore elbows, again

Level III pumping is for many another good preventative of the sore-elbow syndrome. Since adding substantial amounts of it to my workouts, I've noticed no local tenderness whatever. I haven't yet figured why the move helps. My best hunch now is the "more muscle hypothesis"—big work shared by lots of groups, thus diluting the strain at the lateral epicondyle. Third-level movements should be jaunty and relaxed, and neither overwed to short- or long-lever movement.

3. Pay attention to what your body tells you. Even moderate exercise probably causes miscroscopic injuries among the muscle fibers involved. These heal rapidly and, aside from mild and temporary local discomfort, are not likely to stall the motivated exerciser. Once an injury and its associated spasm reach our consciousness there is a warning, an inhibiting effect that cancels the pleasure-in-motion we normally get from our workouts. In effect, if it hurts, stop.

4. Shun or bypass inhibiting injuries. The Heavyhands repertoire provides good alternatives. As an example, when I've overdone punching with heavier than typical weights, I feel the characteristic soreness at the outside of my elbows. In effect, I have mild tennis elbow, two of them, in fact, because my work is symmetrical. Warned by that ache, I switch to short levers like pump 'n' run moves for my workouts, uninhibted by any sensation of discomfort. In a day or two, restored, I can return to a full range of combinations, wiser for the experience and less apt to repeat the overuse. Injuries sustained during exercise are on the whole highly localized, so that the contraction of adjacent muscles may continue painlessly.

5. Being too cautious can injure you. Ofttimes a muscle is stiff simply from unusual usage, like the sore arms we came to expect as kids every spring when our enthusiasm overrode good judgment. The next day it was painful even to toss a baseball, but we knew that we could "work it out" after a few minutes of throwing. And so it is with the garden variety of stiffness encountered during Heavyhands exercise. Soon one comes to intuit which hurts require rest and which can be safely worked through. At times your best guesses will be wrong, whereupon you simply rest up or bypass the hurt. There is a well-recognized danger in being overconservative. Habitually "resting" rather than mobilizing leads to further limitation of motion, which ultimately means more pain with any activity.

6. Weekend heroics produce lots of injuries. Many who work out at modest levels of intensity and duration on weekdays may try to cram in as much extra as possible on days off. Indeed, there is some sound physiological justification for this. There are indications that runners have maintained high levels of oxygen-consuming capacity by a *single prolonged* run each week. Studies also point to reduced incidence of injury when runners work three or four

Jumping and morning foot pain

Most jumping involves the balls of the feet. There may be some morning spasm in the sole of the foot, especially near the heel. It's mostly true in beginners, and can be helped a good bit by alternately lifting and depressing the toes so as to stretch the calves and anterior shin muscles, holding each position for 20 to 30 seconds. In any event, the discomfort is usually self-limited, disappearing within a few minutes once you're up and about.

Time-out from exercise

I don't know that a holiday from exercise is always a bad idea. I managed a few of these when swimming and running were my pet aerobic preoccupations. At nearly fifty-seven I can't chance the long layoff that at twenty-one wouldn't have fazed me. Now I covet fitness, one might say. Heavyhands allows me to train more intensively than most young people without risking a sidelining injury. I start each workout supremely confident that I will not injure. Most of my sessions are rigged to keep me at 90 or so percent of my VO_2Max. There are literally dozens of combinations that keep me where I want to be physiologically. I'll never quit. Not because I find exercise inordinately pleasurable — I simply can't afford to abandon the life-style it affords me. I don't want "holidays."

Pitcher's arm

As an erstwhile aspiring pitcher, I sometimes ponder the precarious health of some very talented pitching arms. I pore over the arithmetic of pitchers' lives: the number of pitches per game; the rest between innings and between games; the outrageous stresses to elbow and shoulder from the assortment of breaking pitches, change-ups, and knucklers. One day I tried to produce a sore arm or two by "mock" throwing alternately, two 10-pound weights for 5 minutes at 100 throws per minute. I sparked a 120 steady pulse, but my arm was limber as a strand of cooked spaghetti the next morning. Then I reasoned: it's not simply the hard work that's injuring our pitchers. It's the shearing forces, determined by the guts of the equation, force equals mass times acceleration; arms whipping toward the plate, accelerating the ball to close to 100 mph by the time the batter whacks at it, can injure. So I tried 200 pitches a minute for 5 minutes with 2-pounders. (A baseball weighs about 5.3 ounces.) My pulse reached 130 this time. Still spaghetti. Ball players may one day avoid layoffs and surgery through Heavyhands training and come off with VO$_2$Maxes better than they currently carry.

days rather than seven days per week. I would guess that experimenters with Heavyhands may run higher-than-average risk of upper-torso injury when they "double up," so to speak, on weekends early in the course of training. This risk stems in part, I expect, from the relatively deconditioned state of the upper extremity.

7. I must stress again the role of strength in the prevention of injury. Short, infrequent intervals with relatively heavy weights, aside from providing aerobic exercise, can help ensure some immunity from injury. Total time invested in these moves can be insignificant. I have seldom used very heavy weights for more than a *5-minute-weekly* total and for two years I've used none at all.

8. Anticipating the future, I am concerned about the invasion of Heavyhands by the human urge to compete. Despite platitudinous modifiers such as "friendly," "casual," and "good-natured," competition may be at the root of many of running's casualties, and I believe a similar fate could befall Heavyhands. Competition can produce an effect analogous to the severe injuries sustained during contact sports that become consciously painful only *after* the game is ended. In any event, group activities tend to lead some participants to be dangerously heedless of their body's condition and therefore subject to workloads that exceed their best training levels. Heavyhands group exercise can be particularly enjoyable if competition can be largely excluded. The interplay of so many variables promotes individualized performances, which make serious comparison with one's fellows farcical as well as dangerous. Even so, it would be naive to underestimate those motives that conspire to make winning so important. To restate the obvious: there can be little wisdom or virtue in making a horse race out of a technique whose very nature seeks uniqueness.

Many injuries occur in response to overt or unconscious needs to *win* over real or imagined adversaries. When that motive takes over, self-awareness and thus safety may dip — at times dangerously. Be honest about your competitiveness. Keeping it in mind can help preserve the joy of pain-free fitness.

COMMON COMPLAINTS AND THEIR ANTIDOTES

CURE FOR TENNIS ELBOW?

The "two tennis elbow syndrome" is probably unique to Heavy-handers and ambidextrous tennis players. I have developed a gim-mick that cures, without fail, my "lateral epicondylitis." I'll pass it on to you and you can try it even if you only have the one-sided variety. Actually you can use it either as preventative or as palliative once you've been smitten. Take one to three rubber bands, the wide ones, about ⅜-inch width or so, and place them around your fingers as shown. Starting from a closed fist, open your hand *hard,* fanning the extended fingers consciously against the resistance

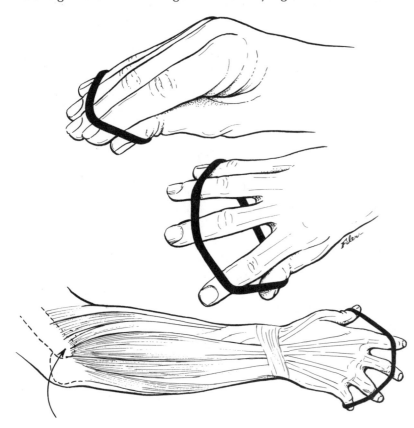

lateral epicondyle

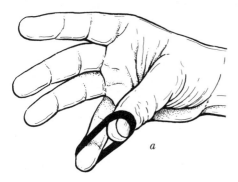

provided by the rubber bands. Add or subtract bands until you can do 20 to 30 repetitions. You will note some muscle activity about your lateral epicondyles (those bony protuberances at the outside of your elbows). That's because finger and wrist extensor muscles "originate" or attach there. Those muscles and their attachments are weak, since they get a little direct work in everyday life. I keep a few bands around all the time — only a minute or two of the exercise seems to do the trick.

TENDER KNEES

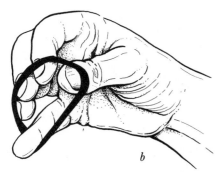

For those who use a lot of backaerobics such as double ski-poling, short-lever jackknifing, pump 'n' walk, and reach in their routines, another localized tenderness may occur. Because these exercises make demands upon the muscles of the thigh front—the quadriceps — there is bound to be more strain upon its tendon. The "quad" tendon "inserts" below the kneecap at the so-called tibial tubercle. So far a mild tenderness has occurred there in a few Heavyhanders who are especially enamored with these movements. It has always been self-limited and the soreness isn't evident unless you press at the point of the tendon's insertion. If such soreness bothers you unduly, switch to more "military" upright movements. Once you are well into your program, this problem tends to disappear.

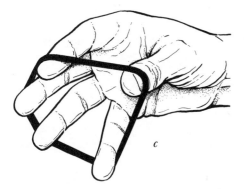

PSYCHOLOGICAL PROBLEMS OF INJURY

Sheer physical discomfort and interruption of exercise are not the only disadvantages of injury. For those who reach the happy stage of "positive addiction," prolonged sidelining may pose actual threats to psychic equilibrium. Depression and anxiety are common symptoms in injured and out-of-commission athletes and exercisers. The personality cannot always readily substitute for the loss of activity. A restive, agitated, "fish out of water" syndrome may follow; preoccupation and a sense of worthlessness may occur. It becomes increasingly important that we fashion exercises that allow for the development of great capacity, with minimal risk of serious injuries.

Engaging in exercise with a high risk of injury may place a pall of a sort on the activity. The performer, aware of the danger of the exercise in numerous and subtle ways, may hold back in training, especially if he or she has already suffered injury. Those who are injured frequently may unconsciously be looking to quit. Some injured exercisers may return to activity with considerably reduced enthusiasm and studiously lowered performance level. This "compromise" response usually falls below desired levels of fitness exercise can produce.

Overall high performance level with maximum sense of freedom and low real risk of serious injury is the ideal. Beyond these obvious criteria, the ideal exercise allows for continuation of some exercise after unavoidable injury has occurred. Our strategy, then, must be multifaceted to provide built-in alternatives without sacrificing any of the essential physiologic components of good exercise.

HEAVYHANDS AS PREVENTATIVE MEDICINE

Sports medicine suffers, as do other medical specialities, from the problem of frequently having to cure that which often could have been prevented. Weak muscles are liabilities simply because their vulnerability to overload is high. Once injured, recovery may be complicated. Pain precludes training. The time required to mend allows further weakening. When training *does* begin again it is often abandoned prematurely, or there's a greater risk of reinjury.

For runners, Heavyhands training reduces the notorious "anterior" weaknesses that lead to injuries. I recommend Heavyhands walking, doing the swagger, pump, and jackknife, and reach-variations once or twice weekly, using the heaviest weights that can be managed for short intervals (5 minutes a week, say). These will do wonders for the hip extensors, including the hamstrings that are so prone to injury. Heavyhands jumps in sensible, graded doses add the vertical strength lacking in so many runners. Double ski-poling will produce back, hip extensor, shoulder, and chest muscle strength and add suppleness to the runner's entire musculature.

Heavyhands kickbacks for hamstrings

I got to thinking about the too frequent hamstring injuries among middle-distance runners, soccer players, wide receivers, and such. Seems that the stretch-for-protection strategy may not always suffice. It occurred to me there's no good overkill tactic to strengthen the hamstrings for the kind of stress they're apt to receive during peak moments of competition. A few leg curls with heavy weights don't do the job and ordinary speed work at the track doesn't provide enough range of motion. So I devised a hamstring exercise that is the equivalent of fast arm-pumps. Doing pump 'n' run-in-place, I kick *back*, trying to hit my bottom with my alternately raised heels. A surprisingly fast pulse initially announces an expectable deficiency in the heart-hamstring duet. You can tune the workload by varying hand weight, pump frequency and range of motion. With light weights I kick back fast, going to Level III and lateral thrusts work just fine too. Do interval cycles (Chapter 16) to get going and try alternating the kickbacks with double-ski-poling in place or insert them into any medley. Don't be surprised if your sprint times, hill running, and hamstring comfort all improve from this prescription.

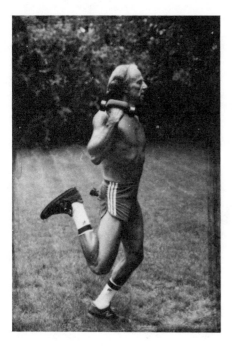

The same prescription will tend to protect the serious swimmer from his all-too-common back and shoulder injuries. Swimmers all need antigravity work, not so much to enhance their swimming, but to fit them out more solidly for their lives out of the pool.

Heavyhands dancing has proven beneficial for a variety of mild injuries associated with sports and exercise. The combination of strength and grace required, the constantly changing patterns, the stretchlike movements, and the psychic effects of music may all help. A half-hour of dance after a hard run that's taken its toll on my blighted left hamstring always leaves me restored and pain-free.

In Heavyhands exercise the distribution of the workload, the diversity of movement angles and planes, and the reduction in the number of traumatic "strikes" make for greater safety relative to the workload level than do conventional endurance strategies.

All this notwithstanding, any exercise ambitious enough to reap rich fitness returns is potentially injurious. One point I cannot overstress: *listen to your body.* Part of the adventure of exercise is finding that narrow zone that lies between fitness and injury. It is a tribute to the central nervous system that many negotiate that "zone" safely for years. Delicate "feedback" signals tell you when to push and when to lay back. But you must learn to pay attention.

A final note about stretching. My experience suggests that the strength-endurance combination along with the *dynamic* stretching (stretching muscles in motion) inherent in many Heavyhands movements will go far to prevent injury. This proves particularly true for those who use Heavyhands as their *primary* exercise. When Heavyhands serves as a filler for runners and other aerobic exercise some static stretching (stretching immobilized muscles) may be a usefully complement. Only plenty of trial runs — erring initially on the side of caution — can structure a program containing what *you* need in the way of the warm-up and stretch elements that make for optimal safety.

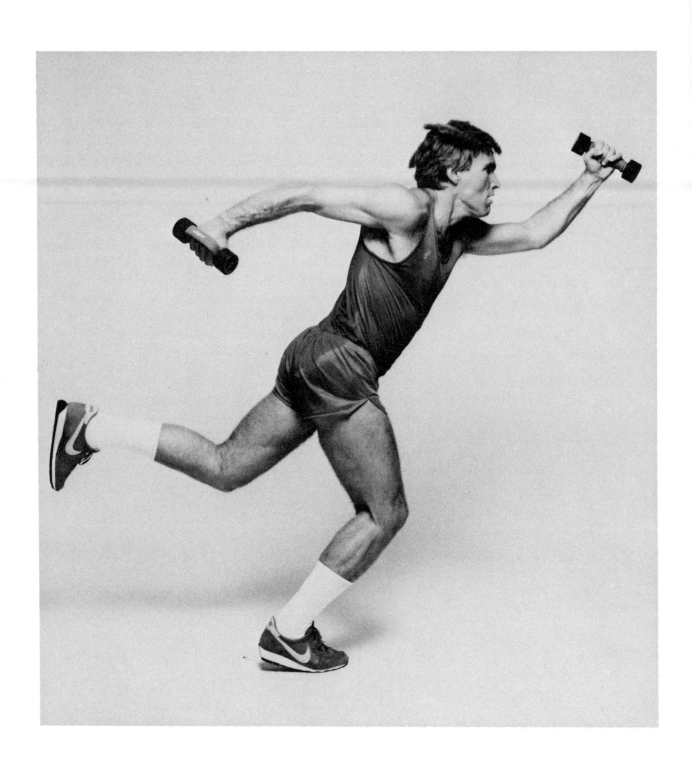

15

Fat: Fact and Fallacy

I TRY TO KEEP my excitement about Heavyhands' impact upon body fat control "scientifically" muted. Such carefulness is well warranted because a wide range of treatment strategies have taken center stage, enjoyed brief acceptance, then faded like their predecessors. It's axiomatic in medical circles that the more varied the "cures" for a given ailment, the poorer the cure rate. And that's precisely where we stand in relation to the relentless, frustrating crusade against extra fat.

Most exercise manuals start out by stressing the inescapable importance of activity in weight control. Most of those hedge their bets by including diet tactics as well. So many books seesaw uncertainly between diet and exercise. This one doesn't! Hardly heedless of the fact that starvation will make you skinny, I'm dead set, philosophically and physiologically, against diet as a primary choice for anyone interested in a good body as a permanent vehicle for their life. In a nation where 98 percent of the diets are doomed to final failure, I can't do much worse. I'll air some of my convictions about the fat problem generally, then end it on a more specific note.

PILLS

Hope has blossomed from time to time. We used to think a pill could do it. For years the appetite-diminishing properties of amphetamines and like preparations were pressed into vigorous, if ineffectual, service. Some bariatricians, those physicians who specialize in overweight, continue to prescribe combinations of chemical agents thought to help the victim of obesity. But research suggests, alas, that the effect, if any, of amphetamine as a controller of appetite is shortlived. Besides, there is a real risk of dangerous habituation.

DIETS

With the decline of hope for a wonderous pill, diet, a less magical panacea, got a new lease on its marketable life. Diet books hit the bestseller list in rapid sequence, each fading as hotter items take their place. Diets have became favorite small talk. Does one count calories or carbohydrates? How do you go the high-protein route without consuming too much fat? What's with vitamins? The role of diet in blood-vessel disease? The place of trace minerals? Bee pollen? Fructose? Natural foods? And since the credentialed experts differ among themselves, what is the baffled customer to do?

Obesity may be compared with aging in that its disadvantages run parallel. Most readers who dabble in matters of health can recite the risk factors associated with overweight as well as I. Hypertension, diabetes, and cardiovascular disease; renal and pulmonary problems; gall bladder and obstetrical complications. The social and employment problems of the obese are well documented. And so it is with aging.

CAUSE OF OBESITY

The important writers and researchers in the field of obesity have all mentioned the role of activity in its cause and cure. The arithmetic is unassailable. If you eat more calories than you expend in activity, you simply will *store fat*, molecule by inevitable molecule — either just beneath your skin or elsewhere in your body. This is one of those unimpeachable bits of logic. A professor I know once tried to convince me that *ignorance* of the facts of nutrition was the chief culprit in the *cause* of obesity. Presented with the realities, however harsh, the heretofore uninformed should, he thought, be quite capable of becoming and staying slim. The fact is, the information spewed by the media nowadays isn't helping much. The statistics on obesity grow worse and promise to continue to do so at an even faster rate. Authorities hint that early in the twenty-first century fully 60 percent of us will be classifiable as obese unless some radical change occurs in our feeding habits.

WHY EVERYTHING WORKS AT FIRST

Behavior modification is a recent addition to the war against spreading obesity. Essentially calculated to organize behavior into manageable parcels, it has enjoyed spotty success. By the way, everything that's tried seems to be greeted by early success. The diet game, played perhaps more enthusiastically in this country than abroad, panders to the Fleeting Hope Syndrome, which is related to the

Fat and energy

Americans cumulatively carry about 500,000 tons of extra blubber beneath their skins. At 9.3 calories per gram, that represents fuel enough to power a fair-sized town or two for a year! More importantly, the subtle to blatant motor disability that extra avoirdupois produces may actually increase our fuel bills: fitness produces both better tolerance for cold and heat and fewer fiddlings with the thermostat.

What's wrong with diets?

Only that most proceed upon a spurious basis which panders to the shortsighted motives of some very intelligent people. One diet fiasco doesn't disturb me. It's the recycled ritual — blind to the past, hightailing it toward an almost certain repeated failure — that makes me worry.

The body-weight question

If you haven't asked yourself how strong, speedy, supple, graceful, coordinated, and balanced you should be — the question of how much you should weigh is probably meaningless!

What should Heavyhanders eat?

The nutritional requirements for Heavyhands trainers do not differ appreciably from those of other endurance exercisers. High-carbohydrate diets — mostly the complex variety: potatoes, breads, rice, cereals, pastas, with little of the refined sugars — are "in" these days. Protein requirements, formerly pushed by nutritionists, have fallen to something below the traditional 1 gram per kilo of body weight per day. Fats should probably be restricted to 15 to 25 percent of one's caloric intake. The trick may be to eat as much as you can without gaining weight. That means plenty of chow and plenty of work. I admit to abject ignorance where it comes to the subtleties of nutrition: the pros and cons of rare minerals and extra vitamins leave me uncertain at best. Where it comes to vitamins, one is faced with an ironic dilemma: if you eat enough food you don't usually need them, and if you're starving there's nothing for vitamins to do, since they are catalysts of chemical processes that involve what you've eaten!

same urge that motivates gambling or other versions of the need to strike it rich. On a new diet kick, touted by friends as surefire, the overplump adventurer seems strangely oblivious of his or her own past failures. Hope springs eternal, often unsupported by solid justification or even the laws of probability. The vast majority of dieters live out their lives delivering sops to a conscience by the act of *trying*. From Mayo, Stillman, and Atkins, to the Drinking Man's to the Scarsdale diets, we shift fickle allegiance from one promise to the next. The diet philosophy plays very heavily upon what the infantile conscience is all about: crime and punishment. Endless cycles of it. Eat and transgress; then diet in guilt-erasing penance. Those mechanisms were lodged in our makeup long before our weight became a worrisome focus. The diet game seems to be another variation of human neuroticism. Marketing resourcefulness simply exploits our constant concern over our health and silhouettes.

WHY SO MANY DIFFERENT DIETS?

That the various dieting strategies differ so and the statistics are so poor tends to make one wonder if dieting will ever solve the problem. The nature of the individual, the seriousness and the duration of his affliction, and his motives are probably surer predictors of a given diet's success than the specifics of the eating ritual being hyped at the moment. Even nutrition, a presumably more scientifically based area, doesn't have all the answers. We know that we *all* need *enough* food to support our metabolism as well as the expanded requirements of growth and the fueling of extra workloads of any sort. And we need vitamins to keep our biochemical apparatus turning out the essentials that we derive from food. How much of these we need beyond what we got in the food we eat is debatable. We need protein because it's an important component of our cellular structure and requires replenishing at some — again, debatable — rate. It's nearly impossible to feed totally fat-free, but too much fat is risky, apparently more in some than in others, because of differences in our genes. And we need lots of water because body chemistry doesn't work without it. And some say we should dispense with "junk food," laden with refined sugars. What *is* important is that dieting for weight loss is only indirectly related to the subject of nutrition. Whatever the specifics of a diet, it's the reduction of *calories* that causes one to shed weight.

The diet innovator concocts some combination of foods sufficiently tolerable to gratify the dieter while holding back the calorie allowance. Diets evidently don't succeed over the long pull. Usually the early "honeymoon" phase of the diet is launched into enthusiastically because the scale indicates rapid weight loss (which is usually derived from water loss).

Within the frustrating game of weight losing, the dieter can prove his system effective. If the diet works — a dubious grammatic construction to begin with — that is to say, if he deprives himself sufficiently, he *loses body mass*. But what were the other contributors? Activity? Depression? Metabolic speeders? Pure grit? Blatant fear of losing something as dear as health or even life itself? With all the factors one could mix into the complicated thing called *motivation, starvation,* however elegantly rigged, appears to *work,* at least temporarily. The "diet" seems to lend authority, medical sanction, and even the fantasy of safety to an operation that runs against the grain of one of our strongest instincts toward survival — feeding.

> **Scales**
>
> A scale is a gadget that measures how hard we are being pulled toward the earth's center. The scale includes a tricky way of converting that force into numbers that apparently have meaning. The act of weighing-in seems innocent enough; simply the need for information about ourselves. After a while the weighing ritual may take on symbolic meaning also: an act of contrition following a bout of gluttony; or proof that we're "trying." Ever watch the deliberate care with which some step onto a scale? As though hoping their worst premonitions won't be realized! Stepping off the scale the corners of the mouth move either north or south. Emotion should be reserved for sterner stuff.

YOU CAN'T BEAT EATING

Let me quickly add another basic theory or two relating to obesity. The mouth and its data-processing equipment are a hard act to beat. By this I mean that our taste buds are the least *ambiguous,* most gratifyingly predictable of our sense organs. When we pop a generous bit of buttery chocolate into our mouths, we come closest to seeking and accomplishing precisely what we set out to do. That chocolate dainty may be the symbolic equivalent of mother's milk — the gratifying, unqualified, deliciousness of the here-and-now taste, the special sensation yearned for and instantly realized, which just can't be beaten or analyzed out of its special, primal pleasure. As powerful as is the sex drive, it is for most a timorous and intermittent one compared to the urge toward three square meals and more.

We all would like to be gorgeous and well fed at the same time. Let's look at the national sihouette for a few depressing moments.

Ideal physiques are scarce as hen's teeth. If 100,000,000 or so of us are not classifiable as blatantly fat, but are within range of the cherished body beautiful, why do we so consistently fail to achieve it? Losing weight for *appearance's sake* doesn't appear to work. Yet appearance looms as the most conscious and compelling motive. Health less so, perhaps.

The dieter about to embark on his journey toward slimmer proportions is not apt to be honest with himself. While his expectations are huge and urgent, they are dissociated from the difficulty he is likely to encounter in getting there. A *number* is chosen from the doctor's weight charts and often becomes a preoccupation — a symbol to defeat or be defeated by; a cause for senseless celebration or equally senseless despair; a benchmark full of magic that makes us victims of fad, tireless investors in sure losers, bettors on the 20-to-1 shot the average dieter is up against. That's the bottom line: only one out of twenty dieters takes — and keeps — weight off.

That would explain the large number of people who *lose* weight compared to the number who *remain* lean. It's a cyclic business and typical of all addictions characterized by a pattern: a strong resolve; early success at self-deprivation; some sort of disappointment; abandonment of the resolve; return with full force to the addiction — at which point the cycle tends to repeat. A food addiction is usually mild compared with other kinds. Think of it. Very few people gain 100 pounds a year. Yet 930 extra calories per day will accomplish that neatly. A few daily mouthfuls of ice cream above one's food requirement can add 25 pounds in a year. And fortunately, not many of us do *that*.

Exercise and risk

It may be said that exercise is somewhat risky business, especially as one approaches the extremes: not at all or too much.

Health cost

Everyone knows nothing useful comes without some cost. Why, then, do we complain so over the modest ante of time and sweat that pays for a life-style that seems too good to relinquish?

EXERCISE AS THE SOLUTION

During the five years of my experiments with Heavyhands I consumed enough food to have gained, conservatively, 250 pounds, based on my prior activity level and eating habits. That means my activity used up 400 or so extra calories each day, on the average. A bit more, actually, because I lost some 15 pounds during that interval. *There was never any conscious attempt to lose weight.* I simply failed at times to eat enough to replenish the calories I lost during my exercise. But since my strength increased as well as my muscle endurance, it is likely that my lean body weight increased somewhat. So, effectively, I was burning skinfold fat that I didn't replace, while adding a few ounces of muscle here and there.

My five-year experience accomplished what every ambitious diet does in terms of pounds. *There the similarity ends.* First off, I was not on a reducing diet. I indulged myself as I never have during my adult life. Prior to the program I had been a typical ten-pound-dieter, sliding upward for a year or so then taking a couple of months to lose it simply by stopping all eating after dinner. My experience during these past five years could have been likened to that of Jean Mayer's rats. Mayer is the famous researcher who established unequivocally the crucial relationship between activity and the problem of obesity. His rats, exercised on a wheel for varying intervals each day, established dietary patterns that accurately mirrored their exercise time. I, too, found myself eating amounts that reflected that day's exercise.

If indeed I was unconcerned about weight loss, what *was* I concerned about? Training. I was busy experimenting with exercise, its effects upon my cardiopulmonary function, my strength, endurance, power, skill, etc. As it turned out, it changed my body structure somewhat.

But while that was happening I did a good bit of thinking about the overall legitimacy of exercise as *the supreme weight-controlling device.* I started with the proven premise that the dieter's overall track record is nothing to write home about. Statistics vary, but finally only between 2 to 9 percent of dieters manage to *keep lost weight off for good.* The fact that most serious endurance athletes become and remain lean is clearly important. I was naturally interested in Heavyhands' potential effect in weight control compared with other aerobic methods.

WORKLOAD PARALLELS CALORIE LOSS

Workloads and calorie loss are, in fact, different expressions for the same phenomenon. We can calculate the mechanical work done in units of distance times force, i.e., foot-pounds. We can measure a working subject's oxygen consumption because experiment has shown that to be a very good measure of how much the *whole body* is doing. It's an easy matter to calculate how many pounds will be

---

Diet and exercise intensity

I have a feeling that Americans are more willing to exercise *long* than *hard.* Keeping score sneakily, my estimates would be that 90 percent of those I watch exercise somewhere below an intensity of 10 METs. True enough, 10 METs is better than nothing, but low-intensity exercise may help explain both the loud grousing over the time required and the erratic weight-loss patterns experienced by some exercisers. Sometimes the "word" exercise takes on an aura of magic. The inexorable numbers, the METs times minutes, are often ignored outright. The simple fact that one has "exercised" does not turn the trick. One nice lady I know was close to despair when her dutiful hour-a-day exercise ritual left her clothes snugger than before. Analysis showed a fast resting pulse and that her "exercises," performed at an energy cost of about 200 calories per hour, left her short of target pulse. The "real" magic of exercise is to be found in the growth of training effects. Consuming calories even at a *slow rate,* 3 extra minutes of munching daily can undo an hour of low-intensity work.

Set-point theory

Laboratory animals — force-fed to obesity — will return to their normal body weights when allowed to eat at will. Similarly, animals thinned by starvation, given ordinary diets, will quickly regain their former body weights. Dr. Richard Keesey advances an interesting hypothesis. Strict maintenance of a given body weight whether above or below the norm seems to be the rule. Huge increases in food intake as well as significant restrictions fail to produce the predicted upward or downward changes in body weight. In animals these "set points" are rather uniform, e.g., one seldom sees a fat giraffe. In humans these well-defended "set points" run the wide gamut suggested by merely people watching from any crowded street corner. Alterations in energy output, i.e., metabolic rate and activity, are the best explanations offered for rigid fixing of individuals to a given body weight over a span of years. We're left, however, with the knotty problem as to why humans latch onto a particular body weight so tenaciously. Whatever the mechanisms, the ability to vary our energy output over the widest range of workloads seems the best antidote to set points that are too high. Given high fitness levels the set point can be aggressively selected and consciously maintained. The fittest among us may thus come to enjoy the weight control commonly observed in laboratory rats!

lost because it's been determined that roughly 3,500 calories is the equivalent of one pound of body weight.

Heavyhanders, by the nature of the workloads they generate, produce greater calorie losses per minute than do conventional exercisers. Running with weights I consume more oxygen than I can without them, by an impressive margin. We discovered that total workload, expressed in terms like strength, muscle endurance, and speed-power, applied to all or nearly all of the muscles, could make a telling difference. Why simply run in place when one could do that with weights, eventually performing larger amounts of work and conditioning more of one's musculature? Why limit oneself to short levers alone when simple experiment has taught us that long levers might produce bigger output per minute as well as other useful training effects? We discovered that generalized strength, endurance, and speed-power were not only boosters of cardiopulmonary functions, they were useful in living — both work and play time — and could do for body-weight control what literally *nothing* in the way of conventional exercise could.

Supplied by the oxygen-transport system, combined strength and endurance tends to *incinerate fat and build muscle simultaneously.* Thus body composition can be ideally altered within the scope of a single comprehensive strategy. A program including both weight lifting and running *might* produce such a change. But the time consumed could become prohibitive and could *not* produce the general level of muscle endurance and cardiopulmonary endurance we're talking about. And the small numbers of repetitions typical of weight training can't dispatch the number of calories Heavyhands can.

OBESITY WILL NOT BE CONQUERED SO LONG AS DIETING REMAINS A NATIONAL PREOCCUPATION

The removal of fat by activity is vastly superior to dieting in a number of ways. The addition of activity to your life as a conscious, practiced, growing project assures you of the kinds of success that parallel training effect. Jean Mayer's rats maintain their body weight by some sort of intuitive feeding behavior. Yet the human cortex, fashioned for poetry and calculus and string quartets, seems unable to solve the problem of regulating its own body's mass.

The accomplished practitioner of exercise may free himself forever from the preoccupation with something that should be as self-regulated as breathing. The function shapes the structure, which is why no one can know, before achieving it, what his ideal weight should be.

THE FICTIONAL END POINT

The fallacy embodied in most weight-reduction schemes is the fictional end point, a magical moment when the travail is over and the payoff begins. Since our physiology and our psyches aren't built that way, since our appetites remain formidable for a lifetime, any program that offers a "promised land" is an almost certain loser. Of course, one can, and will, opt for another diet, preserving the belief that a "right answer" exists, somehow, somewhere, out there.

If in the course of dieting someone drops to the yearned-for weight, nothing in particular happens to herald the event. After a brief acknowledgment by more perceptive friends, the matter is brushed aside. Stripped before his mirror, the "successful" dieter appears not strikingly different or beautiful, but quite himself, somewhat shrunken. Surface improvement has been disappointing, appetite remains demanding, and the weight is regained once more. When the scale tips near the top of their typical gain-loss pattern, the number takes on a frightening significance: symbolic loss of love, health, youth, or a combination of these may produce panic in some. So, again, they dutifully swear off indulgence, decide to be "good." The process typically aborts for one reason or another and then repeats again and again.

RATIONAL BODY WEIGHT AND THE NEUROTIC FAT PAD

Why do we so consistently settle for anything but what I call *rational bodyweight*? Much of the multibillion-dollar spa-emporium business flourishes around the issue of *looks*. Indeed the few extra pounds almost all of us carry probably don't increase health risks significantly in most instances. And overeating is not the problem, either. Poising our body weight 10 to 15 pounds above the "rational," most

A weight in hand is worth twice as much on the body

Researchers recently learned that holding a given weight in the hands makes for twice the workload produced if the equivalent weight were part of the exerciser's body. Pumping the weight is, of course, another matter. Weights attached to the feet exact six times the work as would that amount of additional body weight. Added foot weight soon becomes onerous, however, slowing the runner to a snail's pace before much has been added. Pumping hand-held iron does it all; it makes for large workloads that prove to be well tolerated for long hauls. For example, 3-pound weights pumped to Level III at a brisk (150 short paces per minute) become the work equivalent of moving 2.5 to 3 times my entire body weight at an identical speed, unencumbered!

The "add" point

The add point in Heavyhands training is achieved when combined exercise becomes a measurable advantage in oxygen transport; when arms plus legs produce greater total work than legs alone can. Nothing dramatic announces one's arrival at the add point; only a gradual sense of everything pulling together more effectively. Some become aware of it when body fat disappears at a noticeably more rapid rate despite no increase in either total training time or feeding pattern. I noticed it when I found that I no longer had to weight-watch.

Are fat and thin opposites?

An academic question, surely. Better put: Is it *useful* to view them as opposites? I think not.

Supposing, for example, we decided to look upon fat and thin as variations on a single theme of "appearance consciousness" rather than as opposites. Muscularity might be considered the opposite of "appearance consciousness," standing for a peculiar style of the mind-body in which *doing* things outweighs the importance of the surface appearance of things. This is not pure whimsy. The people I know who are muscular types are the ones who seem most immune to the capricious woes and pleasures that "fat consciousness" has become these days.

The problem isn't simple. Old preoccupations just like old shoes aren't abandoned without a tinge of grief and are not easily replaced. For many, body fat may have become a whopping symbol — too dear simply to cancel. In many people I've studied, it has seemed at times a cross to bear, an unconscious spoiler of dangerous beauty, a badge of helplessness, a "reason" for loneliness and invisibility, and even a body-clay to be fashioned with enthusiasm and determination. But if appearance must remain a high priority item, muscle definition might be the most useful "preoccupation." To gain those valued "rips" or "cuts," the high rep format of Heavyhands is the premier tactic and the heart is not neglected.

of us *keep it there*. The decision to diet is prompted when our weight rises above our more typical overweight condition.

Do we really prize our looks as much as we claim or do our taste buds simply override everything else? As a psychiatrist I believe we've a lot to learn about ourselves from the study of this stubborn deviation from a bodily condition we apparently prize but seldom achieve. I call it the problem of the *neurotic fat pad*. As a nation we have focused our attention on that intolerable, but fixed, layer of blubber. We flirt with it mentally, knead and massage it, label it variously, starve it periodically, replenish it, gape at it, worry incessantly over it, and in the last analysis seem to maintain it with almost religious fervor. People without it are readily countable: the serious exercisers, those with wasting or catastrophic illness, the congenital hyperactives, the compulsive starvers. Almost everyone else carries the omnipresent fat pad, usually around their middles, as a shibboleth of the "good life" managed unwisely.

I think the 10 to 20 pounds we store beneath our skins is the equivalent of other *inertial problems*. As a nation we learn to read, steady out at 300 or so words per minute, and *stay put:* we develop any of our activities to a certain level of performance, let them grow into our stereotyped definitions of work and leisure, and seldom reorder them consciously. The training effect, the keystone of body fitness, seldom pervades our lives. Our stubborn acceptance of sameness makes us curious prey to fads. Most diets may be defined as fads having to do with food and body contour. A fad is a form of altered behavior that, among other things, grants us a brief sense of belonging to our social order. Fads, by their very nature, come and go, often before their validity, or lack thereof, is established. People who indulge in fads don't usually learn from the experience, and making the manipulation of body fat a central concern is a sure, salable gimmick. Recycled problems guarantee future sales. Again, I would predict that so long as the motive holds sway, we've small chance of beating obesity, short of a national famine. I'd suggest that the treatment of individual and national obesity proceed in three stages:

WHAT'S TO BE DONE

1. Diets must be recognized simply for what they are. We should view them as temporary, stopgap means at best, seldom *lasting* solutions. Even when they do work, the "lean body product" derived from dieting exclusively must be acknowledged to be second rate. The more activity is used to solve the problem of weight control entirely, the closer one approaches nature's way. In the interest of health, diets should be employed judiciously when the cardiopulmonary apparatus and/or the neuromuscular system cannot handle the workload required to control weight effectively. Incidentally, even many cardiacs would *not* require diets using those criteria.

2. The total abandonment of dieting for the purpose of weight control. This would exclude only a few medical problems. Activity would become the accepted preventative of obesity in all but the few glandular disturbances which require appropriate medical management.

3. During this final phase the concept of weight control itself *would simply have disappeared as a conscious motive.* Understanding of the problem would have evolved to the degree that control of body weight would constitue an implicit routine, seldom an explicit concern. Like Jean Mayer's exercising rats, nutrition would become intrinsically associated with activity. Scales would disappear for the most part.

We are a long way from the science-fiction Nirvana of Phase 3. And we've small chance of arriving there so long as fat reduction continues to epitomize the way to achieve the best body possible. By touting slenderness we *avoid* what is *infinitely* more important. Built into the obsessive drive for the body beautiful are the excuses that hasten the return to the "normal" 10 to 20 pounds of excess weight, that typical aftermath of the "successful" diet. The lean "new body" image usually misses the goal—the beautiful body—by a sad margin.

The slowest muncher can consume calories far faster than the fittest jock can lose them chugging away on a fast treatmill inclined steeply uphill. But, suppose one could develop a work capacity of 25 to 35 calories per minute, or more, at least for short, multiple intervals daily. The 10- to 20-pound-overweight group are rarely, in fact, compulsive eaters. At 20 pounds over whatever is "right"

Heavyhands and "negative work"

When the forearm flexes as in our pump motion, the biceps and other muscles shorten during their contraction and move our bones. When the raised hand is then lowered, the lengthening biceps, resisting the tug of gravity, performs *negative* work and is contracting "eccentrically." This happens during Heavyhands exercise especially when rather heavy handweights are used. Then, of course, the frequency of motion is on average *slower* than what we can manage when we choose very light weights.

Negative work has been estimated to be about one-third of positive or "concentric" work. Interestingly enough, eccentric work strengthens a given muscle very nearly as much as positive work though it uses less energy (negative work consumes less oxygen, for instance).

Suppose we take two 1-pound weights and pump them to Level III alternately 200 times a minute. Allowing for the estimated arm weight, we calculate the energy requirement of that work at roughly 5 calories per minute.

But in the laboratory, measuring my oxygen uptake, I found myself using at least 15 calories per minute during the exercise described above! Why the huge discrepancy? I suspect that at such great hand speeds (up to a maximum of close to 70 mph) the bargain of negative work becomes instead a massive expenditure of energy. At such a frequency gravity is little help. The elongated contracting biceps doesn't ease the weight down; triceps pushes it — faster than grav-

cont.

ity's pull can. Then, of course, great energy is expended in braking the hand's rapid motion at both top and bottom of their excursions.

The result: three times as much work as conventional physics would predict. This phenomenon, this inordinate consumption of oxygen at high "pump" frequencies, can be done by legs too, as you will appreciate when you run at frequencies approaching 300 steps per minute. But the legs can't move 3 feet vertically and Mother Earth, not muscle, stops the downstroke without nearly the labor and calorie loss. This special effect, so well developed in advanced Heavyhanders, is unsurpassed in shedding pounds or producing overhead smashes on the tennis court.

We've decided that this sort of high-repetition work in Heavyhands exercise is a unique process. So we distinguish between its conventional cousins — negative or concentric work — by calling it simply "down work." Its most evident application comes in fast striding (120–140/min) with pumps to level 3 or higher. Those numbers force the exerciser to pull the weight down fast to get ready for the next cycle. Down work is one of the explanations for the surprising aerobic power little arms can generate.

for them, they have collected, usually over years of very ordinary eating, some 70,000 extra calories. Over ten years that's only about 20 calories above their energy output per day! One daily 3-minute session of Heavyhands running in place would have prevented it, and produced an annual loss of 10 additional pounds credited against the ever-present tendency to overeat.

There is something ironical about the consistent exerciser's success with weight control. More often than not the serious exerciser is not conscious of the problem of weight control. It may be that if he *is* motivated to exercise purely to dispose of fat, he's less apt to succeed. If his goal in exercising is to attain some reachable state of motor improvement, he'll continue to lose fat for reasons that remain present long after his initial success at weight loss.

If he's training to reach a better level of fat-losing efficiency, that might make sense. I'm not suggesting that the exerciser need be oblivious of the effect of his work in the matter of weight control. He may use that knowledge at the *conscious level* now and then. But that is not the same as the endless preoccupation, the worrisome, guilt-ridden, ego-blighting course that faces 19 out of 20 dieters.

BODY COMPOSITION

Weight control is really a misleading expression. *Control of body composition* is more accurate. This implies more than simple reduction in body mass. The claim of Heavyhands in relation to body composition is clear: *The largest overall change of any known exercise form, i.e., the largest combined reduction in body fat and increase in lean body weight per unit of exercise time.*

METHOD	FAT LOSS	MUSCLE LOSS	MUSCLE GAIN
Diet	+ +	+	0
Weight Lifting	+	0	+ + +
Running	+ +	0	+
Heavyhands	+ + + +	0	+ +

There is some evidence that indicates that Heavyhands, through its high-repetition format, may also pry fat loose from its location *inside* muscles. Indeed, the double-pronged effect that increases strength and endurance simultaneously may be best suited to accomplish that. Without a lot of biopsies it is difficult to prove, but it is generally assumed that sagging muscles are caused in part because their muscle cell structure has been contaminated by islands of fat—the "marbled" effect the butcher boasts of in his choicest steaks.

ACTIVE OR PASSIVE CONTROL

What could motivate us to find a body style that suits us enough to stick with it? We could divide life-styles generally into roughly two categories — passive and active. Dieting is passive. The state of one's fat deposits reflects the lifelong balance of energy. When input exceeds output of energy, fat increases, and the reverse also holds true. But you can't modify fat's behavior. You can't train it, or sculpt it. You can only add or subtract it from the body. It has no active function. Aside from some metabolic functions, it participates in our lives passively.

Not so with muscle. When activated through training, its function changes willy-nilly depending on the paces you put it through. To a varying degree you can negotiate the shape, size, and functions of each of the muscles individually, then push the heart pump with its new power and have it receive oxygen-rich nutrition for its labor. Muscle participates, in a sense, in our every thought and motion, our every emotional exchange. It is an enormous contributor to what shapes our personality type — our decisionmaking, our aggressive behavior, our capacity to give and to love. And its development, in every respect we've repeated here so often, is the *best determiner* of the destiny of the nuisance fat pad.

As we noted before, people who are 10 to 20 pounds too heavy don't usually eat all that much. Three doughnuts per day beyond caloric balance will gain you 106 pounds per year! A pound gain per year requires roughly 10 extra calories per day. Over a period of years enough to make us fat, but hardly what you'd call gluttony. Ten calories of exercise can be accomplished by most trained people in 30 vigorous seconds or less.

Using our musculature allows us to control the fat pad far better than any diet. Only by achieving a body composition that's right

---

A typical Heavyhands week

MONDAY
Three 5-minute intervals of jump with lateral thrusts spread irregularly through the day.
20 minutes of pump 'n' run in the evening.

TUESDAY
30-minute consecutive medley in the evening, including:
  a. 10 minutes of stretch-strength-striding to Level III;
  b. 10 minutes of pump 'n' run;
  c. 10 minutes of double ski-poling.

WEDNESDAY
A light-fast 25-minute pump 'n' run followed by 5 minutes of double ski-poling.

THURSDAY
Shadowboxing for 25 minutes plus 5 minutes of stretch-strength-striding to Level III.

FRIDAY
Heavyhands dance for 30 minutes.

SATURDAY
Pump 'n' walk for 30 minutes.

SUNDAY
30-minute Heavyhands medley.

Total training time: 3 hours and 35 minutes
Calories: 3800 (which would translate into an annual weight loss of over 50 pounds — *without dieting*)

Changing silhouette standards

I hear by the professional grapevine that the definitions of normal weight are beginning to drift upward. That means your insurer is less apt to "rate" you as a bad risk at a given poundage than he would have a couple of decades ago. Likewise, at age fifty or so, many laboratories will include a 330 blood cholesterol as "within normal limits." Definitions of normal are apt to correspond with what, numerically speaking, is "average." If indeed our national health is slipping here and there, individuals must consciously resist the hypnotic appeal of lessening standards.

Fitness and fat one more time

To risk repetition in an important area: Fitness produces calorie loss in sundry subtle, often subconscious ways. The compulsion to repeat ourselves may stem in part from the fact that our skills are too few. New tools produce an ego itch to use them. Strength-speed-power and muscle endurance with enhanced oxygen transport should be viewed as equipment. Once equipped, we humans tend to seek opportunities to break away from that ego-crushing compulsion to repeat. We become implicitly and explicitly more active, more ways. The heat thus generated pares us inevitably toward leaner readiness.

for us and our unique assignments in life can we avoid the *passive drift* that is the basis of 10- to 20-pound obesity.

WEIGHT AND FUNCTION

Ordinary weight gain is imperceptible from day to day largely because the gradual increase *doesn't create any particular anxiety over loss of function.* A 10- to 15-percent increase in body weight will not affect ordinary motor patterns in otherwise healthy people. But if we train conscientiously, we automatically begin to associate enhanced function with body structure. Fitness becomes a series of valued functions: our endurance or wind, our ability to move rapidly, gracefully, and powerfully. Slight variations are noticed and serve as a signal to regain what's been lost.

While I disagree with the diet philosophy, I also realize that *any* activity that results in loss of fat is, in effect, a *diet.* If you perform 660 calories of extra work in the form of exercise per day and lose 3 ounces in the process, you must also have deprived yourself of that much additional caloric intake. Because Heavyhands produces the largest calorie-per-minute intensity, it is the best means for shifting from deprivation (diet) to activity (exercise). That makes it the quickest, surest way to maximize body-composition control.

Walking at the rate of 3 miles per hour, it takes 44 minutes to lose an ounce of fat. A daily hour of that will lose about two pounds a month providing we don't "cover" the mileage with extra consumption of food. But slow walking usually will not produce pulse rates adequate to train the heart and will effect only minor changes in either muscle composition or function.

I'm convinced that almost anyone healthy enough to tackle the existing aerobic methods can train himself or herself to employ Heavyhands at the rate of 15 or more calories per minute loss in prolonged sessions of from 20 to 120 minutes, and as high as 20 to 30 calories per minute in briefer, more intense intervals, depending upon the bodyweight of the exerciser.

The editor of this book began Heavyhanding as he worked on the manuscript. Early in his training he calculated he was good for a 15-calorie-per-minute intensity for prolonged sessions of 20 minutes or more. In briefer, higher-intensity work he hit 20 to 25 calories per minute. Doing 30 continuous minutes, four times a week, he cruised at 15 calories per minute — 450 calories per session. On the three remaining days he practiced Heavyhands odds and ends in a number of irregularly spaced, high-intensity (15–30 calories per minute) intervals of 5 to 10 minutes. He shed twenty-five pounds in five months without changing his eating or drinking habits. His weight watching became *interested* rather than *anxious*. His running pace quickened a gratifying 20 percent in the first six months of his training on an unbelievable low weekly total of less than 10 miles! His cruising caloric output closed in on 20 calories per minute. Beyond the matter of weight control and redistribution, his training strategy nicely demonstrates the principle of the "spread" of Heavyhands training effect. Combined work not only produced high calorie output; it improved the effectiveness of training at other specific exercises — in this instance, running.

The Heavyhands method should change your attitudes toward food. Without diminishing your lust for life's delectables, you stop viewing food as an enemy, a temptation, or a *weakness* associated with suffering in the form of sporadic deprivation or outlandish physical labor, or both. Instead, you'll perceive food as *fueling* the work that improves you. That the fueling process is pleasurable is a bonus effect.

SPOT REDUCTION

A word or two on the issue of spot reduction. You are wrong if you believe your 30 daily sit-ups, however performed, will flatten your tummy. The best bet for a slim waist is reduction of the body fat pad which tends to arrange itself around your middle. A friend and colleague who has just recently begun Heavyhands picked up a couple of weights in my living room and started a series of lateral raises (long levers), enthusiastically flapping his wings. He volunteered that he does this frequently while watching television, and had noticed that his belly was shrinking. "I think it's because my abdomen tightens each time I raise my arms." Now there may be a grain of truth in what my friend says. He may inadvertently contract his abdominal muscles with his raises, which would indeed

---

You're a marathoner!

When you've become even fitter and remain sufficiently ambitious, you can work to a 15-MET level that will place you on par with the best of marathoners. And if you have 180 mintues to "ante up" to your program — a lot less than most training marathoners do — the fat-loss figures will stagger you. Sticking to the diet that had kept you at balance (net change 0), our 154-pound Heavyhander will "defat" at the rate of 50 pounds a year. At that rate only a fatter grocery bill will ensure visibility for long.

Walking off 50 pounds

Presuming an average body weight of 154 pounds — 70 kilos — you can convert a 3-mile-per-hour stroll (3.5 METs) to 10-MET pump 'n' walk by pumping 1-pounders to Level III at about 130 stride-pumps per minute. One hundred and fifty minutes per week, five 30-minute sessions, will lose you the equivalent of a half pound of fat per week. That rate would "cure" about 98 percent of the world's obesity problem in two years by losing more than 50 pounds. Or doubling your exercise, you could consume 1800 extra calories' worth of healthy delectables while producing desirable shifts in body composition as well as an expanding assortment of motor skills.

strengthen them. Actually his encumbered wing flapping is what's responsible for the incineration of belly blubber. For most people, the muscles of the abdominal wall are *least* able to help in the reduction of the paunch. Bellyaerobics, however, will help achieve the valued flat abdomen.

Aside from the healthy advantages of leanness, it is virtually impossible for you to exercise well while fat. Excess body fat is simply a mechanical impediment and, as a result, it is likely that obese people avoid even *thoughts* that would lead to activity. The total effect on the life-style, viewed cumulatively, is hard to imagine. More important, once the would-be exerciser wants to lose flab so that he can move better, rather than to achieve some dreamlike silhouette, he's virtually won the battle of the bulge.

AN IMPORTANT CAVEAT

Because Heavyhands is so effective at consuming calories, it can conceal potentially dangerous nutritional sins. My wife and I had a rude awakening recently when our blood chemistries revealed elevated cholesterols. This flew in the face of research that suggested exercisers enjoyed lower blood fats than nonexercisers. We had taken our success at body-composition control as an invitation to indulge at the table. We immediately embarked upon a rather stringent low-cholesterol regime. Ten days later our combined cholesterol reduction was 33 percent. Too much dietary cholesterol had been the culprit. Moral of the story: successful weight loss through exercise doesn't always mean you can eat all the eggs, butter, and bacon you want.

Exercise may lower some of the blood fats, but it can't always be relied upon to keep pace with the consumption of unusually large amounts of animal fat. The cholesterol level may not respond readily to exertion. An unconstrained meat-eater could be headed for eventual blood vessel troubles. Anyone interested in this problem should read Nathan Pritikin's work for a perhaps extreme but nonetheless thought-provoking position dealing with nutrition, exercise, blood fat and survival.

SOME SPECIFICS FOR USING ACTIVITY IN BODY COMPOSITION CONTROL

To be more specific about the advantages of Heavyhands in body composition control let me summarize some of the glaring differences between diet and exercise in this regard. I prefer to call these methods respectively deprivation-dominated and activity-dominated strategies for shaping the body. That's because neither method is pure: if weight is lost, *some deprivation* is involved, even with good exercise; and even the most rigorous "diet" is supplemented by the activity of everyday life, regardless of how little its intensity and duration.

Let me divide the differences into physiologic and psychologic categories. Even here clean separation is rather artificial: mind and body are most often a blend of functions.

To lose an ounce

If you've the heart and muscle it takes to manage 15 METs, you can divest yourself of skinfold fat at the rate of a full ounce of fat in sessions lasting from 8 to 15 minutes, depending where your body weight falls in the range between 50 and 100 kilos. And you can do it dozens of ways because your oxygen transport, having reached a 15-MET load by Heavyhanding, can throw four or five hundred muscles into the process.

PHYSIOLOGIC DIFFERENCES

DIET DEPRIVATION EMPHASIS	EXERCISE ACTIVITY EMPHASIS
1. Weight loss consists of both fat and muscle tissue.	1. Predominantly fat loss.
2. Some loss of working capacity.	2. Little or no loss of working capacity; it may increase sizably.
3. More chance of nutritional deficiency.	3. Increased food intake lessens likelihood of vitamin, mineral deficiency.
4. Activity may be consciously reduced to avoid appetite increases.	4. Activity welcomed as well as appropriate appetite increases.
5. Maximal weight loss limited to that which is produced by total starvation.	5. No theoretic limit. Limited by intensity times duration of exercise possible.
6. Increase in "relative" VO₂Max simply by weight loss. These gains may be in part "lost" when muscle tissue is lost.	6. VO₂Max may increase by three methods: by reduction of total body mass, by increases in lean body weight (muscle), and by training effects.
7. Failure to reap general rewards associated with fitness training: better health.	7. Many body systems upgraded: cardiopulmonary; musculoskeletal; digestive; central nervous.

PSYCHOLOGIC DIFFERENCES

DIET DEPRIVATION DOMINATED	EXERCISE ACTIVITY DOMINATED
1. Diminished oral gratification may be associated with irritability and depression.	1. Feeding behavior tends to parallel energy output; may lessen need for adjacent oral needs, i.e., alcohol, tobacco.
2. Preoccupation with food; considerable guilt, shame, anxiety over "transgressions."	2. Normal hunger-feeding cycle; variations from day to day depending on activity level.
3. Dieter haunted by awareness of low overall success rate; excess body preoccupation.	3. Body structure thought of in terms of functional serviceability.
4. Tendency to be less objective about body image.	4. No need for depressive distortions; body interest rather than hypochondria.
5. Binging digressions common — often accompanied by depression and abandonment of diet.	5. Freedom to binge guiltlessly because of confident attitudes toward activity. Extra eating may be seen as "fueling" planned extra activity.
6. Typical denial of the harsh realities of calorie arithmetic.	6. A developing intuition about the interaction between food intake and the workloads required to metabolize same.
7. Preoccupation with scale weight as magical "end point" to suffering associated with diet.	7. Concern shifts from additional fat loss to new ambitions related to activity.
8. Interpersonal complications—defensive reactions foisted upon loved ones frequently.	8. Psychic pluses, e.g., confidence, creativity, aggressive thinking patterns; problems solved *outside* the self.
9. Eating may be increasingly perceived as a bad activity, as punishment.	9. Feeding and activity seen as intrinsic parts of the function of "doing."

Sweating and weight loss

A recent note in the *Journal of the American Medical Association* suggested the importance of sweating in the conditioning process. The author indicated that each gram of water lost through sweat is accompanied by more than a half calorie of heat loss. A liter of sweat — not an uncommonly large loss during prolonged workouts in warm, humid weather — would lose 600 or so calories beyond that predicted by the work itself!

If your body fat excess exceeds 20 percent or so, or if your cardiac status or health is in any doubt, your doctor should *always* be consulted. For most people, I see no particular wisdom in starting out on a deprivation-dominated strategy, then switching gradually to an activity-dominated strategy. But I have no strong objections, either, especially in those over forty with very poor response to the 1–10–100 test (increases in heart rate of 40 per minute or more).

How long it should take to gain ideal body composition is complicated and varies with the individual. I prefer to leave that an open question — since few can predict either what their activity requirements will be a year hence much less their body's changed architecture at that time. Weight *changes* will amount to fat losses minus muscle gains. For most the latter will be relatively small, but these small increments of muscle mass *will make tremendous differences in appearance when coupled with significant reductions in skinfold fat.*

If deconditioned at the outset you *cannot* lose weight *rapidly* through *activity.* Moreover there seems small point in agonizing over it. Slow, steady losses at first are what's needed. As the intensity and/or duration of exercise increases, the fat losses will happen faster. I encourage patients to abandon their previous preoccupation with scale weight. Once a reasonable intensity level is established, given time, fat can be dispatched at a rapid rate. However, for most, that is *never* necessary. One to two pounds a week is *fast* fat loss, and a year is a precious short time to sculpt a body you will want to keep for a lifetime.

If your present weight is more than you want it to be, but you're not gaining any more, you're at energy balance — input and output are on average, equal. *Any exercise* you add to your life without adding more food will cause you to lose weight. Walking a mile in 20 minutes will lose you roughly 100 calories, about 5 calories per minute; and 35 miles a week, 5 miles every day, would lose 3,500 calories or one pound. I see nothing wrong with such a program actually. Thousands of people have lost weight effectively precisely that way. But it takes very disciplined person to walk 100 minutes a day, every day. Five-calories-per-minute intensity isn't much and I hope you're not thrilled by that level of fitness as a permanent thing. Depending upon your age, your heart, your skeletal muscles, and your determination, you should have no problem raising your intensity to 10 or more calories per minute. A 500-calorie-per-day program — losing you a pound every week you do it — would then require 50 minutes a day.

As you remember, at least 300 calories should be lost in your 30-minute fitness prescription eventually. That can be accomplished neatly by any of the following sample prescriptions:

Quick weight-MET-calorie converter

This chart will enable you to calculate your calorie loss per minute by knowing your weight and the MET level of your exercise. The numbers listed at the right opposite your weight multiplied by the number of METs you're doing will be close to the calorie cost per minute. Example: If you weigh 176 pounds (80 kilos) your calories per MET fall right between 1.25 and 1.50, or 1.375. At 8 METs you'd be using 11 calories per minute (8 × 1.375 = 11 calories per minute).

Pounds	Kilo	Cal/Min/MET
55	25	.5
66	30	
77	35	
88	40	
(95)	(43)	.75
99	45	
110	50	
121	55	
(125)	(57)	1.0
131	60	
143	65	
154	70	
(156)	(71)	1.25
165	75	
176	80	
187	85	1.50
198	90	
209	95	
220	100	1.75
231	105	
242	110	
(251)	(114)	2.0
253	115	
264	120	

Calorie costs of Heavyhands jumping

Heavyhands jumping is a nifty way of shooing calories in bunches quickly. Jumping while lateral thrusting weights can come close to being a 50-50 exercise (arms and legs contributing equally to the workload). This can be achieved even when using little weights if you get the tempo high enough. The calorie cost of the exercise varies with the individual, naturally, because arm-length variations make for different energy requirements per jump-thrust. But jumping five minutes with 1-pounders at 150 jumps per minute ought to net you 12 METs; 11–13 calories per minute at the very least.

Long and easy beats the calories

Ordinarily, when I train I use 3 to 3.5 liters of oxygen a minute, a fair amount for a little old man, I think. But some days, following an especially acute bout of gluttony, I go long and easy, cruising comfortably at 2.5 to 3 liters. At that rate I can conjure new problems, identify birdcalls, and observe the scene, without the distraction of my own breathing, and lose only 2.5 calories *less* for each of many minutes of exercise.

300-CALORIE EXERCISES IN PLACE AT LEVEL II, FOR A 154-POUND SUBJECT

Pump 'n' walk	4 pounds	30 minutes	130 per minute
Pump 'n' walk	3 pounds	30 minutes	150 per minute
Pump 'n' walk	2 pounds	30 minutes	170 per minute
Pump 'n' run	1 pound	30 minutes	200 per minute

These are approximately 10-calorie-per-minute intensities — a bit more if you're over 150 pounds, a bit less if you're lighter than that.

Now you can easily burn off an additional 200 calories in the form of strength and speed intervals at somewhat higher intensities. For instance, you may wish to exercise at 12.5 calories per minute by increasing the frequency by 25 percent, with the weight that loses 10 calories per minute. Four- or 5-minute intervals at that intensity distributed throughout your day will add the 200 calories of extra loss that amounts to close to 21 pounds a year fat loss.

Remember these additions are part of your fitness strategy and will incidentally alter your body composition for the better. As your per-minute intensity increases, you will intuitively add other movements at increasing intensities that will *not feel more difficult* by the time you're ready for them. Once your silhouette is about where you think it ought to be, there are endless combinations of Heavyhands METs times minutes that will maintain both your appearance and that slow pulse, your badge of excellence in terms of oxygen transport.

By now you'll have guessed I'm not enthralled by calorie counting — whether they be ingoing or outgoing calories. If you enjoy counting or are drawn to it inexorably, do it, by all means. Or if your interest in matters physiologic makes numbers appealing, that's only to the good. From the standpoint of fitness and its relevance to body mass and skinfold fat, the only thing you ever need count is your pulse. After that the clocks and chemistries of body processes really do it for you. And after you're well enough into Heavyhands that various body signals become accurately translated as numerical values — such as heart rate — your counting days are over. Your calorie pulse, which brings *real time* and your *work intensity* together, will serve well as an intermittent check — useful perhaps in making you aware of your progress and keeping you *realistic* about your eating habits.

LOSING WHILE YOU SLEEP

Another way of looking at strategies for controlling body composition is to decide to lose *all* your weight during sleep. If by bedtime you used up all the calories you had consumed that day, in a year you'd lose roughly 65 pounds. That's because your body metabolism goes on during sleep, though at a lowered rate. But then, your intake is *zero*.

Simply count your calories. Figure what you've used up in work and leisure, add your 30-minute strategy, plus enough intervals to make up the difference, and sleep soundly knowing you're losing about 3 ounces before breakfast. It adds up.

If you're in the 10- to 30-pound-overweight bracket, have been that way a long time, and have dieted a number of times, pay attention to things like workloads, muscle groups, and movement repertoires. Forget about scales, pinch tests, clothing sizes, or dropping 10 pounds in time for Cousin Suzy's wedding. As your mind drifts to muscle and movement — the hardware and software of activity — fat, those passive globules that will fuel your experiments, will dissolve along with your habitual worry over it.

USE YOUR TELEVISION SET

If TV has, as some contend, contributed to our national obesity problem, it may ironically become its eventual antidote. Within the space occupied by an 8-foot cube, Heavyhanders can duplicate the caloric loss of a cross-country run, a hard swim, or a long bike ride, without missing their TV's best offerings. Television time is perfect for physique control. For advanced Heavyhanders, many of whom will achieve a 15 or more calorie per minute exercise intensity within a year, there are almost no limits to caloric loss, so long as time is available. For instance, eight 10-minute intervals can be squeezed closely together within an evening's viewing. With the use of Heavyhands interval cycles (Chapter 16) literally hours of moderate-intensity work can be performed with remarkable comfort. These cycles will become favorites for those converted to activity rather than deprivation emphasis. And they are excellent fitness producers. Pump 'n' run and double ski-poling are superb for TV. Four pairs of various-sized weights are stationed beneath my set.

Heavyhands naturals for television watchers

The following moves work especially well for TV watching, since they allow the viewer's eyes to remain virtually fixed front:

1. Pump 'n' walk and pump 'n' run in place
2. Punch 'n' dip
3. Lateral thrusts with pelvic thrusts
4. Lateral raises and side kicks (arm and leg long-levers)
5. Punch 'n' kick
6. Dips and shrugs

Any of these can be pushed to your maximal comfortable steady state. And, of course, different programs couple differently with these exercises. A football broadcast, for instance, can work well with any of the in-place Heavyhands repertoire, because the "meat" of the action may be concentrated in about 15 minutes of actual play-time spread thin over three hours. An ambitious Heavyhander can do a hefty week's training in an afternoon in front of his television, without missing a play. There's a bit of skill involved in shrewd TV exercising. You learn to sprint intervals during commercials, slower moves when keying on dramatic moments, how best to move when listening for important news details, etc.

The evening news, frequently all I ever watch, gives me a solid half-hour to discharge my obligations to my body.

WEEKENDS

Weekends are good for physique control *à la* Heavyhands. Most weight is gained during leisure, and weekends are especially dangerous when it comes to gluttony. So if you *lose weight* on a Sunday, you're way ahead of the game. One way is to dispatch each meal with equivalent exercise. If you eat a 300-calorie breakfast and a 300-calorie lunch, doing a 30-minute session in midmorning or before breakfast and another during midafternoon, you can greet the dinner table fearlessly. Once you begin to sense the work equivalent of a bite of rich dessert, you will likely moderate your most freakish food penchants. And you will also learn that a vigorous interval before meals will probably *not* increase your appetite.

Keep in mind that it will not be hard for you to *up* your caloric output through *arm work.* If you can increase arm work intensity by 5 calories a minute, you'll be adding over 15 pounds of dietary freedom to each year of your life. That is, if you exercise 200 minutes per week. And that doesn't count your formidable leg drivers, either.

As your fitness improves and you lose fat, your sinewy hardware will surface. You'll like the look that says you're built for action. When that happens you'll enjoy the best of both worlds: the ability to move in ways you've never moved before, and freedom to enjoy your beloved appetite. You can eat what you need and manage, while working toward fitness, to *need plenty!*

I believe that people who feel consummate control of their body structure, via activity, begin to eat more sensibly. The psychological corollary of that is that senseless eating, the blatantly self-defeating kind, may be a reaction to our lifelong frustration and conflict over food. When nourishment comes to mean a pleasurable fueling of life's work and play, you've arrived.

If you must diet, plan to do it only *once more.* To help make that a reality, start your Heavyhands strategy, planning to increase its intensity while you *reduce* the rigorousness of your dieting. If you plan to stay lean by following the tired dictum that advises you to "change your eating habits," you're betting against large odds. As an exerciser, you can finally capitulate to a habit which was never a bad one to begin with. Successful, conscientious dieters are always ambivalent; they love food and hate the restraint with which they must confront it daily.

DIETING IS PROGRESSIVELY LESS EFFICIENT

A couple of facts of life uncovered by experts in the field of metabolism and nutrition are worth considering. Dieting tends to be-

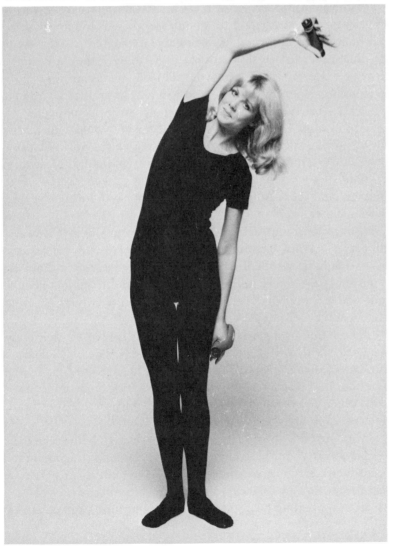

come a *less efficient* operation as it is repeated over the years. Apparently bodily sensors tighten the metabolic belt and make a little food go farther in supplying our needs. The *diet* loses effectiveness, you could say, as the body's metabolism becomes *more efficient.* A similar thing happens during the course of a prolonged diet. The amount of body fat lost daily tends to diminish from week to week, though the calorie intake and activity level remain fixed. Our instincts, served perhaps by our chemistry, seem intent upon avoiding starvation even if it means keeping us fat. So the dieter, ironically, seems to get less for his dieting zeal as time passes, an interesting twist for the behaviorists to unscramble.

Exercisers get a better deal. As the intensity of their strategy builds they become more *efficient* weight losers, *inefficient* husbanders of consumed victuals. Their average metabolic rates *increase,* unlike the chronic dieters whose rates inevitably fall. One fact tends to balance things somewhat: the obese exerciser enjoys a diminished appetite, the lean and active crave and consume in proportion to their exertion.

The moral gained from these facts of physiology says it bluntly — exercise is the way to become and stay lean and to eat worry-free.

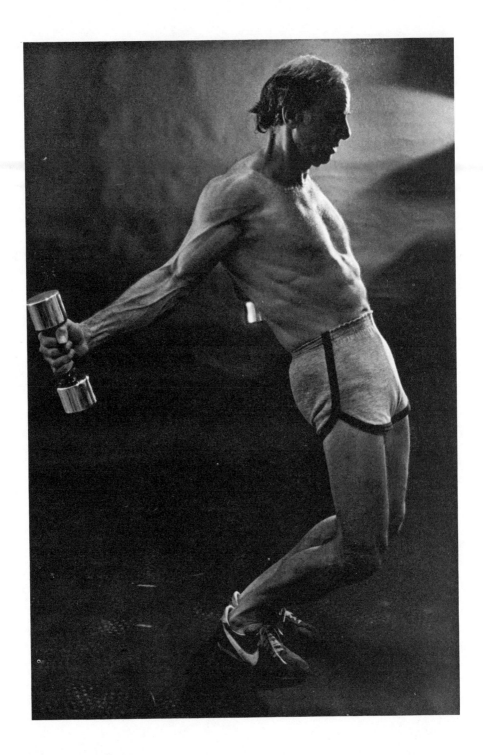

16

Heavyhands Intervals and "Cycles"

INTERVAL TRAINING IS a form of exercise in which brief periods of intense work are relieved with periods of rest, and the "cycle" is repeated over and over again. There is plenty of reason to use interval training in Heavyhands. Some physiologists believe this kind of training produces greater levels of fitness with less investment of actual working time. My findings after hundreds of experiments with Heavyhands intervals suggest that one can perform larger *total* workloads using them than exercising uninterruptedly.

I'll explain. Three years ago I did some pump 'n' run at 200 steps a minute to arm-weariness, which occurred after 18 minutes. After enough rest, I started in again with the same weights and tempo. This time I worked 18 seconds, rested 12, and repeated that "work-relief" cycle each half-minute for 2 hours. Since I worked 60 percent of the time, at the end of 2 hours, I had done 72 minutes (.60 × 120) of work at an intensity equal to that which had me pooped after 18 consecutive minutes of it.

For a few weeks I included such "cycles" frequently. I used them for special varieties of high-intensity exercise, strength, or speed-work — poundages or frequencies that I couldn't manage comfortably in long-endurance runs. Gradually I pushed on to higher percentages of work, like:

> 20 sec. on–10 sec. off cycles = 66.6 percent work;
> 22 sec. on– 8 sec. off cycles = 73   percent work;
> 24 sec. on– 6 sec. off cycles = 80   percent work.

As hard as it may be to believe until you try it, a few brief seconds are enough to restore the so-called ATP system — the energy-chemistry that recharges contracting muscle fibers. The heart-lung machinery doesn't balk either. I once devoted a solid three months to Heavyhands cycles of no more than a 2-hour-weekly total, relief time included. At the end of that time, my resting pulse was unchanged and my strength and speed were up a notch or two.

CYCLES SPEND CALORIES

Aside from the fitness factors — strength, endurance, speed, the contributors to workload — Heavyhands cycles use *calories* at a spectacular clip. For the exerciser intent upon the loss of fat and the addition of muscle, these "cycles" are the way to go. I fully expect Heavyhands intervallic cycles to become the standard for all-out exercise-oriented body-composition control. It's simply the most convenient, quickest way of doing the most work for the longest cumulative time yet devised.

In very fit Heavyhanders, 80 percent work–20 percent relief cycles, given proper weights and tempo, are quite comfortable. The return of the pulse after each work interval is so prompt that the 6-second relief gives the feeling of a fresh start. The 24-second work doesn't push the pulse out of the target range when the cycles are "right." If weight, frequency, or work–relief ratios are too much, a few cycles will send you toward oxygen debt — at which point you merely ease up on one or more of the work elements. Soon your intuition about cycle construction will allow you to choose your tempo, weights, and cycle ratios in a number of combinations that bring you to the same pulse rates.

Ratios of work to relief time for beginners should be geared for more rest, naturally. One way to track your progress is to keep

Constructing interval cycles on the move

You can take any two Heavyhands exercises on the move and convert them to use as interval cycles. Just select one that's palpably easier than the other and alternate them as work-relief cycles. I do that frequently with stretch-strength-strides and pump 'n' run. Furthermore, by juggling the workload factors (i.e., range of motion and frequency), I can decide which one will be work, which relief, during a given outing.

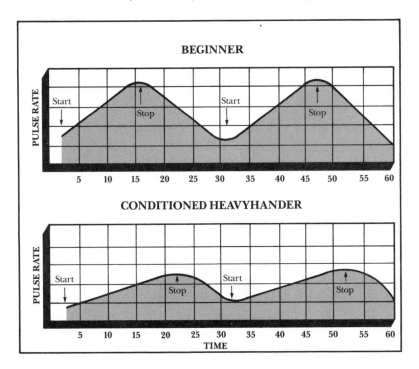

tempo and weights constant, gradually inching toward larger proportions of *work time*.

You will recall that the characteristics of the heart-rate curves in the conditioned state differ from the ones produced by those less fit. Conditioned Heavyhanders, for a given workload, produce a smaller pulse-rate increase and quicker return than do beginners. Thus a larger proportion of work-to-rest is feasible for them.

Television watching is perfect for Heavyhands intervallic cycles. Well-trained Heavyhanders can do the equivalent of a hefty week's workload during a Sunday afternoon of football watching. Just set your metronome or "pacer" watch, if you own one. A sweep-second clock plus a metronome makes counting steps unnecessary and comfortably allows you to enjoy the picture and sound.

I began my Heavyhands intervallic cycles with pump 'n' run. Since then I've used dozens of moves. All of the Heavyhands calisthenic group are suitable, as well as bellyaerobics (Heavyhands style), sports moves, shadowboxing, and dance work well performed cyclically.

CYCLING TO NEW MOVES

Intervallic cycles are a logical way of introducing new moves into a calisthenic medley. Practice them this way for a few minutes for several days — then they will slip smoothly into your routine. Working at high intensities, the strength-speed development will make you more graceful when doing a particular move more sedately over longer durations. You can really feel this happen. Work out in vigorous pump 'n' run cycles in place one day, then do pump 'n' run on the move with half of the weight next day. As one interested in things psychological, I used to suspect that sense of "lightness" was purely psychic "self-deception" until I realized that my demonstrable, objective performance was improving, too.

Evidence is accumulating that intervals may also be less apt to injure. The 72 minutes of work I squeezed into my aforementioned pump 'n' run "marathon" was easily enough work to have produced several injuries. Those relief moments, however brief, may allow

Interval cycle chart for 30-minute exercise

MOVEMENT FREQUENCY (PER MINUTE)	WORK-TO-RELIEF RATIO	REPETITIONS (EACH 30 SECONDS)	WORK (SECONDS)	REST (SECONDS)	PERCENT OF TIME WORKING	TOTAL WORK (MINUTES)
150	.5	25	10	20	33	10
150	1.0	38	15	15	50	15
150	1.5	45	18	12	60	18
150	2.0	50	20	10	67	20
150	3.3	57	23	7	77	23
150	5.0	62	25	5	83	25
175	.5	29	10	20	33	10
175	1.0	44	15	15	50	15
175	1.5	53	18	12	60	18
175	2.0	58	20	10	67	20
175	3.3	67	23	7	77	23
175	5.0	73	25	5	83	25
200	.5	33	10	20	33	10
200	1.0	50	15	15	50	15
200	1.5	60	18	12	60	18
200	2.0	67	20	10	67	20
200	3.3	77	23	7	77	23
200	5.0	83	25	5	83	25
225	.5	38	10	20	33	10
225	1.0	56	15	15	50	15
225	1.5	68	18	12	60	18
225	2.0	75	20	10	67	20
225	3.3	86	23	7	77	23
225	5.0	94	25	5	83	25
250	.5	42	10	20	33	10
250	1.0	63	15	15	50	15
250	1.5	75	18	12	60	18
250	2.0	83	20	10	67	20
250	3.3	96	23	7	77	23
250	5.0	104	25	5	83	25
275	.5	46	10	20	33	10
275	1.0	69	15	15	50	15
275	1.5	83	18	12	60	18
275	2.0	92	20	10	67	20
275	3.3	105	23	7	77	23
275	5.0	115	25	5	83	25
300	.5	50	10	20	33	10
300	1.0	75	15	15	50	15
300	1.5	90	18	17	60	18
300	2.0	100	20	10	67	20
300	3.3	115	23	7	77	23
300	5.0	125	25	5	80	25

joint surfaces, tendons, ligaments, and muscles to restore themselves in time for the next flurry of activity. Along the same line of reasoning, Heavyhands intervallic cycles may be a good way to reintroduce an injured leg or arm after a lay-off. Cycles may neatly avoid those critical levels of overload that injure.

Sometimes I divide my workouts into a lengthy endurance interval followed by a sequence of intervallic cycles. So when working 30 minutes, I may go 15 minutes at something like fast-light ski-poling, then do heavy pump 'n' run cycles with the rest of my time. Next time around I might reverse the procedure, devoting half to heavy long levers like double or alternate ski-poling then some very fast-light pump 'n' run. I included the chart on page 230 for your convenience.

THE BONUS

In previous chapters I've indicated how much weight you will lose by doing a given exercise, at a specifc pace, with a certain amount of iron for a given period of time. The calories (and thus pounds) expended have been calculated directly from the workload produced by the exercise. In actual fact, you will lose more weight than the figures indicate. The reason is simple. The moment you stop doing a 10-MET exercise your body does not instantly return to rest (remember, 1 MET). You are no longer pump 'n' running, but your metabolism continues to race along at a much higher rate than at rest. Of course, this is true with any activity, but the high-intensity workloads of Heavyhands, particularly of cycles, exaggerate the effect. The big bonus of Heavyhands, particularly of intervallic cycle training, is that your calorie (weight) loss gets a free ride. How much of a free ride can't be predicted: it depends upon the intensity of the work you just completed and your own condition. But for most people, the free ride is substantial.

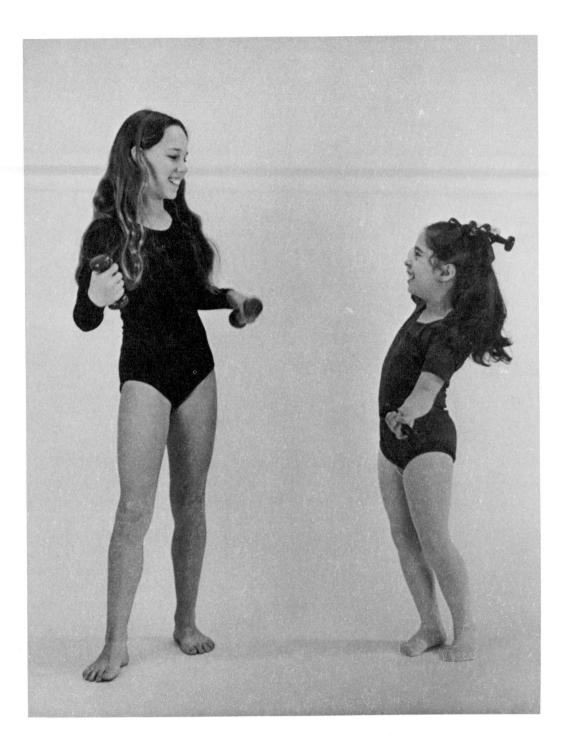

17

Exer-psychology

SO THERE YOU HAVE IT: the results of a lot of experimenting — mine and others — with exercise accompanied by those ever-present little weights. I believe Heavyhands is *the* best single-package exercise. But exercise, as we understand it today, is a relatively new idea. For various reasons most people either avoid it or, even if initially attracted, soon give it up.

Back to those two thousand or so books on fitness. I often wonder about the fate of self-help books, especially those on exercise, and, more especially, those that introduce a new method. The reader may feel somewhat tentative, even anxious. Exercise, like the castor oil of our grandmother's era, is acknowledged as good for us but anticipated with dread. Of course, there could be pleasant fantasies — soaring notions of newfound health, beauty, and function. But launching into something new in exercise is bound to feel risky.

Here's why. Once you absorb the contents of most books, the job is done. You may use the information you've gleaned now and again in one of a thousand ways during your life, in casual conversation or in mixing paint, if that's what it was about. With books about exercise, most certainly the aerobic kind, the *easiest* part of it is the act of *reading*.

It's clear why the reader of an exercise book can become anxious. He spent good money for relatively uninteresting reading that makes outrageous demands on his time and energy, and that then leaves him sheepish and guilt-ridden if he doesn't follow through. And if he does abandon the project, he may never know just what prompted him to do so.

There are too many casualties among would-be exercisers. Plenty of us start but the dropout rate is high. As a psychiatrist, I should be right in my element discussing the erratic motives that propel us toward and away from good exercise. Though there can be little doubt that psychologic factors are most responsible for the fickleness of the exercise motive, the dynamics of that fickleness are far from clear.

It is obvious that every exercise, however well contrived, is affected by the fact that *not* doing it is easier. While educators rhapsodize over the inborn instinct toward activity, the maturing human often seems more intent upon rest. Inertia is, after all, a fact of life. How else can we explain the awesome numbers who quit exercise programs that promise longer and better lives, social acceptance, body beauty, better moods, and better mentality?

I cannot afford to be blasé on the subject of motivation. It's the blood, bones, and guts of any exercise system. Heavyhands, however finely tuned, shaped, or expanded to your special needs, will halt as soon as you go into psychologic "neutral." Motivation is the most vulnerable link in the complicated chain of events that will get you fit and keep you that way forever.

The simple and repetitious nature of current aerobic methods may be a cause of slack motivation. Traditional wisdom nevertheless dictates: "Don't make waves. We've gotten him to run when we never thought he'd walk. Load him down with a couple of iron weights and he may just never move again!"

Heavyhands takes a strong but risky stand here. We're saying *more* may be *better* from the psychologic as well as the physiologic side. If you decide that what seemed interesting yesterday has become unutterably difficult or insufferably dull today, no one will be there to argue with your best objections, or give CPR to the last gasping quivers of your intention to exercise.

Nor will I take much conscious pleasure in saying, "I told you so," once you've copped out. I wrote *Heavyhands* partly because I was so profoundly frustrated by so many people's willingness to quit exercise, some even after they'd made good progress. If we knew how to get through the motivational maze that confronts exercisers at any stage in their development, I wouldn't be writing this. The psychology of *sports* has, incidentally, lured many writers: there is a special attraction to competition, leadership, team cohesiveness, and things like that.

But the psychology of exercise has been given rather shabby treatment overall. There's been too little analysis as to why we *do* or *don't* exercise and almost nothing cogent about how to prevent quitting. The lion's share of exercise psychology turns out to be personal reports of the performers describing their own experiences. The academics who have systematically studied the "emotional responses" to exercise seem least convinced of its long-term psychological benefits.

Despite the fact that you have bought or borrowed this book, and have read at least this far, I would be willing to bet hard cash *against* your strategy's long-range survival. I have a poor track record as a bettor, and I also know how feisty some people become as soon as you bet against them, but you can't argue with numbers

---

A few factors that lead to quitting

1. Unrealistic goals
2. A chronic history of sedentary ways
3. Depression
4. Injury, sometimes self-inflicted by over- or underexercising
5. Physical "symptoms" during exercise: anxious breathlessness, abundant sweat, dizziness, muscles aches, headache
6. Overcompetitiveness — an outsized need to be number one regardless of a lot of harsh realities
7. Boredom — an irrational expectation that "difficult" and entertaining are apt to be synonymous
8. An envious spouse or some other "other"
9. Hypochrondia — the addiction to the need to complain about one's body
10. Aloneness
11. Embarrassment related to poor coordination or simply the felt silliness of it all
12. Guilt, when exercise is categorized as fun and play.
13. Intelligence, if you've been taught to believe anything from the neck down is plain dumb.

Does exercise really energize?

Can there by any doubt? Lord Kelvin defined energy as the capacity to do work. Total work to exhaustion, the total number of bricks one can toss into the truckbed before the system is obliged to stop, can increase by tens of thousands of percent. Witness the jogger who struggles initially to finish 100 yards but who, two years later, completes the marathon, some 46,000 yards and a 46,000 percent increase! Arm increases are even more astounding because of the arms' typically deconditoned state at the beginning of Heavyhands training.

What is fatigue?

"What made you stop?" I ask when someone's movement grinds to a sudden halt. "I was tired." "Where?" The question sounds naive at first blush and the answer would seem obvious. Fatigue is no simple matter. It seems that a psychic component or "set" becomes an established limit that defines "enough" in terms that aren't always immediately clear. Is it pumpbellows tired, general skeletal-muscle tired, localized-ache tired, dehydration tired, or bored-stiff tired? Do we quit hysterically upon reaching some predetermined, perhaps unconsciously inscribed work total or intensity level? As creatures of habit, are we afraid to extend ourselves? One thing is sure: good training guarantees a spontaneous revamping of our outmoded ways of estimating our tolerance for exertion — hence our fatiguability.

and they suggest your odds for sticking to exercise of *any* type are poor.

Actually, things may not be quite so bleak. None of the students who've remained long enough to gain the feel of Heavyhands have seceded so far. Early resistance is our worst enemy. Those who weather the early symptoms seem to gain staying power steadily.

Nonetheless this *is* a book and not the same as a one-on-one tutorial. Let me just run through a few caveats, tips, and free associations gleaned from clinical experience with the knotty problem of motives vis-a-vis exercise.

The high dropout rate among exercisers suggest beginners' motives may leave much to be desired. Today's eagerness, ambition, and resolve may slacken rapidly if the initial motives were built on an unstable foundation. Here are a few of what I call motivational traps. Ironically, they serve to get us started, but may later convert to convenient excuses for quitting.

THE TOO-MUCH-TOO-QUICK TRAP

If you require fabulous images of yourself as the body beautiful to make you exercise, your exercise program is already an endangered species. Goals should be plotted but kept close enough to what you are now so that they are attainable within the foreseeable future.

THE SINGLE-FOCUS TRAP

Since most goals are mixtures of solid ideas and fuzzy fantasies, becoming overfocused upon something you want dearly from your exercise may leave you a bit disheartened and ready to quit when it doesn't live up to expectations. Consciously find multiple reasons to exercise, being sure to make them all reasonably within reach.

Don't denounce any fitness factor as something *you don't need.* A desire to accomplish something — a number of repetitions, an increase in hand-held weight, or some kind of grace or skill — may surface from unconscious sources and become so symbolically insistent that you will push yourself to attain it. Take advantage of these peculiar and frequently irrational drives. Their only danger is that they may get you into an all-or-nothing, now-or-never effort.

Acknowledging and accepting some of your tawdriest, most ridiculous plans can help you continue through those shaky early days. Which leads to the notion that self-observation during exercise can be a fantastic source of *self-knowledge*. This, or any exercise for that matter, puts you through a very complicated body-mind obstacle course; observing your response to various challenges and stresses is an excellent way of meeting yourself in a different context. And you should become better and better at it. It's the kind of intimacy with yourself that will help keep you injury-free on the one hand, more adventuresome on the other. What's best about it is that there are often important translations from the body language of exercise to the larger business of living.

THE BOREDOM TRAP

Be bored if you must but try not to think it as a repeated incantation. Here I'm concerned about boredom's lethal nature with respect to the exercise habit. One question should be confronted directly and immediately. Ask yourself if you need to enjoy every moment of exercise. While I've advised you to seek multiple reasons for exercise, it would be a childish mistake to expect every moment of exercise to be blissful in ways that few moments *outside* of exercise are. Remember that one thing you *never* get when you don't exercise is whatever you hoped exercise would provide. Once you've decided that your body is an essential part of you and worth your investment in it, you shouldn't be blighted much by boredom. Boredom's signal, a vital part of intelligence, can make an adventurer of you, in fact. It might be a good idea for us to consider exercise as we would other motor acts that we *elect* to perform daily. Once we *elect* to do anything we seldom complain of boredom. Exercise is boring because we, as poor self-proprietors, don't really feel authors of the act of exercise. Elite runners never complain of boredom. We learn boredom when, as children, we decide that the chores Mama doled out were not what we'd prefer to be doing just then. Somebody else's wishes instilled into us have a great chance of becoming a bore. Once you've identified with exercise, the exercise becomes part of *you*. And none of us seriously believes *we're* bores!

Zapping boredom

1. Avoid using the *word* itself — those inner mutterings can be dangerously hypnotic.

2. Control your exercise. Plan roughly beforehand. Mix movements aggressively. Be your own best *constructive critic*.

3. Maintain work intensity. A good workout may produce sundry discomforts, but boredom is not one of them.

4. Stay curious and get knowledgeable: about *your* body's peculiar responses to exercise. Interest is one of boredom's most potent antidotes.

5. Improvise and experiment. No one can be the movement architect for your body that *you* can be. Improvisation is to movement what sightseeing is to travel. Neither is boring.

6. Laugh at your failures. Humor is generally incompatible with boredom.

7. Exercise aggressively and frequently precisely when you're bored with *other* things. That will cure both boredom and the defensive notion that exercise, in particular, is boring.

8. Use music. Few complain of boredom when simply listening to what they consider good music. Adding exercise to target and you're doubly immunized.

9. Think of exercise as a skill. While practicing a difficult passage at the piano or hitting nine buckets of balls at the tee, no one carps about boredom despite the number of repeats.

10. Listen to exercisers' complaints around boredom with interest. Understanding their plight will bring new insights to your own struggle, which is, after all, a universal blight on the lives of culturated folk.

THE TIME TRAP

I'm frankly nonplussed by the people who can't exercise because they haven't time. Do they mean their bodies aren't important to them or is their *time* simply *more* important? Perhaps they're dismissing the body generally as an ersatz institution of some sort, quite separate from mind. It turns out that the winners of Nobels and Pulitzers are often quite active people who somehow *find* time to exercise. Freud, who usually worked on two manuscripts at once, always had time for vigorous exercise. The time exemption is one that worries me as a doctor. I ask myself, What next will they discover they haven't time for? What's most intriguing and so utterly frustrating is that exercise, in its own way, *creates* time — longer life and, once fit, less time devoted to exercise. Those who skip exercise may refuse to understand that fact—perhaps as a convenient defense. Oddly enough, the *boredom* and *time* excuses are often used by the same people. One would think they'd mutually exclude each other, because time hangs heavy upon bored people and people who haven't any time shouldn't be bored.

THE BEAUTY TRAP

People repeatedly tackle prolonged diet and exercise routines that are truly dreadful, just to make a good appearance for two hours at some future social event. Few of us, alas, are willing to sort myth from reality in the matter of beauty. Many who exercise for its pure cosmetic effect would probably never start if made aware of the harsh facts. The beauty seekers are sometimes in for disappointment because they seek the unattainable through methods that simply don't work. When the flawed logic surfaces, many choose to quit good exercise because it didn't accomplish what it *couldn't* have in the first place. If improved *function* were prized more than physical change, we could tolerate better the fixed physical characteristics nature bequeathed us.

THE QUICK-CURE TRAP

Exercise is said to be a good antidepressant. We're not sure how that happens or if it happens for the same reasons in every case. Depression, of course, can scotch exercise, too. Exercisers tend to

---

Why is exercise an antidepressant?

No one really knows exactly. Monkeys seem to understand intuitively the relationship between activity and health. The group often physically jostles a depressed member, as though to shake the victim free of a blue mood. And most often it seems to work, according to expert monkey watchers. Some years ago, researchers noted an increase in adrenaline-like chemicals in the spinal fluids of hospitalized depressed patients after they exercised on a treadmill. Even so, the issue can't be simple: people respond variously to activity. We need to learn a great deal more about what kinds of people respond how to which kinds of exercise.

Beta endorphins and exercise

These so-called opiates of the brain have received a lot of attention recently in connection with the good moods that come from exercise. Most studies show increased blood levels of endorphin during exercise. Oddly enough, the resting endorphin levels may be *lower* in some habitual exercisers. There is more to be learned, obviously, about the chemical tie-ins between exercise and mood.

be more dilligent when things are going well and their performance tends to improve then, too. I generally advise patients who are severely depressed not to push things too much until they are less destitute. I do believe that the tendency toward moderate recurrent depression improves gradually in habitual exercisers. But exercise doesn't work miracles and will be abandoned quickly by those who expect it to.

Up until now we've been troubleshooting, providing you with some protection against the common pitfalls. If you are going to become an exerciser — which means you're going to exercise for the rest of your life — you should know about some of the positive ways you can help your exercise and the ways your exercise can help you.

PRACTICE

I notice that the word "practice," frequently used in sports, seldom appears in connection with exercise. A ball player in a slump may practice hitting for hours to regain his timing. Most sports demand practice, but we don't think in terms of practicing most noncompetitive aerobic exercise. In sharp contrast, intent upon conditioning, the exerciser is captive to an endless repetition of his routine, because most popular aerobic strategies don't emphasize *skill*. I think that's important. Skills, those cooperative ventures that bind mind and muscle, are valued so by humans that neglecting the opportunity to develop them in exercise could be a major cause of dropping out.

For runners who compete, the nuances of running assume great importance. And it is probably true that competitive runners are *least* apt to abandon it as exercise. I'm not suggesting that exercise need be competitive in order to preserve the urge to practice. In fact, skill, and the practice that develops it, can be a part of a solitary routine or group activity in which explicit competition plays no conscious part.

Seeking more complicated versions of movement gives exercise new meaning, and fitness is taken more for granted. As the target pulse becomes a background cadence rather than a conscious preoccupation, exercisers are able to devote themselves more to

Functionalism in exercise

The individualization of exercise always presents a fascinating though difficult problem. Given the core requirements, upgrading of oxygen transport, control of body composition, motor freedom and skill — the nuances of training should be in synch with what we do and what we intend to do. It's a wonderful measure of body-mind integrity — a physique honed to the explicit needs of its host. The obverse — those calamitous mismatches of "hard- and software" — often suggest a personality that has quit the cause of self-proprietorship.

Heavyhands and Gestalt

The Gestaltists would doubtless have plenty to say about Heavyhands exercise. They teach that the whole is *not* simply the sum of its parts. Arm exercise, then leg exercise is *not* the same as pump 'n walk. Simultaneous work makes it a different game. That's why moving pictures say it better; they are not hidebound by the sequential unfolding of the print medium, which might be a clue to the performance of complex exercise with the joy of abandon. Once you've got it, it's no longer arms and legs and trunk. It's all *one* action.

Collecting progress

Can our inordinate passion for collecting extra things be converted to a yearning for new function? If not, I suspect we are not long for this universe. Perhaps the relentless search for one's limits is itself a bit neurotic. I'm merely convinced that we can "care" for each other more effectively when we *take care* of ourselves. A 10-percent increase in individual energy output — easily within reach — would dwarf the combined effects of the Renaissance and the Industrial Revolution.

Training and exercise

Some might consider the distinction to be hair-splitting. For me, training connotes a sense of growth, a conscious intention to improve. While exercise can be almost anything from static yoga to sprints-to-exhaustion, it includes everyone who isn't dead-set against the idea. The catch-all "exercise" may account for the swollen numbers of Americans who get counted by pollsters. Trainers pursue particular functions, implemented by thought-out plans or strategies, and may be more realistic about expectable progress. Just a thought.

practicing skills, knowing their oxygen transport will take care of itself. The laws of physiology should, as time passes, free the exerciser for more creative pursuits. The free-form exercises in Heavyhands dance and shadowboxing were inserted with that in mind. Even the calisthenic moves can be ingeniously choreographed, making improvisation at some level part of every session. Ideally the dutiful, by-the-numbers aspect recedes, replaced by freer expressive movement, somewhat different from session to session — without ever neglecting the fitness factors. Practice also makes you more specifically and consciously the proprietor of your exercise — less oriented to chores which, after all, someone else cooked up for you. That state of mind may be the best guarantor of continuing exercise. Practice implies growth and humans simply don't perform well or enthusiastically when growth stops. Since exercise is for most of us an elective, zero growth may bring us perilously close to termination of the program. If the *practice of practicing* is developed through the medium of exercise, its effects may radiate to other activities. In somewhat idyllic fantasies, I see a world where the urge toward practice would become an essential character trait and growth a conscious goal along the entire life cycle. If, while exercising, you happen upon a new movement variation, refine it, and include it in your practice, your indoctrination into the Cult of Exercise will be established.

I suspect that practice is a natural human instinct. Unfortunately, it may be lost early in life when we're told too often to do it. That's a good example of how developing humans may deprive themselves of superb traits in the process of defying authority. The exerciser has the opportunity to revive the practice option, this time as an adult elective.

PLEASURE

Most people new at exercise seem genuinely surprised to find themselves *feeling* better. Sometimes it's not clear whether the good feelings are linked to the exercise itself or to a general realignment of attitudes that often comes with *anything* new. Researchers in the field seem uncertain still as to what these claims mean and how long they're apt to last. Some believe the initial "pleasant surprise" converts to a more sedate pleasure or becomes associated in its lasting form with the excitement of competition or the attainment of levels of performance. Mind and body types vary; some are less apt to "take" to exercise than others. And most have highly specific tastes where it comes to body movement. This is particularly true in the case of dance, where it seems people respond overtly with either enthusiasm or frank reluctance. When nondancers come to enjoy dance, I think a special psychic miracle occurs. Once converted, these people take on a sense of body freedom that simply defies description.

Those less inclined toward the pleasure of movement may find the going very arduous at first. And hearing about others' pleasure in their own exercises doesn't make life easier. The pleasure motive can become mixed with competition. Sometimes a kind of one-upsmanship becomes a contaminant, especially in those who, less than proud of their *performance,* extol its *emotional advantages.* Those with less motor aptitude may feel shut out, different, and may stop before they've gotten under way.

If you don't consider yourself graceful, focus first on oxygen transport, pulse counting, workloads, and things that are more independent of skill and grace. Take *your* pleasure in what you *know* is happening for the better in you. It's a mistake for those of us who are on the awkward side to expect to glean everything from exercise that our coordinated friends do.

Pleasure that comes early and easily is a bit suspect anyway. In the usual course of events, good kinds of pleasure — the substantial variety — continue to mount as the various sorts of rewards accrue. Pleasure for most of us turns out to be part of the *goal* and part of the *process,* not an "up-front" given. Take your time and don't be frightened off by those who are drippingly effusive about their first moments of exertion. The pleasure of exercise is as variable as your mood and your muscular performance. It can't be sensibly likened to ice cream, orgasm, glorious sunsets, or Beethoven sonatas. If you're not an expert exerciser, part of the adventure should come in the discovery of the unique array of pleasures it can provide you with.

The psychotherapeutics of dancing

I'd like to see an enormous surge of interest in dance, not as a spectator-oriented art but a combination of sophisticated physiology and what's left of our primal instinct toward active expression. Resurrected in the form of a freewheeling ritual, the practice of dance could help obesity, malaise, other poisonous moods, hatred, sexual inhibition, humorlessness, atrophy of various parts of our body-mind anatomies. The terror some of us experience in relation to dance may be related to the expectation that once opened to its charm, we will never hold still for proper "adulthood" again.

Overspecialization — one more time!

Could it be that this penchant for working a few muscles into overspecialized exercise is laced with an assortment of magical thoughts locked in the unconscious? Are the skinny upper torsos of the typical marathoners a kind of conscience-sop? A few studies have shown elite runners to have arm-work capabilities *lower* than sedentary types. Is this a result of unwitting but studious neglect? And isn't it interesting that the real "structuralists," the body builders, dutifully work *every* muscle group as though fearing to leave anything out. Runners who never flex a sinewy quad or hamstring also don't seem to mind that their arm-shoulders appear to be terminal. Perhaps all this may be remotely related to the fact that few, in my acquaintance at least, have embraced two or three religions *simultaneously.*

EXERCISE AND INTELLIGENCE

Exercise can make you more effective mentally. Body movements may be regarded as pieces of intelligence just like facts and vocabularies and logic. And I think the inclusion of the upper torso in an exercise program makes that more likely. The brain's connections with the upper extremitiess are numerous and the latter's movements enjoy an obviously wider range of movement capabilities.

In terms of oxygen transport, a high VO_2Max — the largest amount of oxygen you can process per minute — tends to preserve your thinking in a variety of situations. I'll explain. Suppose your work capacity is 20 METS — a high level to be sure. At rest (1 MET) you are working at 5 percent of your capacity. If your MET capacity, however, were 7, just sitting would tax you to the tune of about 15 percent of your capacity. Walking at 4 miles an hour, the problem changes drastically. The person with 20-MET capability feels no sense of exertion. At 4 miles an hour, a 150-pound person with 7-MET capability is close to the end of his rope, so to speak. What feels like a stroll to one is a huge effort for the other. Inevitably when you're functioning close to your physical limit, attention is focused on your body's travail. So even at a 15-minute-per-mile pace, two people with equal intelligence at rest would be all but out of rapport if their fitness levels were that mismatched. Another way of saying that fitness tends to "preserve" intelligence. Bodily preoccupations have a way of preempting everything else, as though nature "believes" the body comes first. Something analogous occurs with dieting. Well into a diet, its effectiveness is reduced measurably. The calorie deprivation that lost you two ounces of fat daily only loses you an ounce or even half an ounce as dieting continues. Body economy spares your starving body by making you more fuel-efficient, even though it's ruining your diet strategy. Interestingly, many of the responses to stress follow a similar pattern.

THE ENERGY GAP

This is another way of discussing the laudable effect of exercise on psychic function. The energy gap exists in all of us. Since thinking

---

Intelligence quotients: fitness quotients

I'm one of those doctors who doesn't hold the IQ in high regard. I think cultures create models of intelligence and individuals live, more or less, up to them. Same with oxygen transport, strength, grace, skill, and motor improvisation. Brains and muscles are just pieces of hardware ready for most anything we might wish to "program" into them. The equipment is being dangerously underutilized. Ironically, underachievers are always ready to blame their *deficient hardware*.

I am optimistic about the unleashing of unheralded energy through combined exercise, but it will not be easy. All manner of resistances will be encountered. Sometimes I muse over the initial reluctance to vigorous arm activity. One pet explanation is that there resides in us a lurking, atavistic anxiety related to giving up our lofty perch on the evolutionary ladder. New research in the exciting field of chemical paleontology suggests we are closer to our lower anthropoid kin than had been supposed. And when I watch with awe a consummate gymnast whirling about the high bar in a one-handed giant swing, I feel hopeful that the resurrection of the talented ape forelimb is not an idle fantasy. Brachiation, which means swinging through trees, is not likely to be restored as a major mode of transportation by modern man! But climbing and ambition are certainly not strangers to human motivation, and man couldn't be man without hands. I've been quoted as saying Heavyhands is the "no monkey business exercise." I may have to cancel that claim!

is easy — consuming infinitesimal amounts of energy as compared with muscular work — mental activity may actually become a kind of refuge we seek in order to "rest." This is particularly true of the more "passive" mental states when we merely receive sense data — such as watching television — or in the passive form of thinking we call fantasizing. In these, the sense of mental effort is quite low as compared, for example, with problem-solving. I believe that, *on average,* people with high work capabilities, in purely caloric terms, tend to resort less frequently and prolongedly to passive mental states. They have *narrow energy gaps,* whereas less-active people tend to resort more to fantasy for their "accomplishments." Which is not to say fantasy hasn't a useful place in our mental lives. But excessive fantasy, substituted too often for action, can cripple. Fitness may bring thought and action into a better harmony. The deconditioned state, on the contrary, widens the gap — so that a person in poor condition may depend more and more often on fantasy for solutions that should be forged in the world of action.

Furthermore, the development of motor freedom tends, itself, to generate types of thinking of a more active sort. A *plan,* for example, is an idea *strongly linked to action.* High levels of conditioning may make for a more effective flow between thinking and doing.

CONFIDENCE

Are exercisers more confident, less neurotic? I have seen patients in whom exercise seemingly wrought therapeutic miracles when "understanding" failed. My guess is that each fitness component finds a mental parallel and they all contribute in mysterious and wonderful ways to what we call confidence. Strength, for example, must carry with it a special sort of confidence that encourages us to seek tasks that require *strength.* Given tools, we humans seem bound and determined to find uses for them. And when we create a new and more effective body through training we seek success by using it whenever possible. Mind inherits body. Body inherits mind. Comprehensive conditioning may reduce neurotic wheel-spinning. The lessening of "general" neuroticism is a more predictable result of exercising than its effect upon *specific* symptoms of long standing. A conditioned individual may thus become gen-

Fitness factors and confidence — a tentative theory

I was interested in concocting a comprehensive exercise package partly because it seemed that each of the fitness elements corresponded to some aspect of our mental life. More explicitly, I think strength, speed, power, range of motion, endurance, flexibility, skill, grace, and spontaneity each came into being because of certain *intentions* which were surely mental. Once developed, these physical functions in turn ignite more of the ideas that begot them and the glorious cycle threatens to spiral heavenward in fortunate souls. A rather maudlin and rhapsodic hypothesis, I'll admit, but I've seen some convincing evidence. Like people who latch onto a paintbrush or cello, or hook a rug — and become overtly "manual" for the first time after beginning an "exercise" that studiously mobilized their hands.

Rest

Rest requirement is an individual problem. Suffice it to say that the higher your fitness level, the stronger your sense of confidence, the more your work-rest pattern will be governed by day-to-day physiologic and psychologic realities. Rigid scheduling that defies fatigue, illness, and high-priority life events suggests lurking self-doubts and magical thinking.

erally less hypochondriacal and depressed, but his fear of high places may remain intact. More important is the fact that his overall improvement seems to lessen the problem posed by the phobia itself.

SCHEDULING EXERCISE

Some people are fastidious exercisers, others are not. I enjoy eating when I feel like it and I treat myself to exercise in much the same manner. That doesn't mean I'm casual about it. I feel I have to keep after it consciously. If you're a neat and compulsive person in all sorts of ways, slot your exercise the same way. Your exercise, a highly vulnerable enterprise to begin with, should remain in phase with your personality. If you're a binging type, you may enjoy long sessions with two or three days off in between. That may not be ideal, but if that sort of thing keeps you at it, that's the way to go. And even though four to seven 30-minute sessions per week are prescribed, you're better off doing it "as you like it" in order to cater to your shaky status as a beginner. Later, you may change. Follow your inclinations so long as they stick with the cardinal rules and keep you as safe as possible from injury.

FEAR

Few people admit to fear as a major deterrent to exercise. But I think it ranks quite high among the emotions that inhibit us. Mostly these fears lie beneath consciousness so they can't be dealt with directly. I locate them by inference. Often people neatly avoid the idea of fear — by using face-saving substitutes instead; they simply "prefer" not to exercise, or suggest that after careful consideration they latched onto meditation as a way of "releasing" tension, or they've "gone" the exercise route and find it a terrible bore and besides, its validity has "never really been established." A clue to the presence of fear is the ironic fact that fear itself may be the *only* thing that finally galvanizes these people into action.

The fear of exercise is not simple. For many it stems from ov-

Exercise and addiction

Each of us is addicted to something. If not to a substance, to a compulsive activity or a maladaptive tactic or even a negative attitude. I often prescribe exercise as a kind of therapeutic addiction that may bump less healthy ones that waste our space, time, and energy. Twenty-two percent of our runners are said to smoke; the percentage falls virtually to zero among marathoners. A serious addiction to a *good thing* may become a benefit.

Collidophobia

I think we come into life, most of us, with an embryonic fear of motion and its consequences. In some the fear blossoms. I've noticed when I double ski-pole on my patio past my lounging dog she doesn't perceive me as the menacing juggernaut I really am! I must avoid *her* with my flying hands because she yawns through the session, obviously unconcerned despite all those near misses. We humans seem to operate with greater anxiety because of our intelligent imagery about what happens when irresistible force meets immovable object. In some the fear of collision may scotch the impulse to move beyond a snail's pace.

erdrawn notions that link violent activity with sudden cardiac death. Many seem to court an image in which they're primed into robust health one moment, panting and blue the next. If a story about a presumably conditioned exerciser who dies suddenly hits print, the fear-ridden victim may use it to verify what he's secretly suspected all along. Some fearful people have genealogies that are loaded with early cardiac deaths. So their fear contains a rational core that may become an obsession. Sometimes a thoroughgoing medical work-up and some simple instruction may prevent turning reasonable caution into self-neglect.

The problem with fear of exercise is that it tends to coexist with the falacious notion that *not* to do it is tantamount to *protection.* I believe that future generations will deal more intelligently with the psychic reasons for avoiding exercise. Perhaps several hours of honest introspection and a whole lot of good information would not be wasted *before any* program is begun. Many start exercise harboring latent intentions to quit. The trial is a symbolic sop to the conscience. *Not* to have tried would have left them guilty or anxious. Having appeased the gods, so to speak, by their mock trial, they can ease out conscience-free.

Not all fear of exercise is related to death. Some may fear the sense of suffocation that occurs in the *anaerobic* state. Many may systematically avoid any exertion sufficient to get them close to that. I have questioned dozens of people who couldn't remember the last time they were "out of breath." Aerobic exercise may push the oxygen-transport apparatus to within a few percent of the anaerobic level. When running at 80 to 90 percent of your capacity, a brief burst of enthusiasm can get you into oxygen debt. Intervals are frequently performed mostly anaerobically. Sooner or later good training should include anaerobic work and confer a sense of familiarity with it and therefore greater comfort while in oxygen debt. It's like swimming under water, another activity that doesn't lure many and probably by reason of that same primal fear. So we come up against another of those ironies that pervade the exercise motive: caution may protect from anxiety, but at the cost of increased physical risk. I see that ill-fated logic acted out again and again. It is a good example of chosing short-range comforts rather than more durable values. The confirmed exerciser may make the reverse sort of trade-off. He insists, in fact, upon dealing aggressively with the present discomforts of training in order to reduce

Brain-mind analogy

Heavyhands research findings say categorically that our oxygen transport systems are seldom used efficiently. The trained heart remains that way, as though waiting for enough work to be put to it. But the tasks of this world are such that only a small portion of our muscle mass makes demands upon the heart's output at *any given moment.* Putting many muscles to work simultaneously, the same heart pump can fuel a lot more work. After a few months of serious aerobic training, the heart becomes very nearly as efficient as it's ever apt to be. After that, it can seldom be accused of underachievement. The best *match* for a conditioned heart is an array of conditioned muscles working together. The heart, with all its persistence (thank God), is a rather stupid organ. Confronted with a poor muscle match, i.e., insufficient mass to consume its offering efficiently, the heart will continue to pump hard and fast, trying to achieve the impossible. The movements with which we measure our oxygen transport capabilities on treadmills and bikes usually tap deconditioned hearts against deconditioned muscles, or relatively conditioned hearts against *a few* conditioned muscles. The millions of conventional exercise cardiograms on file don't begin to reflect man's highest work potential. Now, doesn't that sound like the school counselors who contend that poor Johnny isn't living up to his bright young mind's potential? Neither hearts nor brains perform up to snuff unless "programmed" by plenty of diverse work. Putting a lot of duets together makes sense, whether we're dealing with nervous tissue or oxygen transport apparatuses.

Obsessive exercise

Only those uncertain about exercise become anxious over missed sessions. The more solidly entrenched your motives, the more willing you should be to skip exercise when intuition and judgment demand. Anything good should be interruptable. Everyone can't play with the iron consecutiveness of a Lou Gehrig. To do so compulsively is merely a sop to one's conscience and has little to do with health.

Doing Heavyhands correctly

It will be crystal-clear to most of my readers that there can be nothing special about the movements presented here. What makes a given execution correct or plain wrong? Sticking with the underlying principles, mostly. Mobilizing lots of muscle mass — many heart-muscle duets, we say — is a top priority consideration, along with keeping to some comfortable target heart rate. After that, things are less obligatory, more loose and elective — choices of muscle groups to exercise, exercise as rehearsal for sport, or inclusion of grace and flexibility in your panaerobic routines. The most flagrant no-no in Heavyhands is continued failure to maximize the arms' gigantic, usually latent, aerobic potential, which turns out to be such a physiologic bonanza for the circulatory system. Another departure from "correctness" is the failure to exploit the legs' musculature beyond the benefits derived from conventional walk-run strategies. The advanced Heavyhander, employing these simple principles, is free of anxiety about doing it wrong, and free to flow his/her instincts toward uncharted movement territory.

his anxiety about the future. By an intriguing sort of mental alchemy some are able to convert the travail of exercise into its emotional quintessence. The plain fact is that subtle shifts of emphasis and hard-to-identify feelings will make or break you as an exerciser.

I have seen a few who made the leap from real aversion to total immersion in exercise. These "reaction formations" are familiar to the behavioral scientist. But they are especially important in exercise becaue they affect the destiny of our very anatomies. Prompted by fear, these exercise fanatics push exercise beyond its physical and psychological advantages. A single missed session can precipitate the symptoms of abject depression or anxiety bordering on panic. It is a new syndrome, appearing in medical literature only recently.

We can also fear our own consciences when we come to exercise. One popular tactic for dealing with a conscience hurting from *not* exercising is to keep the intention to do so on the mind's back burners. Certain personalities feel expiated so long as their *spirit is willing*. The reluctance of the flesh doesn't faze them much, especially if they continue to serve sincere notice of their ambitious plans to family and friends. The *good intentions ploy,* as you can see, tends to widen the energy gap.

EXERCISE AND BODY PROPRIETORSHIP

This is a different sort of motivational flaw. There are many would-be exercisers who neither lust unrealistically toward improbable goals nor use flabby excuses to avoid exercise. These are the people I call nonproprietors of the mind–body. Actually they know of and believe in all the touted reasons for exercise. They may recite them as fluently as their doctor does. They openly confess their foolishness in not getting started. They are excellent salesmen who never use the product they peddle.

This category of nonexercisers is troublesome precisely because they offer no argument. They agree *too* readily and seem, if anything, especially motivated. They kind of perch themselves on the edge of beginning. If you ask what holds them back you get two stock answers: they either "don't know" or "just can't bring" themselves to do it. The word "just" in this syntax is translatable as "simply" or *not analyzable*. It means that they have not considered the underlying reasons for their inhibition and aren't particularly eager to receive help with that. Incidentally, these folks usually use the "I don't know" or "I just can't" routine in many other sectors of their lives.

There are large numbers of nonproprietors about. To some extent we're all victims. It's like taking the Fifth where it comes to honesty with yourself. It's the attitude opposite of self-actualization, that ultimate in self-proprietorship described by the late Abraham Maslow.

I do believe that nonproprietorship is a variation on the theme of dependency, that nemesis of the human animal that comes from our extralong development. And I think we're peculiarly prone to "body" nonproprietorship. It's as though our minds grow and differentiate while our bodies, in a sense, continue to belong to Mama. A false, even dangerous sense of security may continue long after Mama is gone; one remains safe and viable without trying — a kind of return to the idyllic days of our infantile omnipotence.

It's hard to scare a good nonproprietor, so we doctors, at our threatening best (worst?), become frustratingly impotent. The patient offers no objection, even chimes in with additional pitches. But the patient's belief lacks the quality of conviction that *motorizes*. The body and mind are split: the adult intelligence understands and believes; the fixated body rests as unconcerned as it was at the breast.

DRIVES AND EXERCISE

Both utter avoidance and excess are as harmful in exercise as at the dinner table. Indeed some very interesting parallels and contrasts exist between the drives toward food and toward activity that may be worth mentioning.

The need for activity is subtle compared with the hunger urge. Only in unusual states does the drive toward action become as compelling in the same sense as is ravenous appetite. But deprivation of food and activity both produce varying degrees of irritability and depression. Both drives can be present as sporadic bursts or as almost constant need. Both can be gratified rather quickly. In the case of feeding we speak of satiety — a sense of fullness that ends the urge; fatigue or some other sort of general muscular depletion reaches consciousness and may halt the motive to *act*.

Should some people not exercise?

A hard one to answer with categoric certainty, especially if you're as prejudiced as I am. Yes, I think some folks might, all things considered, fare better without exercise. Leaving out those for whom infirmities, even mild ones, make exertion dangerous, some people mix with exercise like oil and water. I worry most about those who "somehow can't," but never manage to excuse themselves cleanly.

Arm resistance

My spies in the community confirm my own direct observations. Despite a book, dozens of illustrated magazine articles, more TV and radio appearances than I can recall, many Americans — having spent good cash on those lovely little red-and-black weights with cushioned strap and handle — *don't use them properly.* Some hold the weight by its strap, which is hard to figure. Perhaps they consider it an iron or a kettle. Some, assiduously refusing to pump the weights, leave them hanging fixed at mid-thigh during their perambulations. Some select pump-stride frequencies like 1:3 that don't give the lusty uppers an even break. One man I know pumps one hand perfectly, keeping the other firmly planted at his waist! Once in New York on our way to dinner I glimpsed a Heavyhander speeding along at around 8 knots, *holding* his 3-pounders in the typical runner's arm carry. Despite my tie and the humidity, I took off in hot pursuit, overtaking the young man three blocks up Fifth Avenue. "How come you're not pumpin' 'em?" I panted. His look told me he hadn't the slightest notion as to what I was talking about. After a pleasant chat and a brief demonstration, he was off again, this time cheerily pumping high and proud. I think that's all it takes. But Millie and I suspect we've discovered an archaic defense in this early "reluctance" to do with arms something analogous to what we've always left to legs. Overcoming that defense could, if my numbers are right, add 15 percent or more to our race's oxygen transport capability!

The taste buds and their connections with the central nervous system, and taste imagery, are part of the appetite mechanism. The imagery related to action is more complex and less localized. In the exerciser there are likely dozens of images that converge as the need to act. Unlike hunger and taste, there are ordinarily no readily identifiable physical sensations that stir the exerciser toward activity.

The instincts to feed and to move play differently upon skill and intelligence. For modern man, feeding has become increasingly "technologized." Cooking has become a valued skill and even the act of taking food has become associated with delicate sensitivities and subtleties of judgment. The exerciser generally seeks the *simplest,* most direct way of achieving what he's learned about the benefits of exercise. So it seems that hunger, by far the stronger appetite, gathers the refinements of culture to it more so than does exercise. It is as though the stronger the drive, *the greater the tendency to embellish.* We see that tendency in the imaginative writings and blossoming freedoms of the Sexual Revolution. Feeding and sexuality remain basically unchanged. The technologies that flourish about them are a series of incitements, titillations, fore and end pleasures, if you will.

Exercise suffers obviously from the lack of incitements such as hunger and taste and the various sensations and electric finales of sex. Exercise, simply put, has no erogenous zones. Or, if it does, they are disguised, complex, highly individual, subtly connected with our fantasy life rather than any immediate sort of bodily pleasure. Racial survival depends heavily upon the instincts to nourish and reproduce. Modern man finds himself in the rather macabre position of both stimulating his appetites and keeping them under wraps.

If exercise may be considered a drive, it is surely the least urgent and therefore least dangerous. Not rooted in structures like orifices and special nerve endings, the exercise "instinct" can play freely upon the highest central nervous functions — where idea and motion meet. So while we don't "embellish" much as belabored exercisers, that option should remain wide open to us.

This potential of exercise has hardly been explored. I think it's because as a race we're still annoyed about having been told to exercise. No one had to sell food and sex. To be advised by the experts of the effects of exercise on longevity, health, and the quality of life without being supplied with immediate gratifications such as those associated with feeding and sex makes exercise a very hard sell. Many have resorted to making promises of quick results as though the exercise hucksters were thinking that to peddle exercise it has to be made as gratifying as its neighbor instincts — those more fixed in the flesh.

I think this unreasonable pandering to the need for instant gratification could prove ultimately disastrous to the Fitness Revolution. It may also explain the enraptured responses of novices who claim feeling states that sound as if they belong more properly to the dining table and the boudoir. I suspect exercise pleasure, in its *best* form, will be more intellectual, sedate, and planned. There's nothing wrong with touting the pleasure of exercise so long as we don't get our metaphors mixed. Exercise pleasure belongs to the real though subdued and more prolonged aspects of activity. Training effects and their psychic equivalents shouldn't be placed in the same footrace with other specialized pleasures. The pleasures of exercise can only be properly appreciated once dislodged from the bad habit of *comparing them* with other things.

This is the crucial issue. Exercise today finds itself in the shaky situation of being poor competition with finer skills on the one hand, and the biologic instincts on the other. Neither fish nor fowl, exercise needs a new identity. It is hard for me to believe, given those endless possibilities combining mind and movement, that the growth of exercise is anywhere near its end point. We notice these days a regrettable decline in the performance of young people's language skills. I often wonder if this isn't the time to push "body language" for all it's worth. Rudolph Lowenstein has suggested that the teaching of drawing very early might enhance education — that words are, after all, merely "pointers" that describe the images we generate. Might not the other nonverbal skills — dance, music, eurythmics, body control — lend a needed boost to mental abilities like language? The miracles of oxygen transport are there for the asking. At the outside, a single year of diligent training can produce high fitness levels in most healthy subjects. After that its maintenance can really become a matter of motor adventure. Not the joy of sex nor the joys of gourmet dining to be sure; rather the joy of motion and skill mingled with the sense of confidence and security that go with continuing fitness. Our work capacities are probably as limited as our visual acuity or the rates at which our nerve

Exercise is for living

The biggest thrill for the purebred exerciser is the joy of application of new abilities. It is the rough analogue of winning at sport or perhaps surviving a grueling marathon. Application is to training what spending is to earned money. Once applications in the real world fall into intimate synchrony with your changing training strategy, you can't quit.

impulses travel. *But within that capability we haven't begun to discover ourselves.*

The tasks of Heavyhands as a method and philosophy are clear: one is to bring us to the highest fitness levels of which we are capable. That's the simpler part. More exciting are the choreographies of body and spirit that will make life more interesting in more ways than any of us can yet imagine. Once that happens, concerns about "exercise" should disappear. Sessions, programs, and strategies strike me the same as do diets and weight watching. They underscore a preoccupied struggle that should one day simply become *part of life.* The conscious combination of high workloads and skill just makes good "psychosomatic" sense. Where that option will lead us only time can tell.

Many are still a long way from willingness to work hard, even briefly, during those hours we tacitly assign to "being leisurely." As time goes on it will become more difficult to remain casual about exercise. Perhaps tomorrow's educators will help promote the virtue of vigor in a world where work and love are impossible without energy.

In Chapter 2 we listed our notions of the advantages of Heavyhands exercise. We repeat them now along with the psychologic accompaniments of those advantages as we see them.

A. *Genderless.* The gender excuse is reduced by bringing each sex toward its optimal workload. Also, Heavyhands contains elements that will attract one sex more than the other, thus preserving sexual identity as it relates to physical performance.

B. *Widest range of workloads.* The pooling of various muscle groups into combined activity is the analogue of "getting it together" in the psychologic sense. Training with expectable rewards is the physical parallel to enthusiastic learning.

C. *Ease of entry for the beginner.* The typical fear of new ventures is lessened by reducing likely early failure. Initial difficulty discourages a number of would-be exercisers as well as those about to try anything new. The fear of failure also serves as a defense, especially in cultures where enormous premium is placed upon "success." The anaerobic "suffocating" feeling that most experience in beginning endurance training may be a physiologic equivalent of panic.

D. *Fewer injuries.* Injuries make for general apprehensiveness, which in turn may result in loss of a sense of freedom and interrupt

---

Exercise: its relation to leisure and work

Consider the plight of those whose work constitutes their most vigorous exertion. If leisure for them means "rest," their maximal steady work capacity will eventually shrink to some deconditioned level not much higher than that called for by their job. I would doubt that more than 5 percent of the working population averages 5 METs over an 8-hour stretch of work. Since *work* as a conditioner is a poor bet, fitness levels compatible with health and activity must be "earned," ironically during leisure.

graceful, effective execution. Movements may become "defensive." Injury in endurance athletes may force layoffs prolonged enough to depress the susceptible ones. When a high level of fitness makes injury more likely, a conflict is inevitably created.

E. *Single package.* Security is increased by knowing no major fitness factor is being neglected. That's analogous to the quality of confidence we relate to being "well rounded." Comprehensiveness in this sense also involves the time dimension and reduces the sense of hurriedness which increases tension. One can "relax," so to speak, knowing that one's effort covers the gamut of fitness factors.

F. *Economy of time.* Timesavers diminish anxiety in a world where many are scheduled to their teeth. Freeing of time and energy for other things may produce emotional highs. Increasing the intensity of exercise per minute of output leaves one with a comforting option where it comes to making time for exercise. Good exercise creates time in a sense, because it effectively increases energy.

G. *Convenience.* This works against the ever-present wish to discontinue that which is felt to be difficult (regression). Inconvenience may discourage many before they get going well. It is a major excuse for those who are shaky about exercise to begin with. The need for convenience slackens as the strategy gains momentum and a sense of permanence takes over. That's true of anything else one takes on, incidentally — things far from the world of exercise.

H. *Weight control.* With freedom from constant dietary worry, energy rescued from depression, preoccupation, shame, and conscious conflict can be invested elsewhere. As success in weight control become apparent, there is correspondingly less thought and energy diverted toward matters that should be as automatic for us as they are for giraffes.

I. *Flexibility.* One feels less hemmed in by stereotyped forms of exercise, where obvious options for change and growth are somewhat more limited. And the sense of freedom and control may aid in making permanent identification with exercise.

J. *Prolonged growth.* The longer growth phase inherent in Heavyhands finds it psychic counterpart in optimistic effort projected over the long term and is the equivalent of the ability to delay gratification.

K. *Extends the accomplished athlete.* Renews interest by supplying new opportunities for growth. Skilled athletes may become blasé and neglect fitness maintenance that seems nonessential to their performance. Ironically, those whose bodily performance is central — as in professional athletes — may become less than optimally fit and enjoy the psychic equivalents of fitness less than do some sedentary exercisers.

L. *Practical.* In exercise "practical" means associated with the activities of everyday work and play. An energy saver again because making difficult things easy provides us with the pleasant psychologic sense of mastery over our personal world.

M. *Noncompetitive.* I view competition as a passive trait insofar as one's competition is allowed to regulate one's performance. By its nature any sport has limitations that were created to make competition exciting. So competition, often seen as an instigator of activity, may also limit growth. Competition means that our activity and our level of success is determined by others. The very nature of freedom rests upon our ability to determine our lives by ourselves.

N. *Psychologic Effects.* Of course that's partly what Exerpsychology is about. The next ten years will produce a mountain of new research relating to mind-body interplay. Already a number of universities have fitted out laboratories devoted specifically to the psychologic aspects of fitness and sports. That sort of investigation will father unsuspected ideas about why we're so often content with less than optimal body hardware, and lots of surprises about the good that accrues from having the best body one is capable of having.

I predict, too, that the more genetically oriented theories about physical capability, the you-were-born-to-be-heroic or -sloblike doctrine will lose ground fast. That change will, of course, rob us of some up-front excuses. Instead we'll enjoy the conviction that our genes supply us, most often, with the built-in right to choose more than enough of what we might want to be.

O. *Other exercise and sports.* One activity is felt to be a rehearsal for others. The "togetherness" within the self may be the parallel to what psychiatrists and psychologists call *integration.* Such interdependence prevents the exercise from being felt as an isolated chore.

P. *Rehabilitation.* The antidepressant implications will be obvious. The intact musculature is substituted in a manner reminiscent of the healthy personality's ability to shift from blocked motives to available channels of function and progress.

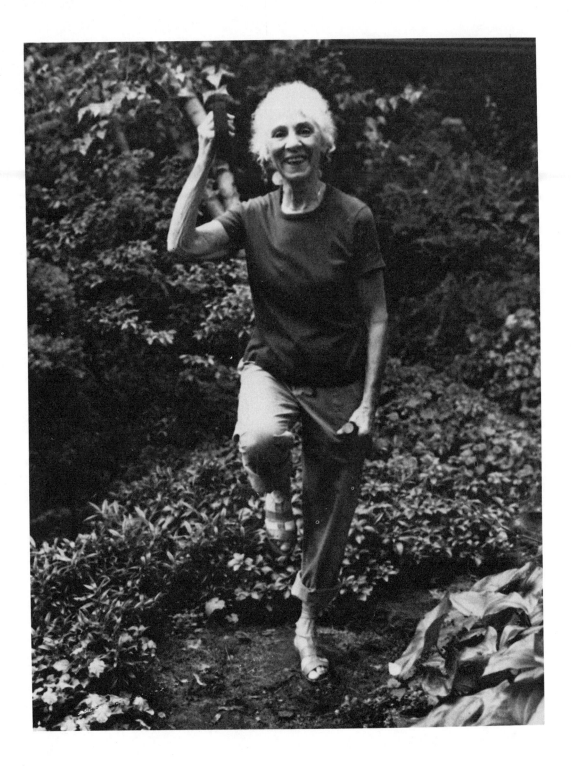

18

Epilogue

I'M NOT SURE how books of this sort should end. Given my preference, this would have been a loose-leaf affair suitable for making hasty deletions and a slew of additions. After all, Heavyhands is supposed to be an "open" system, so what would be more appropriate than an "unbound" format?

And I think it appropriate that we quit as we began — with apologies. These final pages have the dual purpose, then, of finishing the book, while leaving its author a tad less guilty and ashamed. My fantasy is that Heavyhands will initiate a lot of elegant research that will raise new questions about combined exercise — and even answer a few of them. For now this is uncharted territory. The terrain appears lush and inviting and safe and exciting; but you're going to be on this "trip" for a long time, I hope, so you can't blame an anxious parent for stuffing a few last-minute items into your duffle bag.

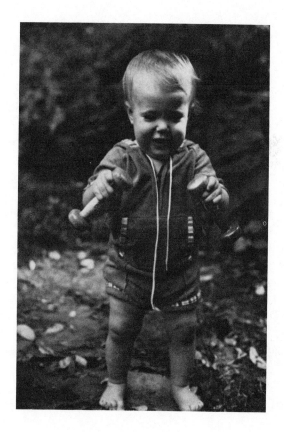

You see, I know at least as well as anyone that exercise comes very easy for some and very hard for many. If the solid reasons for doing it weren't increasing in such profusion, there could be no excuse for this kind of final nagging. Maybe one of the best reasons for adopting exercise is that you don't want ever to regret *not* having seriously considered something that could have made your life — in the broadest sense of the word — better. When one day, those people who are slim from action outnumber those who try to dispatch fat by some fancy form of starvation, we'll have turned an important corner. Our improved appearance will be the smallest of our gains. Work, the kind measured by foot-pounds, shapes bodies and minds that have huge appetites for doing. And that can't be bad.

So here's the last of the tips and warning and admonitions and seductions.

STRATEGIZE

Most exercise systems offer neat programs — step-by-step recipes for gaining fitness. I prefer the word *strategy* to "program." Programs connote for me tight little scheduled directives (things funded by government or fed into computers). Strategy has a more aggressive, individual, thought-out ring about it — for me.

Strategies should be organic, freewheeling plans. Unique bodies teamed with unique minds generate unique strategies, common sense would dicate. The imperative "strategize" gets closer to what we're after. Its impact upon attitude can't be placed on a wall chart or printed schedule. No special game plan — it is the plan to plan *endlessly*. It has no precise word equivalent. It means something like going at it with intelligence and interest. It's a kind of enthusiasm that survives the troughs and peaks that accompany all learning. It's excitement that may ebb and flow somewhat, but never stops. It may latch onto a new focus at any moment — now a discovery, now a resolve, now a challenging impasse, now a reflection upon things past, now a reworking of strategies suddenly and clearly outmoded. Strategizing, like weight watching, conscience, the work ethic, and love, becomes *real* when it leaves our mouths and permeates our selves.

Heavyhands repertoire

Every Heavyhands repertoire should contain an itinerary of movements that are performed with various degrees of competence: like an artist's studio with canvases at various stages of completion. A good model of the growth process generally, one would think. A pastiche of things hard and easy at the extremes reminds me of the contraction and relaxation of muscle.

FLEXIBILITY

Like body suppleness — range of motion — the freedom to change your exercise strategy to match changing needs and outer realities is crucial. Adaptability is another word for it. Adaptability requires energy and produces energy. That may not be obvious at first. It works like this: as your technique improves it fits a wider range of *inner states* (thoughts and moods mostly) and *outer situations* (space and time realities, departures from ideal environmental conditions, injuries). A hill and depression would be examples of outer and inner blockers of performance. Practice makes it easier to continue despite them. Practice *requires energy*, and that makes for better skill at negotiating the slopes and blue funks of life, which in turn makes you a more energetic person. Heavyhands training increases your adaptability by the range of new problems it provides!

Viewed in that light, a new muscle soreness, the aftermath of an experiment with a new movement, becomes a *discovery*. You've in effect discovered a new function and structure that can, once practiced, become a new source of energy and adaptability. If you prefer to think defensively, you've created a new immunity — destroyed an unsuspected vulnerability. Because it strays from stock planes and angles, free form Heavyhands exercise is a good way of locating chinks in your exercise armor. Any new move you happen upon, practiced a few times, can jell into a permanent calisthenic addition. Move is to muscle what thought is to brain. The endless interplay of both makes whole people.

BODY SAVVY

Sigmund Freud once said the first ego was a *body* ego. Translated, that suggests the body is, from early on, much of what we're about. Any exercise can, willy-nilly, teach you a lot about how your body copes with the stressful paces through which you put it. I've said that nonproprietorship is a scourge. But proprietorship is more than an attitude — your body is your territory and the Music Man had it right when he declared "You gotta know the territory."

Under body savvy I include the kind of intelligence that comes from the feedback one receives from the body placed in variety of peculiar circumstances. Exercise is a good place to learn about your body because physiologic responses are culled from extreme or near-extreme tasks.

Around 1960, Borg, a Scandinavian physiologist, devised a scale by which a subject estimated the vigorousness of his exercise at a given moment. You surely will come across the Borg Scale for RPE (rating of perceived exertion) if you read much in the field. But though thousands of experiments have been performed around the world, it's still a bit of a mystery as to just *how* the work level is telegraphed to consciousness. Borg originally measured his subjects' responses against heart rates and found them proportional. But the heart rate per se doesn't tell us *how hard* we're working — it's simply a dependable and understandable *accompaniment* of hard work.

Other investigators found other factors to be better "translators" of the fact of hard work to our central nervous sytems: the volume of air expired per minute, or sensations from the working muscles and stretching tendons. The levels of lactic acid and adrenaline like substances in the blood during exercise have been investigated too.

Most of these researches employ a statistical rather than an individual approach — how *mankind* knows how hard he's working rather than how Sue differs from Herb.

There is some evidence that Heavyhanders will estimate their work levels somewhat differently. Runners I've worked with are often shocked at the high heart rates they achieve at relatively low estimates of their exertion (Borg Scale). They're also shocked at the high oxygen uptakes they generate at low RPEs. Some researchers have noted that the AT (Anaerobic Threshold — the workload at which anaerobic responses suddenly begin to occur) is significantly higher during combined exercise of arms and legs. So we may not be far from a firmly established, physiologic justification for Heavyhands.

In the meantime, body savvy for you is the sum total of smarts you can generate that keep you training safely but sufficiently, and with a healthy gap between you and injury. Your self-proprietorship is your own. Given a heart, lungs, and muscles in common, we tend to read their complex messages differently. *How* we read them is in turn determined by the specifics of our personal history, our fears, our conscious and unconscious aspirations.

Still another caveat on high blood pressure

If your blood pressure is high or borderline, steer clear of much strength-dominated work in your Heavyhands workouts. Err on the side of *littler* weights, even though you can manage to steady out at your target pulse with heavier ones. Particularly for lengthy sessions, go fast and light as in pump 'n walk to level 3. That mobilizes more muscle mass and tends, we believe, to lower the so-called "peripheral resistance" that makes pressure in the arterial tree high. High-swift pumps with little weights will make you stronger for 97 percent of the chores everyday life extracts from you. As your pressure drops, you can gradually add in strength sprints for short intervals at first.

More on exercise and blood pressure

There is a fairly constant relationship between the intensity of exercise and its effect upon blood pressure. Lab studies suggest that the systolic blood pressure (the higher of the two numbers by which blood pressure measurements are notated) elevates somewhere between 7.5 and 12 millimeters of Mercury per *MET*. Thus a 10-MET workload, like running a mile in 10 minutes, would typically *raise* the systolic somewhere between 75mm and 120mm Hg. Our studies, confirmed now by several investigators, indicate that pressure elevations, with four trained limbs working rhythmically, are significantly *lower* per MET of work than with conventional exercise. If this is validated to the satisfaction of the scientific community, Heavyhands will become the choice exercise for millions with resting high blood pressure who often are found to have *exaggerated increases* in pressure at given work levels. Again, it must be understood that these desirable effects come with *gradual* training. Initial attempts at pumping weights high and fast are apt to produce relatively high blood pressure readings. Training effects parallel human destiny generally: Strain lessens as the system adapts to stressors. The rationale side of the masochism of exercise comes in the joy of mastery. Training effects prove it *was* worth it.

Experiment during exercise. For instance, don't settle for a fixed breathing pattern until you've tried several. Learn to guesstimate your heart rate from the frequency and depth of your breathing. Try holding your breath for a second or two at the end of inhalation. Some say that may help ventilation — the efficiency with which oxygen and carbon dioxide are traded between lung and blood and back. Each exercise, each combination of weights, frequency, and range of motion deserves scrutiny. It's fun too, and makes you expert on the only exercise you'll ever observe from *within*.

I know I've lingered long on pulse counting in Chapter 3. By now I expect you're expert enough that you pulse-count rarely — probably only when you're up to something different and can't quite predict your cardiac response to it. I'd bet many of you can estimate your heart rate within 10 or 15 percent by merely sampling two successive pulse beats. You should now extend your awareness. Pulse-take when you're Heavyhanding in hot weather and high humidity and you'll find it higher than usual. You may notice differences in the quality of your felt pulse when you shift from leg to arm emphasis and vice versa. Note premature beats, irregularities that may warn you of too much caffeine, too little rest, or anxiety. Let faster than usual resting rates move you toward the low end of ambition for that day's workout if you *must* exercise at all.

Formulate your workouts to anticipate special demands you intend to make upon your body in the future. Emphasize strength, speed, or range of motion. Push muscle groups you'll need in *ways* you expect to need them. Return to the exercises you long since swore off. That way you learn that your body can adapt in *unexpected* ways. I've known many who turned up their noses when invited to double ski-pole. Can't say I blamed them either — it's hardly your conventional ambultory move and is apt to cause gawkers to stop in their tracks. Several of those original abstainers now do the move to the near exclusion of the remainder of the Heavyhands repertoire. Read physiology and kinesiology (the study of muscles and their actions). Proprietorship means not sedately relegating the knowledge of body structure and function to professionals. You have a *right to be an expert in self-help* regardless of the diplomas you have or haven't. Your survival, measured both in clock time and life-style, may depend more than you know upon an aggressive approach toward super health. Body savvy doesn't mean worrisome watching for the first inkling of symptoms and panicky phone calls. It means lessening the risks by being better than what the books are willing to call *normal* or *average*.

THINKING ON THE MOVE

Sometimes I think those who prefer their exercise in the form of sport are not motivated solely by the love of competition. Our big brains, by far the best cerebral hardware in the animal kingdom, are made for thinking. Most aerobic exercises are not as demanding as court sports, for example, where instant responses of an infinite variety are called for. The exerciser is apparently willing to trade the thinking adventure of competitive sport for the exquisite control, comparative safety, and the physiologic result he gleans from the repetitious grind of training. Anyone who moves to either the games-sports or the training extreme *exclusively* becomes a loser in a sense. I needn't repeat the old saws about the ravages of over-specializtion. Heavyhands makes the choice unnecessary: (1) it provides the best conditioner, within its comprehensive package, for the athlete; (2) it does that with a smaller time expenditure than other aerobics; (3) it provides, within the method itself, elements that, while not games, nonetheless have the psychic flavor and provoke thought patterns that are associated with those of games. I'll be more explicit about the last point because it is so important.

We are *curiously dependent* upon those with whom we compete. The ideal arrangement would be one in which our adversary brings the fiercest competition and skill to the game then loses to us inevitably! The winner emerges with more than a victory — he has upped his pride a notch by usurping a portion of the ego of his opponent. That's why losing hurts some people so — it is as though a portion of themselves had been lost, however valiantly they struggled to win.

For psychiatrists, the problem is even more complicated. Some people lose despite colossal skill; for others relative mediocrity seldom stands in the way of winning. Psychic factors, in other words, may take their toll on those who expect to derive fitness from sports.

Heavyhands exercise may be likened to sports in that practice

---

Exercise and aloneness

I know a lot of people who don't like being alone. Reading is probably the most popular single antidote to that painful aloneness which becomes synonymous with "lonely." Exercise is probably the best way for active people to deal with loneliness. Some have probably become exercise addicts unknowingly in order to beat the pain of loneliness. A few have even discovered *themselves*, finding they're not half bad company.

and skill are essentials and mastery is never complete. Your "opponents," so to speak, are the various resistances you encounter to becoming the "you" you *thought* you wanted to be. The "game" amounts to winning over the *self-defeating elements* that tend to block growth for all of us. Of course, I'm prejudiced professionally and philosophically, but I think this kind of winning is where it's at.

It turns out that your opponent is always in *your* head. He or she is merely the memory of who you used to be — the only opponent in the world whose defeat makes real sense, and the only game in which no one gets hurt.

Many will argue that nothing can replace an in-the-flesh opponent to defeat or be defeated by. True enough, but then that's only *one kind* of game. Since few games require, for example, ultimate levels of oxygen transport, then all conventional games are limiting to that extent. Since all games capitalize on one or a few components of fitness, *no* game can produce comprehensive fitness.

One reads of the fantasies that are said to course through the minds of distance runners, channel swimmers. So often their thoughts are projected *away* from the activity itself, as though attempting to distract themselves from a painful chore — or perhaps a painful spot in the body. I've read of counting rituals and other number games — killing time we call it.

Once one adds the arms and the trunk in combined exercise with the option to change often without stopping, the exerciser thinks *into* the exercise rather than *away* from it. Boredom exits the same way. Now you are truly alone with yesterday's self with no opponent eager to shape your next idea. The most evenly matched pair possible!

I've found that each variety of the Heavyhands repertoire spawns a separate kind of thinking. Doing ambulatory medleys outside, I shift frequently between self-observation and scanning the scene. At pulse rates from 120 to 140 I'm more the observer. From 140 up I tend to slip more into myself, monitoring this and that, making fewer visual forrays into my environment. I have redesigned equipment en route, planned pictures that needed to be taken, thought up countless variations on movement themes. Yes, and I have, hundreds of times, sworn never to Heavyhand again!

The free forms — shadowbox and dance and combinations of them — produce in me a peculiar sort of thought. It's as though the body does it all — leads the cortex. Music combines with space in interesting ensembles. You couple yourself to the music to be artistic and graceful — to the surroundings to be careful. *It is never boring.* I don't know how many runners and swimmers dance. I would very much like to know. Some of the prominent runner-writers have confessed that music and dance are, for them, turn-offs. For me music is conspicuously absent from my runner's mileage. I've threatened to take it along as an electronic earmuff companion of some sort. Often I hum against the pace. A good aerobic practice, incidentally.

GRACE

Remember to shoot for gracefulness. Yes, your heart and lungs will do well without it, as will your muscles. But many of these movements can be beautiful when practice brings a second-nature quality to them.

What are the components of grace? Strength for one. Strength smoothes the stiff, jerky quality from a complex movement. Strength allows consecutive nerve-muscle connections to surface as silky sliding transitions from one set of contractions to the next. Sometimes a mirror helps. More often it's the reduction in self-conscious concern about *parts* of the movement. The golf swing analogy is as good as any. So long as you are flitting agonizingly from your foot position to your extended left arm to the arc of the backswing to the hip rotation to the wrist break to the follow-through, you are a bit like the schizophrenic centipede with multiple simultaneous destinations. Better to work deliberately over a new move until you groove it. Then practice and new strength will iron it smooth. Also heavy and light variations, several practice frequencies, and edging up the range of motion will increase grace. I think, too, the *more* you work a given muscle or group into a number of movements, the more graceful *each* will become. Again music is a help.

I figure gracefulness will help spare you from injury. Graceful movements are performed somewhat short of our limits. If you've run on a treadmill to exhaustion, you'll know what I mean. Just before you've *had it,* a kind of flailing helplessness, awkward disconnectedness takes over your body-mind. When I learned I could syncopate better using more oxygen in combined exercise than I could working the hell out of a couple of limbs, I knew Heavyhands had the makings of an ultimate kind of exercise. I could maintain some semblance of grace, working with four limbs, for a couple of hours — at workloads that had me run ragged within 2 minutes of leg work! Secretly, I believe the inclusion of gracefulness will help make exercise a permanent installation in your life as effectively as will upgraded oxygen transport. Few dancers quit, I'll bet, even though their VO_2Maxes aren't often heroic. Grace lends a sense of belonging — there it is again — proprietorship to your movement behavior. And that might just be a large clue as to what makes a person stick with exercise. They stick when their sense of worth increases as a rough parallel to the training effect. So an increased VO_2Max, mixed delicately with grace, might be what the doctor–choreographer of tomorrow will prescribe.

TOGETHERNESS

Heavyhands is categorically the best aerobic exercise for two people. I read only recently that the rate of divorce among marathon runners is about 3.5 times that of the rest of the population. That might have to do with the reduced togetherness that happens when one spouse runs 100 to 200 miles a week preparing for long races.

Physiological differences make togetherness between any two people difficult to come by and that problem is accentuated when males and females try to exercise together. Take two young people pared to muscular leanness and married to each other. They want to run together. With equal training, the male's VO_2Max will be enough higher than his wife's that either he must take it easy or she must labor or both, for them to keep company en route. The compromise may be good for their marriage but their training won't be optimal. A group of five or even ten people can pump 'n' run in a tight cluster for miles, each right on target. Juggling size of handweight, stride length, frequency, and pump-height level, there is simply no problem.

I bring up togetherness as a reason in itself and in relation to another issue. Some Heavyhands beginners will adopt it because its a good way to stay fit *indoors*. They are the ones who don't relish

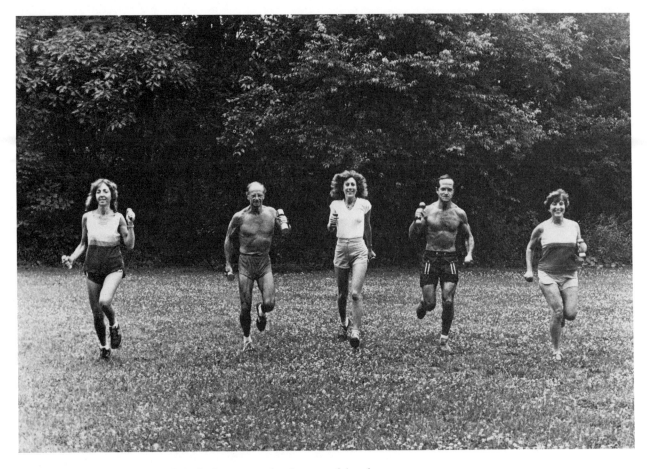

making a public display of their fitness aspirations and inadequacies. Jogging was a real problem for those of us who are shy until enough hit the road that we suspected correctly that we'd be ignored.

But ski-poling and pump 'n' jackknifing, and lateral thrusts on the move and Level III walking won't be regarded as conventional behavior for a little while yet. And while most of these can be accomplished nicely out of sight, it would be a mild shame not to enjoy the option to go outside on a brilliant spring or fall day. A Heavyhands group makes it okay. Other outdoor exercisers can seldom find anyone who matches their own physiologic profile precisely enough — much less a group. Going at it as quadripeds, a group can be utterly heterogeneous physiologically while moving along at the same pace. The same, of course, holds true for group

Groups and Heavyhands

Some people will never embark upon an exercise strategy that doesn't involve *group* participation. And calling man a gregarious animal doesn't quite explain *why* exercise groups are so popular these days. From my own classes, I've collected an offbeat hunch. It may be that the exercising group enjoys a special sort of communication. It is obvious that more work means less talk and so good exercise may beget communications of the nonverbal variety! And it does seem so with our group. A nod or a smile or a hackneyed salutation emitted between fast breaths may be quite enough. And when one thinks of it, these paragraph-length litanies — profound dueling, I call it — may be precisely where many relationships come acropper. Strangely, at the end of a year of communal sweating to the sound of music mostly, we all feel we know a great deal about each other! The group is so clearly intent upon motion that we barely notice *what* anyone is wearing. What we *do* notice is a movement that's an obvious departure from the usual, or some member's frequent absence. It's tempting to call this a refreshing regression to a kind of tribal state in the service of the ego, but I'll resist that temptation for now. For those who have come to believe nothing has meaning unless transcribed into language, an exercise group can be a mind opener. From the psychoanalyst's view the obvious reduction in anxiety may come from the *relief of the need to make talk.*

Heavyhands dance, where handweights make it possible for everyone to bring his or her own workload prescription to the music.

TEACH HEAVYHANDS

Something may happen to doers of anything once they turn teacher. Or perhaps something may alter in the doing of something that may create the impulse to teach it. However it works, the role of teacher could confer a permanence to the thing taught in the life of the teacher. Responsibility may be part of it. Teachers are parent surrogates of a sort, since the prototype of teaching must be what happens between the parent and the human most in need of information — the infant.

TIPS FOR PUTTING WORKOUTS TOGETHER

These came from several years of accumulated experience from other Heavyhanders and myself. Some may be good rules of thumb for you. Don't fret if they all don't seem to suit you. You will soon find yourself sliding into *patterns* and even those will seldom become permanent fixtures. Body-minds in training approach each session with subtly altered body hardware and attitudes. A few of these have been suggested in the body of the text but bear repetition in this quick, final review.

• If you have no pet aversion among them, try to include some in-place or on-the-move pump 'n' walk, some Heavyhand jumps, and one or more exercises that involve body flexion (jackknifing) in every session.

• If any exercise leaves you sore each time, especially in the same spot, either dismiss it outright for a while or perform it with weights that are clearly too light for you. Some find it useful to plug those exercises into the session relatively late rather than early — to get the benefit of well-warmed muscles. Or repeat the exercise several times during the session, always quitting well short of even a suggestion of strain.

• Some runners find themselves stiff in leg and hip following modest (5 miles or less) sessions, even with plenty of static stretching, before and after. If that describes *you* approximately, start early in your Heavyhands career to specialize in double ski-poling on the move. Preferably, work both heavy and light during each session. Try to get to fairly heavy weights. If you're very strong and have no particular back problems, you may find yourself eventually able to manage as much as 15 percent of your body weight in each hand at a cycle of frequency of 35 per minute! Also, if you're not as supple as a ballet dancer, finish your ambulatory sessions with double ski-poling and chances are good you'll go home less taut than you were at the start of the workout.

• Jumping medleys are of particular importance to runners, because all running contains that omnipresent vertical component. Since hills are a nemesis for many runners and since most runners jump poorly without special training, it seems sensible to practice that vertical component rather aggressively. I think my jumping medleys are why my running times continue to improve on insignificant mileage — less than 2 miles a week average — as I near sixty. Jump slow and fast, 120 to 220 per minute, juggling the size of handweights and the type and range of upper-torso accompaniment. There's no excuse for seasonal deconditioning once your repertoire includes these, especially if your TV is in working order!

• Initial experience with new exercise is seldom wholly gratifying. The risk of soreness is great, and clumsiness makes it less than an ego trip. So caution is always wise early. Oversized weights seem to be the most frequent offenders, followed by overfast tempos and overextended durations. Essentially, overdoing anything prematurely is what injures. And *all* overuse injuries can occur while your pulse rate is well *below target!*

• If you're on a hot roll with a particular exercise, don't be afraid to ride it for a while. This love-at-first-contraction syndrome assails all of us and nothing is lost by succumbing to it. Just be sure to garnish your workouts with an assortment of your old friends to keep them from growing stale. You will probably go through periods — less graphic perhaps than Picasso's, but every bit as meaningful for you — during which you tend to specialize in new movement territories. It's all part of the game.

• Working in the hot sunny outdoors is tempting and gets you tan "at pulse." But when in tropic climates or in hot, humid, breeze-

O_2 pulse, the anaerobic threshold and the fun zone

We've said or implied ad nauseam that lots of muscle-heart duets trained to top work capacity increases the efficiency of oxygen transport. This is Heavyhands' chief claim. When that happens, the combined exercise O_2 pulse — oxygen or calories used per heartbeat during combined exercise — increases, often strikingly. We have noted that these orchestrations of muscle and heart *delay* the elevation of lactic acid in the blood that signals that the O_2 transport mechanism is, no pun intended, running out of gas. Now, there is surely a relationship and it surely requires further study between this delay and the exerciser's sense of effort. Elevating the anaerobic threshold increases the fun zone; i.e., protects one longer from feeling belabored as the exercise intensity is steadily increased. In particular, the respiratory rate and depth remain lower longer at higher workloads. This is important for those who insist that fun should be a prime requisite for the "good exercise."

less air, throw away your ordinary exercise strategies. If you don't, you may just awaken to the face of a paramedic and the business end of an IV bottle. Heat exhaustion and stroke are real risks. Drink two to three ounces of water often and not only if you're thirsty, especially when going *long*. The better to be safe than sorry admonition is as wisely applied to hot weather as anything. I frankly don't ever feel impelled to execute at high levels of oxygen consumption when it's hot. Attempts at serious sessions have proven unsatisfactory. Working at my usual intensity I don't last long and when my RPE (rating of perceived exertion) is comfortable, my pulse is way below my usual. So when I'm after intensity in July and August, you'll find me jumping or pumping to the background hum of air conditioning.

• If you're a wise Heavyhander you can avoid not only serious injury but most mild discomfort. The longer you're at it — armed with higher MET × minutes levels and higher oxygen pulses — the *less* pain you should encounter. Never do, and don't even *think* in terms of, those oneous *few extra reps*. It makes no sense with Nautilus or Universal machines and even less when you're into combined, high-repetition exercise. When you're doing something new and different, *don't do it for long* no matter what your level of enchantment. Especially true of belly and back muscles, the caveat holds good for any limb muscle pulling through unconventional angles. Indeed you'll want to add these to your repertoire because they make you stronger overall, reduce risk of injury, improve flexibility. But do it one minute at a time, sort of sneaking it, without hysterically painful fanfare, into your exercise mix. Just adding 30 seconds daily would have you at 15 minutes of it in a month, probably more than you need anyway.

• Don't abandon your legs because you've become hypnotized by upper-torso progress. With legs the trick is to push their capacity along conventional lines until you've pushed that duet to within 90 percent or so of its potential. If you've trained seriously as a runner or biker, you may well be there already. Now add in other components. I prefer *vectors*, really — qualities and directions of activity. Jumping will do for legs what running never could. Lateral long-lever moves (Calisthenic No. I) will strengthen hip abductors as other exercises don't. Strength walking (heavier-than-usual weights) will make your legs effectively able to cope with a body weight you never intend to inflict upon them. Ski-poling and other jackknifes, like the reach, will give you those convex anterior thighs (quads) that make you gobble up hills and stairs. Working on the toes, heels, and flat on your feet, you'll be a better runner for it, and a safer one, too.

• Begin to work plenty of 5- and 10-minute intervals into your strategy. They are largely underrated in training methods. They are wonderful for work breaks if your job allows for it, and are perfectly positioned as regards time and intensity to bring respectable levels of both. Our schedules are so often cast such that a 30-minute aerobic session is quite impractical while a 10-minute quickie was the best I could cram into my day, yet my resting pulse continued its almost funereal 38! And when again time permitted I readily could go to 2 hours of double ski-poling without a hitch. Five-minute intervals at high intensity is super exercise, since it virtually gets you steadied out. They will condition you for longer work, build tolerance for time more anaerobically tinged, and in multiples, will incinerate much fat.

YOUR ULTIMATE BODY GOALS

Come to grips with the question: What is the ultimate body for me? It's not an easy one and requires some sober reflection. The answer cannot come from purely pictorial sources. Picking your body ego ideal from *Vogue* or *Esquire* could be a mistake. Think of what you *do* in everyday life, what you *used* to do (especially if you're fifty or better) and what you *would* do given the time, money, and skills you'd like. Then simply discard the first two since they are and were incredible examples of underachievement! Multiply the fantasied third image by five or so and you've a modest model to shoot for!

Start with fat. That's the easiest body component to manipulate, though from looking and listening you'd be tempted to doubt it. Compared to it all other tissues are difficult to impossible to change. Your viscera (i.e., pancreas, liver, spleen, thyroid, etc.) you hope will stay put — because changes in those are apt to be of the unwelcome variety. Bones do better with activity because with it they tend to mineralize optimally. For your blood, you can use iron compounds that may constipate you faster than they fill your vascular tree. Skin you can negotiate: if you've got extra amounts the

Aging and Heavyhands

Purists and academics remain carefully noncommittal on the subject of exercise's effect upon longevity. As consumers of the exercise marketplace, we are confronted with a perplexing knot of findings. "Good" exercise helps remove factors known to increase risk: lowers blood pressure; lowers "bad" blood fats, while increasing the good kind (HDL); helps diminish skin fold fat, insulin requirement in diabetics. So while we *know* exercise reduces risk in multiple ways, no one is ready to say that reducing these risks will keep you alive longer. Studies show that exercise can lower the likelihood of developing coronary heart disease. Coronary heart disease is our number-one killer. Still, we can't say with elegant finality that exercise will keep you alive longer! And, to boot, as one expert put it, no one has shown that the oxygen toxic theory is invalid; i.e., that aerobics may not make us age *more* rapidly. Generally speaking, one may add, it is easier and safer to declare a tactic unproven than proven. Since that final answer may be long in coming, the consumer is really alone with the decision. The real question is, which is riskier — waiting for the truth or not waiting for it! If I could be shown that those who choose *not* to exercise use time more effectively overall than exercisers, I'd somehow feel better about it.

plastic surgeon can lop and tighten it for you. Muscle is where our destiny really beckons. Here the sculptor in you can take over. You can, with intelligence and diligence, change its size and shape and as you know by now, alter its functions to an enormous degree — literally hundreds of percent. So everyone quite naturally wants the *best* muscle possible — and *all* muscles look pretty good. Its what we stuff between them and our skins that makes us recognizable at a distance!

How *much* muscle do you want? Physiologists speak of "excess muscle" probably meaning that amount which encroaches on the efficiency of oxygen transport. Weight training is the best manufacturer of muscle. If you aspire to hulkish proportions, big weights with few reps is *the* answer. But trained to overgenerous proportions, you may find you can't do many reps, especially if you do them fast and continuously. Yes, you *can* lift your Datsun's back end, however, and will when seized by that irresistible impulse.

There are really few occupations, outside of professional competitive sports, that make good use of gargantuan strength. So the decision to lace your frame with bulky muscle that is a burden mostly and an asset occasionally is a very serious one. Once you've opted for outside skeletal muscle, your VO2Max has been automatically clipped, because your heart's output can't possibly cover many reps involving your pushing *you* around.

The best body, where it comes to good work, is the strongest, smallest body you can finesse through life. And I'll lay odds that no single system can produce that as well as Heavyhands. And no *combination* of systems either. I must say I'm disturbed by the women who emit the sounds of burgeoning nausea when it comes to their muscle mass. It has become fashionably feminine to go on record as a despiser of muscle. Now, it is about as reasonable to despise muscle as it is to want more of it than you can carry gracefully. And you might as reasonably despise spleens. Muscles make up the organ of movement, and you can't ever enjoy great movement without the anatomy that goes with it.

Again it is clear that confusion reigns and it's mostly over the issue of looks. Most of the exercises in this book could be performed to phenomenal advantage with weights that don't exceed one pound! What happens to muscles exercised to heart's target at enough METs times enough minutes over many years? In terms of weighable, measurable meat — almost nothing. The changes are mostly of the internal kind — muscle chemistry alters in very demonstrable ways. These chemical changes are visible mostly not in the silhouette of their host, but in the new patterns of movements that changed the chemistry in the first place, and which in turn come to be fueled by those changes. So the big changes in shape are apt to be wrought in lots less fat for both ladies and gents. Men are merely, by virtue of their hormonal disposition, more able to make bigger, stronger muscles.

A word about the *look* of muscularity. We actually only use the word muscular when muscles, whatever their condition, *show*. So muscularity refers mostly to the thickness of skinfold fat that covers muscles. But well-exercised muscles, even small ones, do have a certain look about them. They become thicker in the center (belly), tapered toward the ends. More fusiform, we say. The separations between adjacent muscles become more evident. Muscularity is a term we only use with fellow humans, as though it's a special trait of some sort. We never speak of a cat's or dog's muscularity. That's taken quite properly for granted.

Now if the look of well-worked muscles of ordinary size, when skinfold thickness is minimal, is considered ugly or even mildly offensive, I'm at a loss. You can't exercise enough to extend the fitness factors without becoming "muscular" and you can't become muscular without this "overwork" we've decided exercise *is*. And since we are quite capable of revising our definitions of beauty endlessly, it might be wise to wed health and beauty in definitions that allow us to enjoy both at once! Making muscularity an exclusive property of one gender could be a dangerous form of absurdity and might become a defense for those for whom *movement*, not *muscularity*, is the rub.

Like anything else the issue of "your best body" should be open ended. Whatever your age, you are too young to take fixed positions in matters of such importance. In physical training, growth and change are inseparable ideas. So long as the cardinal rules and protective caveats are obeyed — the body will emerge better for the experience. There is a gradual melding of function and structure which is what "best bodies" must be about.

A LAST FEW PARTING SHOTS AT THE FAT DILEMMA

Start with the premise that you're beautiful enough whatever your weight — that you never aspired to win beauty contests, and those who win them haven't solved all of life's problems, either.

Your motor system, on the other hand, if not describable as downright ugly, is probably a veritable shambles. If you *can't* move well, you *don't*. As you diet more, move less, muscle atrophies ever so slowly and you're pushing the possibility of fitness closer to a place of no return.

If you resolve to lose weight *fast and once and for all,* the chances are you're building castles in the air. Figure wisely that the most successful people in the world have become emotionally and bodily bankrupt playing Russian roulette with dieting.

You can't simply *become thin.* You must *learn* to be thin. Learning takes time. If you beat the time rap and lose fat quickly, you become "pseudo-thin," a model for the still camera and data to prove it *was* possible for anyone who happens to care.

Shoot for *nothing short* of sinewy muscularity — death of fat; birth of rippling activity. Think of yourself at 16 frames per second! Make movement your mantra, not a certain number of pounds or inches of hip or waistline. Only properly induced muscularity will make your weight loss a permanent victory, and one that becomes a dynamic launcher of many more victories.

Don't even try to lose weight *fast.* A single pound per week is a fantastic, blinding, rate! I urge patients *consciously to delay* weight loss until sufficient Heavyhands technique has been acquired and then to begin, slow and easy, to cover intake excesses with groups of 5- to 10-minute intervals. Ironically, the exercisers who watch their food intake within range of practicality almost enjoy the deprivation. The fantasy is that they're "pushing muscle through fat toward their body surface" rather than feeding on fat deposits with small regard for what's beneath them. Remember that 98 percent of fast losers by the diet route are able to do it *each time* they try!

HOW MUCH EXERCISE?

Heavyhands exercise can be performed every day and several times each day. The days of rest usually recommended may be more necessary with exercise that is more stereotyped. Heavyhands' shifting emphasis lessens the load on particular muscle groups. Thus, the more versatile your moves, the fewer days off you require. That's of interest in body composition control and also for those who feel something is missing on days they don't get to exercise. Most Heavyhanders I know do *something,* if only for a few minutes, *every day.*

Progress in Heavyhands ordinarily follows the familiar sigmoidal (S-shaped) curve:

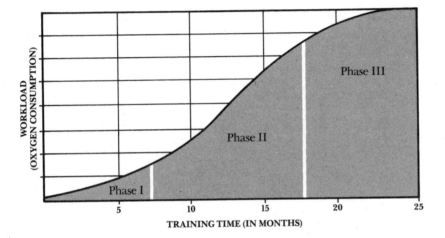

Workloads or oxygen-consumption rates rise slowly at first (Phase I), then explode sharply upward (Phase II), then tend to level to a flattish slope (Phase III). The Phase I lag may be due to the understandable difficulty in mobilizing lots of muscles to the unusual character of the work. The Phase II spurt is doubtless due to the immense *educability* of the upper-torso and trunk muscles, and Phase III may announce the approach of one's genetic limitations.

During Phase III excellent maintenance of fitness factors is possible with investment of surprisingly little actual exercise time. Indeed, at 2 hours or *less* per week, real but modest gains may

---

How fit is fit?

I call this question dynamic because the answer is apt to change while you formulate a response. Fitness spawns more fitness requirements. The parallel to learning is seductive. Knowing increases the thirst for knowledge. Movement greed is as real as other forms of human greed. It simply hasn't arrived at popular consciousness yet.

continue to occur during Phase III. We don't know yet what combination of METs times minutes makes for the most efficient maintenance of one's gains. It is probable that both extremes — high intensity (quite anaerobic short intervals) and very prolonged, lower intensity work, are *expendable*.

Once the need to dispense calories is no longer a large concern, your exercise time can probably be pared to somewhere between 1½ to 2 hours depending upon its intensity, leaving ample time for other activities.

The philosophers of the world will not run out of things to ruminate upon so long as the distinction between mind and body continues to pose fetching questions. For instance, when we say "I," do we mean *both* body and mind? Our minds can be as private as we choose; but the body is far more public, whether we like it or not. I have found it convenient to consider people's bodies as shared between the Self and the World. That shared proprietorship sets off a lot of changing ideas tinged with varying emotional colorings. At moments we seem proud and pleased to be our body's owner. Other times that pride may shrink to the steadfast denial shown by the stroke victim who is dead serious when he announces that his paralyzed leg *isn't his!* The option of making oneself *able* in every sense of the word is really a double duty. Social units the size of families or the size of nations might work better if individuals considered themselves the property of others as well as their own responsibility. Healthy forms of shame and guilt *should* be felt when our body, that community property, is neglected: shame for our *failure* to achieve our best; guilt for having *deprived* ourselves and our fellows of what we might have been.

Appendix

Workload and Calories

Here are a series of MET values and the exercises that will generate those intensities.

5-MET SUGGESTIONS

WEIGHT	EXERCISE	LEVEL	FREQUENCY (per minute)
1 pound	Pump 'n' walk	II	120
1 pound	Pump 'n' walk	III	100
5 pound	Pump 'n' walk	I	100
1 pound	Punch 'n' dip		100 (25 four-punch cycles)

7-MET SUGGESTIONS

WEIGHT	EXERCISE	LEVEL	FREQUENCY (per minute)
1 pound	Pump 'n' walk	II	140
1 pound	Pump 'n' walk	III	120
5 pound	Pump 'n' walk	I	120
1 pound	Punch 'n' dip		120
3 pound	Pump 'n' walk	II	110
no weight	Double ski-poling		25 cycles

10-MET SUGGESTIONS

WEIGHT	EXERCISE	LEVEL	FREQUENCY (per minute)
no weight	Jumps with lateral thrusts		140
no weight	Pump 'n' walk in place	III	150
no weight	Pump 'n' jog	II	180
no weight	Double ski-poling		45 cycles
1 pound	Pump 'n' step heels 12″ from floor	III	130
1 pound	Lateral thrusts — jumping		120
1 pound	Punch 'n' jump		100 (25 four-punch cycles)
1 pound	Double ski-poling (4-step cycles)		35 cycles
1 pound	Double ski-poling in place (2-dip cycles)		40 cycles
1 pound	Pump 'n' walk (3.5 mph)	III	120
1 pound	Pump 'n' jog (4 mph)	II	150
1 pound	Shadowbox (50-50 hop-shuffle with hand over hand)		120
1 pound	Dance (50-50 short-long lever)		120
1 pound	Pump 'n' jog in place	I	200

13-MET SUGGESTIONS*

WEIGHT	EXERCISE	LEVEL	FREQUENCY (per minute)
1 pound	Pump 'n' walk	III	160
2 pound	Pump 'n' jog	II	200
3 pound	Pump 'n' walk	III	140
4 pound	Pump 'n' jog	II	170
5 pound	Pump 'n' walk	III	120
5 pound	Pump 'n' walk	II	150
10 pound	Pump 'n' walk	II	100
15 pound	Pump 'n' walk	I	150

*approximate values

MET VALUES FOR SPECIFIC EXERCISES

EXERCISE	FOOT LIFT HEEL-FLOOR DISTANCE	WEIGHT (each hand)	PUMP HEIGHT (level)	FREQUENCY (per minute)	MET VALUE*
pump 'n' walk in place	12″	1 lb	I	100	3
pump 'n' walk in place	12″	1 lb	I	120	3.5
pump 'n' walk in place	12″	2 lbs	I	140	4
pump 'n' walk in place	12″	3 lbs	I	120	4.5–5
pump 'n' walk in place	12″	1 lb	II	100	5.5–6
pump 'n' walk in place	12″	2 lbs	II	100	6
pump 'n' walk in place	12″	2 lbs	II	120	7
pump 'n' walk in place	12″	2 lbs	I	150	8
pump 'n' walk in place	12″	1 lb	II	150	8

MET VALUES FOR SPECIFIC EXERCISES

EXERCISE	FOOT LIFT HEEL-FLOOR DISTANCE	WEIGHT (each hand)	PUMP HEIGHT (level)	FREQUENCY (per minute)	MET VALUE*
pump 'n' walk in place	12"	2 lbs	II	160	9
pump 'n' walk in place	12"	3 lbs	II	140	9
pump 'n' run	12"	1 lb	II	200	10–11
pump 'n' run	12"	2 lbs	II	200	11–12
pump 'n' walk	12"	2 lbs	III	150	12–13
pump 'n' run	12"	4 lbs	II	200	13–14
pump 'n' walk	12"	3 lbs	III	150	14–15
pump 'n' walk	12"	4 lbs	III	150	15–16
pump 'n' walk	12"	5 lbs	III	150	16–19
pump 'n' walk	12"	8 lbs	III	150	19–22

BOXED-IN AREA = 1–10–100
*All values are approximate

DETERMINING THE MET VALUE OF ANY EXERCISE

Once you begin thinking in terms of METs you may wish to use those numbers to rate your Heavyhands calisthenics, ambulatory or free-form exercise. Obviously, it would be impractical to chart the MET value for every exercise for each of its variables and for every body weight in a book of this size.

First choose an exercise of known MET value. Note your pulse rate after 5 full minutes of exercise. If, for instance, a 7-MET exercise brings you to a steady 130 rate after 5 minutes, you can use that information to estimate the MET value for *any* exercise if you know what *steady pulse rate* it produces.

Since workload and pulse rate are proportional, some simple arithmetic is all you'll need. You are really answering the question: "How many METs (X) are generated at a given pulse rate if I know that a 7-MET exercise generates a pulse of 130?" Supposing you exercise at a steady pulse rate of 170. We'd set up the question this way:

$$\frac{7 \text{ METs}}{130 \text{ Pulse}} = \frac{X \text{ METs}}{170 \text{ Pulse}}$$

The answer is obtained by simply cross multiplying:

$$130 \times (X) = 7 \times 170 \text{ or,}$$
$$130X = 1190$$

dividing through, X = 9.1 METs, your workload at a pulse of 170.

After a few such calculations you will come to know how many METs coincide with various pulse rates at which you "steady out" during your workouts, e.g., 8 METs = 120, 10 METs = 150, 12 METs = 180, etc.

THE CALORIE PULSE

The interested reader can readily convert their "steadied-out" pulse into a calorie counter that really works. You need to know two things: your body weight in kilos and your *steady pulse* after, say, 5 minutes of some exercise of *known MET value*. It's all based on the fact that one's *oxygen pulse* — the number of cc's of oxygen used per heartbeat — remains fairly stable *over a range of heart rates*. While your steady heart rate increases with the workload, your oxygen pulse will actually vary little at heart rates between 120 and 150. So if we know your oxygen pulse and your steady pulse rate, simple multiplication gives us your oxygen consumption per minute and calories are only one simple calculation away from *that*.

Here's how to measure your oxygen pulse. Take one of the exercises from the appendix or even the 1–10–100, which incidentally has a MET value of about 5.5. You'll remember that each MET corresponds to 3.5cc of oxygen per kilo of body weight per minute. If your 1–10–100 gets you steadied at a pulse rate between 120 and 150, we can calculate your oxygen pulse. Supposing you weigh 70 kilos and your 1–10–100 finds you at a pulse rate of 130 at the finish (5.5 METs — the 1–10–100's workload, times 3.5cc for each MET — gives you 19.25, and that times 70 for each of your kilos equals 1347cc of oxygen. That's how much oxygen someone your size uses when working steadily at a 5.5-MET intensity. If you divide 1347 by the steady pulse rate (130) you get 10.36, rounded off 10.4, your oxygen pulse. Given that number you can quickly compute your oxygen consumption by multiplying your steady pulse rate by 10.4. For example:

pulse rate		*oxygen consumption*
120		1248
130	× 10.4 =	1347
140		1456
150		1560

To convert oxygen consumption per minute to calories, divide the first two digits by 2. Thus a 1400cc consumption equals 7 calories per minute (14 ÷ 2 = 7). Now a quick review:

(1) Determine your weight in kilos by dividing your weight in pounds by 2.2 (for example, 154 ÷ 2.2 = 70 kilos).

(2) Do an exercise of known MET value for 5 or more minutes, then count your pulse immediately. Select an exercise at which you steady out between 120 and 150.

(3) Multiply the MET value by 3.5 (e.g., 7 METs × 3.5 = 24.5), and that in turn by your weight in kilos (e.g., 24.5 × 70 = 1715).

(4) Dividing this figure (oxygen consumption per minute) by your pulse (e.g., 1715 ÷ 150 = 11.4) gives your oxygen pulse.

(5) Multiply any heart rate at which you exercise steadily by 11.4 to obtain your per-minute oxygen consumption. For example, at a pulse of 180 your oxygen consumption would be at least 180 × 11.4 = 2052.

(6) Divide the first two digits by 2 to obtain the rate of calorie loss per minute at that pulse rate.

You will, of course, want to recalculate your oxygen pulse every so often. It will hopefully change rapidly at first and continue to change so long as your work intensities increase.

Knowing my oxygen pulse for many exercises is around 30, I know that I use 3 liters of oxygen each minute at a pulse of 100 and that means 15 calories per minute or 900 calories per hour. After a while you'll find yourself automatically thinking calories per minute during the very act of taking your pulse.

ACKNOWLEDGMENTS

There are many to thank. One can only strive to keep appreciation abreast of indebtedness. *That* energy flagged frequently, I confess, during the past three years: my gratitude is more than tinged with apology. The inverse square law applies in such matters, of course; those closest are apt to be hardest hit by one's poisonous moods!

Valuable technical help came in many forms from many sources: Montefiore Hospital provided the use of a mass spectrometer; with it came the knowledge of my friend, Dr. Miroslav Klain of the Department of Anesthesia, who showed us how to use it. The medical library and its staff at Montefiore under the direction of Gloria Rosen, along with Lorraine Serviss, scouted the literature. Devine Providence Hospital through the kind permission of Dr. David S. Huber supplied sophisticated equipment coupled with the skill of Lisa Schramm; Ivy Walsh, R.N., glued electrodes to me and monitored my gyrations with cheerful expertise; Louis F. Sander gave with enthusiasm. I must also thank the Waters Instrument Company, and my associates at Instrument Development Corporation. I am especially grateful to Dr. Allan J. Ryan, editor in chief of *Physician and Sports Medicine,* for both his special brand of patient encouragement and the hard information I required all too often. Dr. David Costill of Ball State University was not too busy to answer my most naive queries or to supply technical tidbits.

Colleague-friends were helpful in so many ways. Dr. Fred Marks for pediatric and sports medicine savvy as well as physiologic data from his own clinical experiments; Dr. Pete Stajduhar, Chief of Staff of the Highland Road Veterans Administration Hospital, for moral support and intensive study and helpful critique of "Exerpsychology." Dr. Ray Goldblum added his own METs-times-minutes along with clinical suggestions. Finally, Dr. Richard L. Kalla who was everything that a multitalented sib surrogate could mean to an aging only child! He provided a spectrum of technical dexterity, sinew, and know-how that has been indispensable over the past five years. I shall be forever grateful.

Thanks to Al Hart, my agent, who was willing to believe in and act in the interest of Heavyhands; Richard and Sue Golomb, who painstakingly and expertly took most of the pictures; many others were taken by Rick Lindner; Ron Filer, my illustrator, for his excellent drawings and for hours spent translating new movements into the stick figures that seemed to come alive; Howard Anderson, a most sensitive industrial engineer, complemented the project by his creative solution of many of our equipment problems.

And thanks to the Neighborhood Gang who came every evening and early Sunday mornings to lateral thrust, double-ski-pole and pump 'n' run pantingly through the streets of Squirrel Hill — in fair weather and foul; to our lifelong and dearest friends, Jean and Saul Chosky, for absorbing hours of my monothematic soapboxing on the subject of fitness; to supportive friends like Russell Patterson, Janet Moritz, Tom Auble, and Jeff Ruttenberg, who were at once advisers and guinea pigs — endless thanks; to Mary Ann and Elliott Meyer for supplying sweet company, lodging, and good grub in New York; to those patients who at times, I fear, *gave* as much as they *got* from me.

Heavyhands was a team effort: highest praise and appreciation belong to the people at Little, Brown; to Peter Carr, head of the Manufacturing Department; to Sue Windheim, for handily putting together the assemblage of word and image we laid on her; to my friend Elaine Richard. Blessings on my copyeditor, Mike Mattil. His prevailing calm and humor and smarts — marks of the quality professional — were just what the doctor and the book ordered.

It is doubtful that many projects could have been as demanding upon their editors as was *Heavyhands.* Roger Donald not only went out on the limb as acquiring editor.

He captained the oftentimes agonized growth of the manuscript; was reassuringly on top of things as canny observer, aggressive organizer, and lusty participant. The author and the reader are lucky to have him.

Thanks to my kids, Debbie and Keith Bailey and Jodi and Rick Lindner, for lots of hours that included everything from carpentry to photography to chart calculations into the wee morning hours, and for their tolerance of my curmudgeonishness!

Last but scarcely least, I thank my wife, Millie, who despite her own hectic work schedule labored with me through some six revisions of the manuscript with nary a whimper. *Heavyhands* could not have happened without her.

Leonard Schwartz
Pittsburgh, Pa. December 1981

TOTAL BODY FITNESS
FROM WARNER BOOKS

RUNNING AND BEING: THE TOTAL EXPERIENCE
Dr. George Sheehan

"George Sheehan is the first great philosopher whose body can run with his mind. **RUNNING AND BEING** examines more than the 'how to' or 'why' of running. It transcends the traditional stereotype analysis of sport and allows us to examine who we are—the runner, the man."
—Bob Glover, co-author of *The Runner's Handbook.*

Sheehan laces his philosophy with practical advice and includes his unique one-day method for determining which sport is best for you. He tells how to prepare for a marathon, how to jog effectively, avoid injuries, and what it takes to compete in a race.

"What particularly endears George Sheehan to runners is his contagious insistence that running is something more than a sport—that it is an activity that offers glimpses of values that are profound."
—James F. Fixx in *The Complete Book of Running.*

Available in large-size quality paperback   (L97-090, $3.95)

RICHARD SIMMONS' BETTER BODY BOOK
Richard Simmons

You can redesign your body—with a little help from the pro! Richard Simmons shows you how to shape up with a slimmer, firmer, tighter body—better than it ever was before! Here is the only book that offers exercise programs for all levels of fitness, tailored to suit *you*. In these pages are over two hundred fully illustrated exercises, individually planned for a workout from head to toe. But first, you'll learn how to determine your body type, assess your level of fitness, begin at your proper exercise level, and separate truth from myth in the exercise program that can transform your body and your life!

Available in hardcover   (L51-263, $16.50 FPT)

IMPORTANT BOOKS FOR YOUR BODY
FROM WARNER BOOKS